CEREBRAL DAMAGE BEFORE AND AFTER CARDIAC SURGERY

DEVELOPMENTS IN
CRITICAL CARE MEDICINE AND ANESTHESIOLOGY

Volume 27

The titles published in this series are listed at the end of this volume.

Cerebral Damage before and after Cardiac Surgery

edited by

ALLEN WILLNER

Long Island Jewish Medical Center, Albert Einstein College of Medicine, Glen Oaks, New York, USA

SPRINGER SCIENCE+BUSINESS MEDIA, B.V.

Cerebral damage before and after cardiac surgery / edited by Allen
Willner.
    p.   cm. -- (Development in critical care medicine and
anesthesiology ; v. 27)
    Includes bibliographical references and index.
    ISBN 978-94-010-4818-7   ISBN 978-94-011-1852-1 (eBook)
    DOI 10.1007/978-94-011-1852-1
    1. Heart--Surgery--Complications. 2. Psychological manifestations
of general diseases. 3. Neurologic manifestations of general
diseases. 4. Brain damage--Diagnosis. 5. Cerebral circulation.
I. Willner, Allen E.   II. Series: Developments in critical care
medicine and anesthesiology ; 27.
    [DNLM: 1. Brain Diseases--etiology. 2. Heart Surgery--adverse
effects. 3. Postoperative Complications.   W1 DE997VRL v.27]
RD598.C399 1993
617.4'1201--dc20
DNLM/DLC
for Library of Congress   92-49816

ISBN 978-94-010-4818-7

Printed on acid-free paper

Table of contents

Preface

Talking to a fellow physician some time ago about the results of coronary bypass operations, we contemplated what we would fear the most if we had to have the operation ourselves. After dwelling some time on major myocardial damage, multiple organ failure and multiple graft occlusion, we decided that the complications to be dreaded most were the cerebral ones. The overt complications with hemiplegia, etc., were bad enough, but, due to their relative rarity, to be taken as a matter of risk. The more subtle complications affecting intellect, memory, personality and emotional life were much more frightening as they seem to be more common, effect parts of the "inner self", are less understood, are less accepted, and may make the patient somewhat of a social cripple.

My friend and I also agreed, that for the more common operations using extracorporeal circulation, cerebral protection was the major remaining perioperative challenge from a scientific point of view. It is surprising that this field has not been more exploited by basic brain researchers. Here they have a brain injury model where we know that a proportion of the patients operated upon will have some degree of brain damage. There is no lack of study objects, the scientific design can be made impeccable with a before and after design, possibly combined with a randomised comparison of various routines or treatments.

Why, then, has this field been somewhat disregarded? I think there are several reasons for this. The function of the brain is notoriously difficult to measure. Working within this field requires an expertise that many medical specialists lack, among them many cardiac surgeons, who are fully occupied in perfecting the cardiac results of the operation. Furthermore, many of the effects of open heart surgery on the brain are subtle, require special knowledge or interest in their diagnosis, are difficult to treat once they have occurred, and may in some institutions be put down to normal, temporary effects of anesthesia, operation and extracorporeal circulation in a very effective and necessary surgical treatment, an attitude that becomes an obstacle to the scientific exploration of this field. There may also be an element of wishful thinking on the part of the surgeon, closing his eyes to cerebral complications in his pursuit of the perfect results.

The present book is a good sign that cerebral complications – and the possibility of lessening them in the future – are taken more seriously nowadays. It is written by some well known authorities in the field, many of whom have devoted years of work to these patients. It is interesting to note that of the 19 chapters, 4 are written by psychiatrists, 3 by neurologists, 7 by psychologists, 3 by surgeons, 1 by an anesthesiologist, and 1 by a perfusionist, depicting the various views by which the brain can be regarded and also giving some idea as to the complexity of the problem.

Reading the book and the contemporary literature, the following conclusions seem to be justified: Open heart surgery more or less regularly brings about symptoms from the central nervous system; symptoms form a continuum from subtle and temporary to obvious and permanent; symptoms seem to be a sign of brain cell injury; there are now multiple methods by which morphology, biochemistry, electrophysiology, and functions of the brain may be followed; the cause of brain cell injury seems to be multifactorial. Hypoxia and hypoperfusion seem to be a common effect of many causes, among them emboli of large, intermediate and small sizes; the main path in decreasing the extent of brain injury seems to be prevention; and the three responsible specialists in persuing prevention of brain injury are the surgeon, the perfusionist, and the anesthesiologist.

Returning to my friend, it turned out that for some years he had had angina pectoris and now discreetly was exploring the outcome of operative treatment. He was operated upon with six peripheral anastomoses and woke up with a right-sided hemiplegia.

Umeå, October 1992   T. ÅBERG

List of contributors

Prof. Dr. med. TORKEL ÅBERG
Head of the Thoracic and Cardiovascular Clinic
University Hospital
Umeå
Sweden

E.H.J.F. BOEZEMAN MD
Department of Clinical Neurophysiology
St. Antonius Hospital
Nieuwegein
The Netherlands

ROBERT J. CHABOT PhD
Department of Psychiatry
New York University Medical Center
New York, New York
USA

Prof. Dr. phil. BERNHARD DAHME
Institute of Psychology III
University of Hamburg
Federal Republic of Germany

Prof. Dr. med. THOMAS EMSKOTTER
Department of Neurology
University Hospital Hamburg-Eppendorf
Federal Republic of Germany

Prof. Dr. med PAUL GÖTZE
Department of Psychiatry and Nervous Diseases
University Hospital Hamburg-Eppendorf
Federal Republic of Germany

Prof. LAVERNE D. GUGINO PhD, MD
Department of Anesthesia
Brigham and Women's Hospital
Harvard Medical School
Boston, MA
USA

Prof. RUBEN C. GUR PhD
Departments of Psychiatry and Neurology
Brain Behavior Laboratory and the Neuropsychiatry Program
University of Pennsylvania
Philadelphia, Pennsylvania
USA

Dr. med. G. HÜSE-KLEINSTOLL
Department of Medical Psychiatry
University Hospital Hamburg-Eppendorf
Federal Republic of Germany

Prof. WAYNE O. ISOM MD
Formerly of the Department of Surgery
New York University Medical Center
Presently Chairman-Department of Cardiothoracic Surgery
Cornell University Medical College
New York, New York
USA

Prof. E. ROY JOHN PhD
Department of Psychiatry
New York University Medical Center, NY
and the Nathan S. Kline Institute for Psychiatric Research
Orangeburg, New York
USA

Prof. Dr. med. P. KALMAR
Department of Thoracic and Cardiovascular Surgery
University Hospital Hamburg-Eppendorf
Federal Republic of Germany

JONATHAN D. KATZ MD
Assoc. Prof. of Clinical Anesthesiology
Yale University School of Medicine
New Haven, Ct.,
Attending Anesthesiologist
St. Vincent's Medical Center,
Bridgeport, Ct.
USA

Dr. med. H-J. KREBBER
Department of Thoracic and Cardiovascular Surgery
University Hospital Hamburg-Eppendorf
Federal Republic of Germany

MARK KURUSZ CCP
Chief Perfusionist
Department of Surgery, Division of Cardiothoracic Surgery
The University of Texas Medical Branch
Galveston, Texas
USA

Prof. Dr. med. L. LACHENMEYER
Department of Neurology
University Hospital Hamburg-Eppendorf
Federal Republic of Germany

Dr. phil. U. LAMPARTER
Department of Psychosomatics
University Hospital Hamburg-Eppendorf
Federal Republic of Germany

PIERRE M. LANDAU MS
Department of Psychiatry
New York University Medical Center
New York, New York
USA

J.A. LEUSINK MD
Department of Anaesthesiology
St. Antonius Hospital
Nieuwegein
The Netherlands

Dr. phil. HEINZ-JÖRG MEFFERT
Department of Thoracic and Cardiovascular Surgery
University Hospital Hamburg-Eppendorf
Federal Republic of Germany

Prof. Dr. med. RUDOLF MEYENDORF
Professor of General Psychopathology
University of Munich
Federal Republic of Germany

STANTON P. NEWMAN PhD
Department of Psychiatry
Middlesex Hospital
London
UK

JOHN C. OPIE MD, FRCS(C), FRCS
Cardiovascular and Thoracic Surgeon
Asst. Prof. University British Columbia (1982–1987)
Western Heart and Lung Surgeons, Ltd.
Phoenix, Arizona
USA

Prof. Dr. med. H. POKAR
Department of Thoracic and Cardiovascular Surgery
University Hospital Hamburg-Eppendorf
Federal Republic of Germany

Prof. LESLIE S. PRICHEP PhD
Department of Psychiatry, NY University Medical Center
and The Nathan S. Kline Institute for Psychiatric Research
Orangeburg, New York
USA

Prof. CHARLES J. RABINER MD
Medical Director, Mesa Vista Hospital
and Clinical Professor, Department of Psychiatry
School of Medicine, University of San Diego
San Diego, California
USA

The Late Prof. Dr. med. GEORG RODEWALD
Department of Thoracic and Cardiovascular Surgery
University Hospital Hamburg-Eppendorf
Federal Republic of Germany

PETER L.C. SMITH MD
The Royal Postgraduate Medical School
Hammersmith Hospital
London
UK

Prof. K.A. SOTANIEMI MD, PhD
Department of Neurology
The University of Oulu
Oulu
Finland

Prof. FREDERICK A. STRUVE PhD
Neurophysiology Research Laboratory
School of Medicine in Shreveport
Louisiana State University Medical Center
Shreveport, Louisiana
USA

Prof. PEKKA TIENARI MD
Department of Psychiatry
The University of Oulu
Oulu
Finland

F.E.E. VERMEULEN MD
Department of Cardiac Thoracic Surgery
St. Antonius Hospital
Nieuwegein
The Netherlands

Assoc. Prof. ALLEN E. WILLNER PhD
Department of Psychology, Long Island Jewish Medical Center
New Hyde Park, NY, and
Albert Einstein College of Medicine,
New York
USA

Acknowledgements

I would like to thank several people who helped to make this book possible:
The late Prof. Dr. med. Georg Rodewald who, by his constant example, keen intelligence, good sense of humor, and wise suggestions, had much to do with the assembling of this volume; the authors of all the chapters comprising this book for their indispensible contribution; Janet Sendar, Psy.D. who was cheerful, intelligent, thorough and patient in carrying out the seemingly endless tasks required to turn a collection of manuscripts into a book; Carol Ritter, Ph.D. who aided in much of the work in organizing this book, during the earlier stages; Alice Stahl, M.D. who provided a first translation of Prof. Rodewald's chapter from German into English; Sally Lauve, Psy.D. who extensively simplified and revised two chapters; Judy Killen, M.S. for much useful advice during the latter part of the revision process; Dr. phil. Jorg Meffert for his unfailing courtesy and helpfulness during the long process of knitting the book together; and finally, thanks to the Long Island Heart Council which helped to support this work financially.

ALLEN WILLNER

PART ONE

Causes of pre- and post-operative cerebral damage

1. The causes of pre-operative psychopathology in cardiac surgery patients

RUDOLF MEYENDORF

To understand the causes of preoperative psychopathology in cardiac surgery patients, we have to go back to the 19th century. The relationship between heart disease and psychopathology was already extensively discussed more than 100 years ago. Textbooks of psychiatry and internal medicine dealt with this question [1–12]. In 1835, Ideler wrote a chapter in his book on mental disease: "Effect of circulatory disease on mental functioning. (Seele)" [13]. Even earlier, in 1818, Nasse wrote a treatise on "Heart and Psyche". In it he tried to correlate the stage of heart disease, psychopathology and post mortem findings [14]. In 1831, Burrows saw a relationship between "irregularities in blood and circulation and their effects on the brain" [15]. In 1844, Jacobi points out the relationship between violent manic states of the mind and blood circulation and Bergmann, also in 1844, describes a case of "mania metastatica arising from the heart". The post mortem findings showed stenosis and thrombosis of the mitral and tricuspid valves [16, 17].

In 1872, Krishaber presented one of the most valuable collections of case histories on psychopathology and heart disease. He described 24 cases as "nevropathie cèrébro-cardiaque" and documented the general physical, neurological and psychopathological state and thus presents patients who seem identical to those in an intensive care unit after cardiac surgery 100 years later. Not only are there states of altered consciousness, auditory and visual hallucinations and delusions, but also phenomena which one only observes after heart surgery if one examines the patient very carefully, such as symptoms of derealization and depersonalization, symptoms of obsessive-compulsive behaviour and at the same time gnostic deficits, pointing out the neurological symptomatology. But furthermore, other phenomena which occur after heart surgery: "Doutes de l'identité de sa propre personne et existence . . . sensations de rève, d'invressse, et de vide . . . abolition des facultes affectives . . . se croit parfois double . . . antipathies et colères non motivée . . . perversion des sens . . . melancolie". In translation: "Doubts of identity of his own person and existence, sensations of dreaming, drunkenness, emptiness . . . abolition of the emotional faculties . . . believes himself sometimes double . . . antipathies and unmotivated angers . . . perversion of the senses . . . melancholy [18].

The mental hospitals of that time, having a great number of patients to compare, try also to relate mental disorders to heart disease. Burman notes "a remarkable relation between heart disease and insanity" [19]. Witkowsky and Karrer recognise a direct relation between heart disease and insanity but believe that heart disease influences only the kind of symptoms of mental disease and is not the cause of it [20, 21]. Greenlees however very clearly correlated etiology of heart disease and mental disease. He stated: 1. "that heart disease occurs with greater frequency among the insane than among the sane, 2. that, not only does heart disease alter the type and delusions of insanity, but also, in some cases . . . the cardiac lesion is, no doubt, the predisposing cause of the insanity, and 3. that, among the sane, heart disease may become so prominent that the physical phenomena exhibited may be those actually of insanity" [22].

Good case histories which are still the most reliable sources regarding the relation between heart disease and mental disease were published at that time: D'Astros in 1881 presents 38 cases and tries to systematize the kinds of psychopathology of organic heart disease. He distinguishes between 1. hysterical phenomena (hytérisme et hystérie cardiaque), 2. physical weakening and dementia (affaiblissement et démence dans les maladies de cœur), and 3. cardiac insanity (folie cardiaque) which may manifest itself through a) hallucinations, b) melancholic insanity (délire à forme mélancholique), c) systematized manic insanity (délire systématisé à forme de manie) and d) insanity with dementia (délire incohérent à forme de démence). We see: D'Astros distinguishes between three major syndromes of mental disease in the course of cardiac disease, which can be applied also to the psychopathology after cardiac surgery: 1. psychogenic (hysteria), 2. productive psychotic (delusion) and 3. psycho-organic (dementia) symptoms. He gives however a very detailed differentiation of symptomatology of organic heart disease as he speaks of "formes d'aliénation mentale, la mélancolie hypochondriaque, monomanie des persecutiones, impulsions des cardiaques" [23].

Mickle, in 1888, wrote an article, "Insanity in relation of cardiac and aortic disease and phthisis". He analyses 336 cases of insanity in relation to cardiac disease with post mortem findings. He separated insanity of mitral valve and aortic valve disease from insanity observed with hypertrophic and dilatative cardiac disease and stresses the fact that insanity does not imply "delirium", but that it involves another category of symptoms, i.e., "melancholy, intense querulousness and delusions of persecution, annoyance, injury", which he associates with mitral insufficiency and mitral stenosis. Furthermore, he enumerates the psychopathology of heart disease in the following way: "Hallucinations of sight and hearing, ideas of delusive character, monomania with delusions as to poisoned food and persecution, delusions about dying or being dead, delusions of conspiracy and of being tormented, delusions that the bodily organs are 'eaten into'". Again we are reminded, that this type of acute productive psychopathology may be observed without any subtle investigation in an intensive care unit after cardiac surgery. But we may find not only these obvious symptoms after cardiac surgery, but also those less conspicuous ones observed also by Mickle in 1888: "A somber emotional dejection or melancholic dread, hypochondriacal symptoms; or else morose, sullen, taciturn states with a marked attitude as of one subjected to annoyance or persecution". Dysphoric syndromes, which are described after cardiac surgery, Mickle describes as symptoms of "querulousness, irritability, ill-temper, discontent, grumbling moroseness".

Besides the nonspecific syndromes, Mickle draws attention to well known entities of mental disease which occur in relation to heart disease such as "persecutory monomania", "delusional insanity", and "melancholia agitata". He stresses the fact that in the majority of cases, insanity followed cardiac disease and only in a few cases insanity was known before the outbreak of cardiac disease [24].

In 1901, the neurologist H. Head wrote an article "Certain mental changes that accompany visceral disease". He presented 62 cases of heart disease and classified the psychopathology. As Mickle already did, he separated "cardiac delirium" from the "much more interesting mental changes" which he divides into 1. hallucinations of vision, hearing and smell, 2. changing of moods with depression or exaltation, 3. suspicion and 4. changes in memory and attention [25].

We encounter the same problem of differentiation of psychopathological syndromes after cardiac surgery. The most important fact that is in these cases is that delirium and a classical exogenic psychosis with clouding of consciousness are separated from paranoid and hallucinatory syndromes with a clear sensorium. Also after cardiac surgery we meet a third major category of syndromes, those with gnostic and memory defects.

The last great treatise on the subject was published in 1910 by Jakob: "Symptomatology, pathogenesis and pathological anatomy of circulatory psychoses" (Zur Symptomatologie, Pathogenese und pathologischen Anatomie der Kreislaufpsy-chosen") [26]. Jakob describes minutely the cardiac findings of 8 patients who developed psychoses in the course of their disease and raises the question, already asked by D'Astros [23], Parant [27], and Fisher [28] as to why all patients with terminal heart disease do not develop psychoses. Jakob does not believe, as the French authors assume, that rheumatic disease is the cause, but rather implicates other etiological factors in connection with an hereditary predisposition [26].

In 1911, Bonhoeffer introduced his concept of "exogenous psychoses" (exogene Reaktionstypen) into psychiatry, implying the uniformity of psychopathologic reactions independent of the various and different causes of known etiologies, e.g., infectious, traumatic, metabolic [29]. Terms like "cardiogenic" or "circulatory" psychoses were no longer favoured as an etiological entity. Nevertheless, even in Germany, where the term "cardiac psychosis" was not favoured anymore in psychiatry, case histories and even treatises on the subject did appear in the following years. The English and French literature also continued to occupy themselves with "cardiogenic psychoses".

Saathoff described 3 cases of aortic valve disease with a psychopathology of anxious confusion, auditory hallucinations and violent outbreaks. Besides an individual predisposition, he sees cardiac failure as a whole as the cause of the mental symptoms [30].

In 1911 a review article appeared by Cotton and Hammond: 'Cardio-genetic psychosis" and a report of one case with an autopsy. A 55 year old woman developed symptoms of anxious depression and delirious episodes with vivid reaction to visual and auditory hallucinations. The autopsy showed a marked myocardial degeneration, chronic sclerotic mitral endocarditis and subacute adhesive pericarditis. Organic heart distress as a whole was seen as a cause of cardiogenic psychosis [31].

Another review article appears in 1921 by Riesman: "Acute psychoses arising during the course of heart disease" [32]. The psychopathology is divided into 5 subgroups, differentiating again those pictures with and without clouding of consciousness, i.e.: 1. Hallucinations, especially rhythmic sounds, 2. confusion, 3. excitation with disorientation, alternating with apathy and excitement, 4. acute mania and melancholia, 5. delusional states, usually persecutory form. "Visceral disease, is seen as the cause of particular diseases of the heart".

Wassermann summarizes again the psychopathology of organic heart disease and depicts syndromes which include symptoms of exogenous and endogenous psychosis, e.g., catatonic behaviour which appeared already in the case history of the 19th century when the distinction between exogenous and endogenous was not yet made. Wassermann believed that biochemical processes are the cause of psychopathology in cardiac psychoses [33].

Hamburger presented 5 cases of "acute cardiac psychosis" with "delirium, acute confusion, visual hallucinations, . . . insomnia, dreams . . .". In all cases he believed that advanced and recurring heart failure, advanced age (47, 49, 64, 66 years) and arteriosclerotic disease and hypertension are the main causes [34]. Left ventricular failure was also seen as the main cause in 1 case of "folie cardiaque" described by Targowla with alternating states of panic and depressive symptoms [35]. Also in this case vivid dreams played a role as in the cases of Hamburger. This is interesting, because after cardiac surgery vivid dreams play a special role (Meyendorf) [36].

Massini divides the psychopathology of organic heart disease into 2 types: 1. delirium with disorientation and 2. delirium without disorientation. Delirium can be understood in this case as an exogenous psychosis. This description of psychopathology is of interest, because he describes the same psychopatho-ophthalmological and gnostic disorders which can be observed in connection with psychoses after cardiac surgery. Massini speaks of optical hallucinations occurring without clouding of consciousness in two ways: 1. in the form of well-formed hallucinations (Gestalthallu-zinationen) and 2. in the form of elementary hallucinations (Elementarhalluzinationen), i.e., hallucinations of unformed objects [37]. After cardiac surgery, visual phenomena may occur in the form of 1. disturbances of visual accuracy, i.e., doubling of contours, surfaces appear fuzzy, waviness of linear components, micropsia, macropsia, upside down vision and 2. disturbances of visual reality testing, i.e., denial of blindness (Anton-Syndrome), visual perseveration (paliopsia) and also visual hallucinations. Visual hallucinations after cardiac surgery may be divided into the delirium type and the spectator type. The first is accompanied by mental confusion and disorientation – not highly organized: dreamlike (Massini delirium type 1 with organic heart disease) and the second is accompanied by a clear sensorium – highly organized: images of people and complex scenery [36].

Leyser writes a treatise on "heart disease and psychoses" and divides the psychopathology according to syndromes which resemble exogenous or endogenous etiology: delirium and confusion on the one hand, depressive, melancholic, anxious syndromes on the other hand. It is noticed that psychoses appear with and without peripheral edema and, besides heart disease, an unknown etiological factor must be the cause [38].

Van Lier described 7 cases of organic heart disease with the psychopathology of anxiety, melancholy, delusion and excitement and believes, that especially "myodegeneratio cordis" and an hereditary predisposition, especially a paranoid and depressive constitution, contribute to the mental symptoms. He distinguished between heart disease, which may occur also among mental patients, and psychoses which follow heart disease [39].

Coombs presents 10 cases of "mental disorder in cardiac disease" and divides them into 2 categories, 1. depression and 2. cardiac delirium which may manifest itself through a loss of memory, confusion to time and space, suspicions of persecution, and great restlessness and excitement (suicide). He believes that through cardiac defects, disturbances of cerebral circulation occur. At the same time he points out that he had reviewed 2000 cases of heart disease and found that in noncomplicated cases, the incidence of mental disturbances is not higher than in the general population. This is in line with observations in cardiac surgery: the highest incidence of postoperative psychoses occurs in cases with cerebral complications [40].

Thiele in 1913 wrote an extensive review article on the subject of "Disturbances of circulation and psychoses". Two points are of interest: first, the concept of etiology and second, the question of different psychopathological phenomena [41]. As to the first point, cardiac failure is seen as one etiological agent which causes anoxemia of the brain which leads to metabolic changes. Currently unknown etiological agents (ätiologische Zwischenglieder) play the role for producing the psychopathologies. As to the second point, it is believed that the question of brain localisation determines the type of psychopathology. I believe that anoxemia is also the first and primary cause for psychoses after cardiac surgery and that metabolic disturbances affecting cellular oxygenation are the cause for any psychotic reaction of the mind.

Gibson argues in his article "Mental changes in cardiac disease" in favor of the hypothesis of anoxemia as a cause of psychoses. He quotes Clouston, who speaks of "cyanotic delirium and cyanotic insanity", which may produce symptoms of confusion, depression, mania and hallucinations. On the other hand, Gibson has no explanation from the cardiological point of view, of

8

why one patient with serious cardiac disease is clear in mind while another shows mental symptoms. He wonders why some may suffer from the grossest forms of cardiac failure and may show no mental change beyond that of gradual enfeeblement of mind. Among 153 patients with heart disease he found 15 = 9.8% with psychotic symptoms. If we realize that in our day the incidence of cardiac psychoses aside from cardiac surgery is only a rare phenomenon we can only ascribe this to the fact that modern treatment of cardiac disease in its final stages is the reason for this reduction of incidence. Even in patients who await heart transplantation we do not observe cardiac psychoses. On the other hand the incidence of cardiac psychoses after cardiac surgery also has gone down. The overall incidence of neuropsychiatric disorders was between 40 and 70% in the 1950s and is today between 10 and 30%, depending on the center and the different operative techniques. The incidence of 10% of cardiac psychoses in 1930 may reflect very well the standard and possibility of treatment at that time [42].

Also in 1930, Stroomann presented 7 cases of cardiac psychoses in the course of heart failure with the symptoms of delirium, excitement, anxiety, delusion and stupor. He again reviews the subject and points out that psychoses may break out very suddenly when circulatory failure occurs but that the actual outbreak of the psychosis may occur as well with the manifestation of cardiac failure as during the course of its treatment. Psychoses may occur with or without edema. In 6 cases of cardiac psychoses there was no involvement of valve disease and in no case there was an hereditary predisposition or mental disease, alcoholism or lues [43].

Spielmeyer and Bodechtel investigated the histopathological findings at autopsy of those cases with cardiac psychoses. The result was that the histopathological changes were alike in cases with and without cardiac psychoses [44, 45]. There may also be no histopathological changes at all at autopsy in cases of cardiac psychoses. Urechia reports one instance of a 50 year old woman with a cardiac psychosis occurring with mitral valve disease. He summarizes the literature of the psychopathology of cardiac psychoses and distinguishes between 1. affective psychoses, paranoid syndromes, nightmares and hypnagogic hallucinations and tendencies towards suicidal behaviour and 2. character disorders in the form of exaggerated emotions, violent behaviour, states of sadness and general suspiciousness. The psychopathology appears during the phase of circulatory decompensation, "et surtout dans l'asystolie terminale" and either towards the end of resorption of edema or before edema appears. Anemia may be a secondary cause [46].

Yaskin, in a review article, deals with the differentiation between cardiac psychoses and cardiac neuroses. The psychotic psychopathology is divided into three types: 1. manic, depressive, paranoid and schizophrenic reaction types, 2. organic reaction types: confusion, disorientation, hallucinosis, persecutory trends and psychomotor excitements, 3. change in the sphere of character: change to a type of conduct foreign to the individual's natural disposition. Three categories of causes are discussed: 1. constitutional pre-disposition and toxic factors: renal toxemia, acidosis, drugs, 2. disturbances of circulation resulting in anoxemia, ie. focal brain signs appear due to arteriosclerosis, thrombosis and embolism. 3. Reflected pain of visceral disease. The concept of reflected pain from visceral disease which finally produces psychopathological symptoms also plays a role in Head's concept of psychopathology [47]

Wortis wrote a very extensive review article: "Cardiac psychoses and the symptoms of anxiety" and quoted very old literature on the subject with figures of incidence of cardiac psychoses. They are: 1, 8, 10, 90%, reflecting the immense range of different figures which reminds one of the early times of cardiac surgery when similar figures were given, depending on the method of registration of symptoms. The psychopathology consists of main and other symptoms. The main symptoms are: 1. confusion, 2. delusions of persecution and 3. anxiety. The other symptoms are: dreams and dreamlike hallucinations, nightmares, becoming overtalkative and circumstantial, visual disturbances, rhythmic auditory hallucinations, and delusions of death and murder. Important to note are the "other symptoms", because the transition of phenomena from dream to dreamlike hallucinations and visual disturbances are typical signs of pathology after cardiac surgery. Wortis describes 32 cases of cardiac failure. Cardiac failure, functional class AHA IIb and III is seen as a main cause of psychoses. It leads to organic symptoms of anxiety (without psychological factors!). There is an absence of other complicating factors! [48].

A multi-etiological view point of cardiac psychoses is presented by Gordon and Cohen who, in a retrospective study, investigate 300 cases of "heart disease" of which 62 (21%) showed "mental changes". These "mental complications of heart disease" showed, according to the records, the following symptoms: confusion (50 times = 81%), delirium (29 times = 47%), abnormal irritability (26 times = 42%), hallucinations (13 times = 21%), mania (6 times = 10%), and paranoid features (4 times = 7%). Of the 62 patients with mental changes, 52 (84%) had cardiac failure, 10 (16%) did not have cardiac failure. Eleven (18%) had a psychopathologic history, personal or family. Other etiological factors were: hypotensive vascular disease, rheumatism, syphilis, arteriosclerosis, coronary artery disease, renal impairment, alcoholic history, and a history of digitalis [49].

Just a few years before modern cardiac surgery began, Rümke described very extensively the psychopathology of cardiac psychoses. He defended this term over other exogenous psychoses (exogene Reaktionstypen Bonhoefer) and contended that in the pathogenesis of the psychoses, heart disease is the conditio sine qua non. Rümke describes very vividly the delirium with confusion and clouding of consciousness, i.e., the obvious organic components of the deranged state of mind, as well as the lucid visual and auditory hallucinations, the paranoid symptomatology, and the characteristic fear and anxiety of these patients, culminating often in the convictions of impending death. He also draws attention to the frequent occurrence of both insomnia and frightful dreams, symptoms which were later attributed to circumstances belonging to the intensive care unit with either sensory deprivation or over-stimulation. Finally, depressions, including suicidal impulses, were pointed out in patients with advanced organic heart disease, a syndrome, that we recognize to be very common after cardiac surgery.

The main etiological agent for Rümke is the change of cerebral circulation with low blood pressure. The hereditary disposition of psychotic decompensation is the second agent. There is no relation to cardiac decompensation: in one patient the psychosis appears before, in another patient during and in a third patient after cardiac decompensation. Rümke stresses the acute or sudden beginning of the psychosis which is a sign of a "true" cardiogenic psychosis [50]. Twenty years later (1960) he deals again with the question of psychology of organic heart disease and stresses again that the cardiogenic psychosis is unique among all other exogenous psychoses [51]. Rümke apparently did not take notice of the appearance of cardiac surgery, otherwise he would have realized that identical syndromes were described in the beginning of heart surgery. In 1948, mitral commisuorotomy was performed routinely when the first papers on the subject appeared: Fox et al.: "Psychological observations of patients undergoing mitral surgery", and Bliss et al.: "Psychiatric complications of mitral surgery". Case histories are presented with the title: "Schizophrenic" or "depressive reactions" which are identical to those of true "cardiac psychoses" [52, 53].

In the 60s and 70s, the literature on postoperative psychoses after cardiac surgery grew enormously. Suddenly articles appeared with the terms "Postcardiotomy delirium", "Cardiac psychoses", or "Post-operative psychoses" in which psychopathological syndromes were described which did not differ at all from cardiac psychoses except for the cardiac surgery. No reference was made to the cardiac psychosis literature whatsoever [54, 55, 56].

On the other hand, the literature on cardiac psychoses aside from cardiac surgery did not subside either. In these articles no reference is made to the psychopathological syndromes after cardiac surgery. Probably psychoses after cardiac surgery were seen as types of postoperative psychosis which also occur after different kinds of surgery. The incidence of postoperative psychoses in other fields of surgery other than cardiac surgery is however very low (0.1–1.0%).

Lueg and Weber wrote an article on "Psychotic disturbances during cardiac failure". They present a case and review the question of cardiac psychoses. Three types of psychopathological syndromes are described: 1. Less severe psychic disturbances such as irritability, psychomotor excitement and suspiciousness, 2. symptomatic psychoses (akuter Reaktionstyp Bonhoefer), and 3. endogenous psychoses: schizophrenic, manic types with a question of whether their manifestation was triggered through cardiac decompensation [57]. Leibbrandt also presents a case of cardiac psychosis and notes that a family member of the patient suffered from schizophrenia [58].

Roger, in a review article, concluded that chronic circulatory insufficiency is a cause for cardiac psychosis and pointed out that the incidence of cerebral complications in heart disease may go up to 35% (116 complications among 343 cardiac patients). He divided minor and major psychopathological syndromes, i.e., nervousness and restlessness on the one hand, delirium and hallucinations on the other hand [59].

Degkwitz presented 17 cases of "symptomatic psychoses" and tried to prove that at the time of resorption of edema, the psychosis manifests itself. Toxic substances may play a role [60].

De Busscher and Matthijs presented 6 cases of cardiac psychoses and described pictures of altered consciousness, amnesia, visual hallucinations, profound anxiety, paranoid melancholia and melancholia with self accusation. They believed that "alterations in circulation" were the cause for cardiac psychoses. They also believed that cardiac psychosis is a psychosis sui generis among all other exogenous psychoses [61].

Lennartz wrote a basic article on "Psychological changes in the course of heart and circulatory disease" and believed that, through heart disease, all degrees of endogenous mental diseases may be triggered [62].

Aresin investigated in a prospective study, 50 cases with heart failure and detected 7 (14%) cardiac psychoses (Herzpsychosen). The psychopathology shows anxiety, psycho-motor restlessness, and hallucinations, mainly visual, but also auditory. He did not find any psychological (psychogenic) causes for the manifestation of the psychoses. There is no relation between a conflict of character and psychosis. He believed that disturbed brain circulation was a cause [63].

Heidrich and Ott described 9 cases of cardiac psychoses. The psychopathology is characterized by exogenous (delirium type) and endogenous (schizophrenic type) disturbances. Hereditary predisposition is believed to be one cause for a psychotic manifestation. The question of autointoxication is raised. In two cases the psychoses appeared without decompensation, in one case during decompensation, and in 6 cases after cardiac decompensation [64].

Hoffmann described one case of delusions of infestation (Dematozoenwahn) occurring during cardiac decompensation which disappeared after implantation of a pacemaker [65].

Meyendorf gives a short review on "Psychopathology in heart disease aside from cardiac surgery" and describes mental changes in organic heart disease (61 patients) and 9 cases of acute cardiac psychoses. There were 45 mental changes (73.8%): 19 depressive syndromes (31.1%), 9 dysphoric syndromes (14.8%), 8 manic syndromes (13.1%), 7 organic brain syndromes (11.5%) and 2 phobic obsessive syndromes (3.3%). The acute psychoses were: 4 paranoid-hallucinatory syndromes, 3 paranoid-depressive syndromes, and 2 delirious syndromes (cardiac delirium with clouding of consciousness and loss of orientation). The 9 patients who developed a classical cardiac psychosis were cases of emergency to whom I was called in the course of 5 years. The 61 patients with organic heart disease were systematically evaluated for psychiatric disturbances [66].

Meyendorf compared the psychiatric disturbances in the course of organic heart disease and after cardiac surgery. The causes of preoperative psychopathology in cardiac surgery patients are basically the same as the causes

12

of post-operative psychopathology. The main cause is hypoxemia. The type of psychopathology depends on an hereditary disposition for a special reaction type. The "exogenous" reaction types can be distinguished only from the "endogenous" reaction types if clouding of consciousness and disorientation plays a role (delirium type). The non-delirium-type of exogenous psychoses can not be distinguished from endogenous reaction types except that they disappear as a rule after a short time. They can be compared however with other psychoses of a very short duration for which no exogenous cause can be found which must be classified however as true psychosis of the endogenous type [67].

References

1. Douty JH. The mental symptoms of aortic regurgitation. Lancet 1885; 2: 336.
2. Eichhorst H. Toxämische Delirien bei Herzkranken. Dtsch Med Wochenschr 1898; 25:389.
3. Gerhardt C. Herzkrankheit und Geisteskrankheit. Wien Med Press 1865; 7: 155.
4. Jaquet A. Über nervöse und psychische Störungen bei Herzkrankheiten. Schweiz Med Wochenschr 1922; 10:145.
5. Joffe H. Geisteskrankheit durch Embolie der Hirngefässe bei bestandener Insufficiensia mitralis. Vierteljahrachr. Psychiatr I Heft, 1867; 57.
6. Kellogg ThH. A textbook on mental diseases. New York, William Wood, 1897.
7. Kiernan JG. Insanity and cardiac disease. Am J Neurol Psychiat 1884; 3:32.
8. Meyendorf R. Hirnembolie und Psychose. Unter Berücksichtigung der Basalganglienapoplexie bei Herzoperationen mit extrakorporaler Zirkulation. J Neurol 1976; 213:163.
9. Mildner E. Spitals-Praxis. Aus der kk. Irrenanstalt in Wien. Wien Med Wochenschr 1857; 46:830; 47:848.
10. Reinhold G. Über organische und funktionelle Herzleiden bei Geisteskranken. Münch Med Wochenschr 1894; 41:305, 328, 355.
11. Saucerotte G. L'influence des maladies du coeur sur les facultés intellectuelles et morales de l'homme. Annal Méd Psych 1844; 4:173.
12. Telgmann J. Toxämische Delirien bei Herzkrankheiten. Dtsch Med Wochenschr 1899; 24:305.
13. Ideler KW. Wirkung der Krankheiten des Kreislaufs auf die Seele. In Grundriss der Seelenheilkunde. Berlin: Theod. Chr. Fried. Enslin-Verlag 1835.
14. Nasse F. Von der psychischen Beziehung des Herzens. Z f psychische Ärzte 1818; 1:49.
15. Burrows GM. Commentare. Weimar, Grossh. Landes-Industrie-Comptoirs, 1831.
16. Jacobi, M. Die Hauptformen der Seelenstörungen in ihrer Beziehung zur Heilkunde. Leipzig. Verlag der Weidmann'sschen Buchhandlung, 1844.
17. Bergmann G. Mania metastatica, vom Herzen ausgehend. Allg Z Psychiatr 1844; 1:574.
18. Krishaber M. Névropathie cérebro-cardiaque. Gaz hebd de méd Paris 1872; 9:323, 342, 371, 422, 434, 485, 550, 581.
19. Burman JW. Heart disease and insanity. West Riding Lunatic Asylum. London, Medical Reports 1873.
20. Witkowski L. Über Herzleiden bei Geisteskrankheiten. Allg Z Psychiatrie 1875; 32:347.
21. Karrer. Über Herzkrankheiten bei Geisteskranken. In Geisteskrankheiten, Erlangen: Hrsg.: FW Hagen. Eduard Besold, 1876.
22. Greenlees TD. Contribution to the study of diseases of the circulatory system in the insane. J Ment Sci 1886; 31:327.
23. D'Astros L. Troubles Psychiques des Cardiaques. Paris: Adrien Delahaye et E. Lecrosnier, 1881.

24. Mickle J. Insanity in relation to cardiac and aortic disease and phthisis. Brit Med J 1888; 1:503.
25. Head H. Certain mental changes that accompany visceral disease. Brain 1901; 14:345.
26. Jakob A. Zur Symptomatologie, Pathogenese und pathologischen Anatomie der "Kreislaufpsychosen" Psychol Neurol 1909–1910; 14:209, 15:99.
27. Parant V. La folie chez les cardiaques. Ann Med Psychol Paris 1889; 7:419.
28. Fischer J. Über Psychosen bein Herzkranken. Allg Z Psychiat 1898; 54:1048.
29. Bonhoeffer K. Die Psychosen im Gefolge von akuten Infektionen, Allgemeinkrankheiten und inneren Erkrankungen. In Aschaffenburg G. (Hrsg.) Handbuch der Psychiatrie. Deuticke, Leipzig, Wien: B: Spezieller Teil, 3. Abt., 1. Hälfte. 1912.
30. Saathoff L. Herzkrankheit und Psychose. Münch Med Wochenschr 1910; 57:509.
31. Cotton H A, Hamond S. Cardio-genetic psychoses. Report of a case with autopsy. Amer J Insan 1911; 67:467.
32. Riesman D. Acute psychoses arising during the course of heart disease. Amer J Med Sci (Phil) 1921; 161:157.
33. Wassermann S. Über psychische Störungen in Verbindung mit den Cheyne-Stokesschen Phänomenen bei gewissen Herzkrankheiten (Die Cheyen-Stockessche Psychose). Med Klin 1921; 17:814.
34. Hamburger W W. Acute cardiac psychoses: Analysis of the toxic and circulatory factors in 5 cases of acute confusion. Med Clin North Am 1923; 7:465.
35. Targowla M R. "Folie cardiaque" et insuffisance ventriculaire gauche. Bull Soc Med 1923; 14:615.
36. Meyendorf R. Psychopatho-opthalmology, gnostic disorders, and psychosis in cardiac surgery – visual disturbances after open heart surgery. Arch Psychiatr Nervenkr 1982; 232:119.
37. Massini R. Über Delirien bei Herzkranken. Schweiz Med Wochenschr 1924; 54:397.
38. Leyser E. Herzkrankheiten und Psychosen. Berlin: Karger, 1924.
39. Van Lier J. Psychose en hart. Ned Tijdschr Geneeskd 1925; 69:2661.
40. Coombs C F. Mental disorder in cardiac disease. J Ment Sci. 1928; 74:305, 250.
41. Thiele R. Kreislaufstörungen und Psychosen. Allg. Ztschr Psychiatrie 1930; 92:208.
42. Gibson A G. Mental changes in cardiac disease. J Ment Sci 1930; 76:632.
43. Stroomann G. Über die psychotischen Störungen bei dekompensierten Herzkranken, speziell über die Zusammenhänge mit der therapeutischen Entwässerung. Nervenarzt 1930; 3:396.
44. Speilmeyer W. Kreislaufstörungen und Psychosen. Z ges Neurol Pschiat 1930; 123:536.
45. Bodechtel G. Gehirnveränderungen bei Herzkrankheiten. Z ges Neurol Psychiat 1932; 140:657.
46. Urechia C I. Psychose post-opèratoire. Arch Internat Neur 1934; 53:563.
47. Yaskin, J C. Cardiac psychoses and neuroses. Am Heart J 1936; 12: 536.
48. Wortis J. Cardiac psychosis and the symptom of anxiety. Am Heart J 1937; 13:394.
49. Gordon A H, Cohen W. The mental complications of heart disease. Canad Med Ass J 1938; 39:517.
50. Rümke H C. Over psychoses bij hartziekten. Ned Tijdschr Geneeskd 1939; 1:728.
51. Rümke H C. Psychosen bij hartziekten. In Psychiatrie II De Psychosen. Amsterdam: Scheltema and Holkema NV, 1960.
52. Fox H M, Rizzo N D, Gifford S. Psychological observations of patients undergoing mitral surgery. Psychosomat Med 1954; 16:186.
53. Bliss E L, Rumel W R, Branch C H H. Psychiatric complications of mitral surgery. Arch Neurol Psychiatry 1955; 74:249.
54. Blachly R H, Starr A. Post-cardiotomy delirium. Am J Psychiatry 1964; 121:371.
55. Abram H S. Adaption to open heart surgery: A psychiatric study of response to the threat of death. Am J Psychiatry 1965; 122:659.
56. Layne O L. Jr, Yudofsky S C. Postoperative psychosis in cardiotomy patients. N Engl J Med 1971; 284:518.
57. Lueg W, Weber R. Über psychotische Störungen bei dekompensierten Herzkranken. Med Welt 1940; 20: 505.

14

58. Leibbrandt CW. Psychose bij stenose van de stihmus aortae. Ned Tijdschr Geneeskd 1949; 93:1875.
59. Roger H. Coeur et cerveau. Hémiplégie, troubles psychiques des cardiaques. Ann Méd Psychol 1953; 111:601.
60. Degkwitz R. Die Verminderung der aktiven Blutmenge bei symptomatischen Kreislaufpsychosen. Nervenarzt 1957; 28:28.
61. De Busscher J, Matthijs R. Les Troubles Psychiques, Symptomatiques D'Alterations Circulatoires D'Origine Cardiaque. Folia psychiat Neerlandia 1958; 61:101.
62. Lennartz H. Psychische Veränderungen bei Herzund Kreislauferkrankungen. Med Welt 1958; 35:1279.
63. Aresin L. Über Korrelation zwischen Persönlichkeit, Lebensgeschichte und Herzkrankheit. In Sammlung zwangloser Abhandlungen aus dem Gebiete der Psychiatrie und Neurologie. Fischer, Jena: Hrsg. Prof. Dr. H. Schwarz. 1960.
64. Heidrich R, Ott J. Exogene Psychosen bei Herzkrankheiten. Psychiat Neurol Med Psychol (Lpz) 1965; 17:401.
65. Hoffmann SO. Rückbildung eines sog. Dermatozoenwahns nach Schrittmacherimplantation – Zum Problem der symptomatischen Psychosen bei Herzkrankheiten. Nervenarzt 1973; 44:48.
66. Meyendorf R. Psychopathology in heart disease aside from cardiac surgery: a historical perspective of cardiac psychosis. Compr Psychiatry 1979; 20:326.
67. Meyendorf R. Die psychischen Störungen bei organischen Herzerkrankungen und im Verlaufe der Herzchirurgie. Internist 1981; 22:24.

2. Cardiac surgery and acute neurological injury

JOHN C. OPIE

Introduction

The brain epitomizes Haldane'e dictum: "Anoxia does not only stop the machine, it wrecks it." Both survival and the quality of the surgical result after open heart surgery depend upon the delivery of oxygen to the brain. The brain consumes 3–5 ml of oxygen/100 g/min, or more than 20% of the total body consumption of oxygen, and nearly 15% of the cardiac output is required to deliver this amount of oxygen to the brain which itself only accounts for 2.5% of the body weight [1].

Open heart operations with cardiopulmonary bypass have proved to be a potent multifactorial hazard for all the levels of the nervous system. The final brain damaging effects of cardiopulmonary bypass are at least partly uncertain and because clinical methods are of limited value in explaining the basic events, investigations must focus on the nerve cell and on the regulators of its metabolism.

Incidence

Neurologic complications associated with surgery of the heart are distressingly frequent enough to be a constant concern to the surgical, anesthetic, and nursing care of the cardiac surgical patient.

The reported incidence of neurologic injury attributable to cardiac surgery has varied from an incidence of 30% reported in 1965 [2], to 53% in 1969 [3], to 44% in 1970 [4]. Following this period, there has been a steady decline in the incidence of brain damage associated with cardiac surgery; more recent reports indicate that the incidence is now more likely to be nearer 5% [5–8]. There are some reports indicating a 2% stroke incidence [9]. The reported decline in the incidence of acute brain syndromes is thought at least in part due to the following:

15

- Improved perfusion techniques.
- Filter (5 micron) use during priming of bypass circuit.
- Arterial line filtration (20 micron).
- Reduced perfusion times.
- Avoidance of perioperative hypotension.
- Treatment of carotid bruits.
- Awareness of the dangers of and how to handle cardiac air.
- Extensive use of hypothermia.
- Cardiotomy filtration (40 micron).
- Venous filtration (100 micron).
- Improved intensive care unit management protocols.

Since the late 1970's there seems to be little change in the incidence of acute cerebral syndromes following cardiac surgery. The general advancing age of cardiac surgical patients may mitigate against the improved technologies.

Presentation

- Altered mental state [2–7, 10]
     Confusion
     Delirium
     Hypoxic-metabolic encephalopathy
     Transient memory deficit
     Altered personality [11]
- Visual impairment [12]
- Voluntary and involuntary movements [12]
- Stroke, mild to dense and extensive [2, 9]
- Seizure disorders (opisthotonos, general and focal)
- Sensory disorders
- Intellectual impairment [7]
- Mononeuritis monoplex [13, 14]
- Cerebellar syndromes [3, 4]
- Brain stem lesions [3, 4]

The majority of patients appear to wake from anesthesia with these effects, although significant defects are observed to develop in the intensive care setting in the postoperative period.

One third of the injuries are focal and half have a likely identifiable cause [10, 15]. Two-thirds are nonfocal and 13% have a possible identifiable cause [10, 15].

Etiology

The pathologic mechanisms causing these cerebral syndromes are not clearly established. The most likely causes of such events are:

- Impaired perfusion (low flow, low pressure bypass) [11]
- Embolization of particulate matter (calcium, fat, platelet aggregations, cholesterol emboli, infected vegetation, atrial myxoma fragments, plastic debris [16], etc.).
- Air embolization (note also right to left or balanced intracardiac shunts and venous air).
- Hypotension
- Hypoxia
- Intracerebral hemorrhage
- Increased age
- Pre-existing renal disease
- Propranolol [17]
- Prolonged extracorporeal circulation
- Perioperative cardiac arrest
- Bubble oxygenators [18] (without a 25 micron arterial filter and bubble trap).
- Existing cerebrovascular disease
- Abnormal cardiac rhythm
- Technical problems on bypass
- Regional blood flow variations on bypass
- Altered blood pressure-volume relationships
- Altered blood composition, e.g., lowered viscosity, gas-hemoglobin affinity alterations, blood gas tensions, hematocrit and oxygen carrying capacity of hemodiluted blood, and blood pH.

There is frequent opportunity for cerebral ischemia to occur during cardiac surgery due to any of the above listed events, and improved methods for assessing and quantifying brain damage during and after bypass are urgently needed. Very few methods exist that can measure brain function during cardiac repair, and those that are available (e.g., evoked potentials, electroencephalography) are imprecise and are not reliable if used to select optimal bypass technique. Newer technologies such as intra-arterial Xenon 133, transcranial Doppler ultrasonography, or the cerebral function analyzing monitor may be useful advances [18–20].

Prevention measures

Avoid cannulating through heavy calcium deposits in the aorta. They may be easily detached and embolized. Select a site if possible where the vessel is soft and pliant. It is reasonable to briefly lower the perfusion pressure by "emptying out" the patient transiently before applying any aortic clamp. This protects the left ventricle from high pressure ejection and allows the surgeon to quickly palpate the aorta for calcium plaques, while it is in a relaxed state and select the best site for the clamp.

Selective cannulation of a branch vessel or the descending thoracic aorta may be undesirable, and in general it may be wiser to use an aortic cannula which is short but long enough to lie in the ascending aorta with its terminal opening near the origin of the innominate artery. Side holes have an indeterminate benefit but are widely available with common perfusion cannulas.

Avoid side clamping of the aorta as a routine for cannulating, but do not hesitate to proceed with this if it is indicated (refer above).

Avoid lifting the heart prior to cross clamping, especially if there is known left ventricular mural thrombus. This can lead to detachment of a major free embolus and catastrophe.

Avoid manipulating the heart with known or suspected atrial clot or tumors, e.g., chronic atrial fibrillation or atrial myxoma. Fragments can embolize from such pathology residing in the left atrium with disastrous consequences.

Avoid unnecessary cardiac manipulation in friable bacterial endocarditis lesions and in prosthetic valve reoperations in which the patients are suffering poorly controlled embolic phenomena due to valve malfunction. Arrange to apply the cross clamp early in the procedure.

Remove free emboli seen to fall into the ventricle and aorta and left atrium when these structures are open.

Flush and aspirate the left ventricle especially during aortic valve replacement procedures. A soaked sponge with a long black thread for identification placed in the cavity of the left ventricle is widely employed, and removed when aortic root and valve decalcification procedures are complete. It acts as a trap and on removal is frequently seen to have caught multiple fragments of noxious debris which may otherwise have been lost inside the interstices of the cavity of the left ventricle only to be fired out at some time later. Calcium emboli have been noted in the retinal artery and have produced delayed sudden blindness after an uneventful operation days before.

Eliminate I.V. tubing air in patients with intracardiac shunts, e.g., atrial septal defects, aortopulmonary windows, etc. This can result in a major systemic air embolus to the patient's brain.

Apply the aortic cross clamp early, prior to significant cardiac manipulation and apply the clamp with just enough force to prevent retrograde bleeding if the aortic root is open, e.g., one to two clicks on the ratchet. It is not necessary nor desirable to use five or six clicks routinely, as this will increase the tendency to damage and fracture the aorta.

Reduce the bypass flows and assume Trendelenburg position (head down) at cross clamp release. Ensure that there is an aortic leak or an aortic vent on high suction at this point. Many surgeons will apply a partially occluding aortic clamp to create an aortic bubble trap distal to a root suction device during active de-airing procedures, and this may help to trap bubbles which will then be aspirated by the root suction.

Transient carotid compression by anesthesia personnel is extensively employed as a possible useful adjunct. However, subsequent carotid release may allow cerebral damage to develop in any case.

Do not assume that intravenous or intracardiac heparin once given will induce a state of total body anticoagulation. Wait for a confirmatory activated clotting time or heparin assay before going on bypass. An accident at this point will likely result in a significant disaster with extensive implications. Inactive solutions, incorrect solutions, extravasation of solutions, or heparin resistance due to antibodies can all occur.

Be meticulous in removing air from the heart at the completion of the procedure. Many variations are used and each surgeon will employ whichever technique they are comfortable with and which works best for them. A sensible approach is that air must be assumed to have entered all structures, even in coronary artery bypass procedures.

Air can be usefully aspirated from upstream structures to downstream structures in sequential order, i.e., pulmonary veins, left atrial appendage, left ventricle, aorta, and repeating the cycle several times with vent suction, several Valsalva maneuvers from the anesthesiologist, and gentle shaking of the heart. The left atrial appendage can be usefully inverted with the surgeon's right index finger with an aortic or left ventricular needle or vent aspirating. The left ventricular apex can be usefully everted while wobbling the heart and aspirating. These procedures stop when no more air is seen to be escaping. It has been a traditional practice to place the patient in Trendelenburg and leave the aorta leaking for several minutes after the cross clamp has been removed and the heart has resumed beating.

The entire hypothesis is loosely based upon the following concepts: That the buoyant properties of bubbles will float them away from the direction of the blood flow, and away from the effects of gravity to the top of the aorta, where it is being vented, and secondly that cerebral vasodilation, as a result of the back pressure generated by the Trendelenburg position, will allow the bubbles to pass through the cerebral microcirculation. However, recent experimental investigations on the effects of assuming the Trendelenburg position and the distribution of arterial air emboli in dogs concluded that the forces of buoyancy do not overcome the force of the arterial blood flow and that the Trendelenburg position does not prevent air from reaching the brain.

This interesting study showed that the large bubbles (0.386 cm) increased in velocity in the blood flow direction up to 30 degrees, and only decreased at 90 degrees (impractical in the clinical setting), and small bubbles (0.237 cm) did not alter their velocity nor their direction of motion and they flowed with the blood up to 30 degrees, and actually increased their velocity and flowed with the blood flow at 90 degrees. No bubbles reached a minimum velocity equal to or less than the velocity of the blood (20 cm/second). To date, the author could not locate any scientific evidence to indicate that the Trendelenburg position, which does dilate the cerebral venous channels, also conclusively dilates the cerebral microvasculature [21]. Thus, both the central hypotheses of the Trendelenburg position in the setting of arterial air emboli have now been scientifically challenged.

Specific emergency measures for major air emboli vary as above but could also include ventilation with 100% oxygen, administration of steroids or possibly barbiturates, and possible temporary retrograde perfusion with cardiopulmonary bypass via the venous cannula with aortic drainage, i.e., transient flow reversal to "back out" the air. In this setting, the Trendelenburg position could have a very useful role. Hyperbaric compression has been reported useful if a chamber is logistically available [22].

Pathophysiology of acute brain syndromes

All brain tissue has a constant requirement for oxygen in order to meet its energy needs. Under normal conditions over 90% of this energy requirement (impulse transmission and membrane ionic gradients) is supplied in the blood and is derived from glucose oxidation [23]. Measured average cerebral blood flow is commonly about 40 ml/100 g/min [24]. Minimal energy storage capacity exists in the brain; therefore, only about four minutes of anoxia can be tolerated at normal temperatures before acute brain syndromes occur. During acute total anoxia and circulatory arrest at normothermia, unconsciousness develops within 15 seconds [25], and electrocerebral silence develops when cerebral venous pO_2 falls below 20 mm Hg – 18 seconds of total anoxia [26].

When local cerebral oxygen transport is reduced, there is uncoupling of flow and metabolism and local lactate acidosis results, with release of creatinine kinase, lactate dehydrogenase, and aspartate aminotransferase into cerebrospinal fluid. The brain specific isoenzyme fraction of creatine kinase, CKBB, peaks between 48 and 72 hours after global brain ischemia. These enzymes have been measured acutely in brain infarctions during cardiac surgery [24]. This may equate to a reduction in blood flow to less than 16–22 ml/100 g/min. This is accompanied by EEG slowing or extinction, and will lead to the development of tissue hyperemic hyperoxygenation or luxury flow (more than 60 ml/100 g/min), if or when blood supply is resumed. The presence of the hyperemia implies compensation for hypoxia and indicates that flow reduction has occurred.

Several factors may be important in this uncoupling reaction and the prominent activators are listed below:

Microvascular blockade due to emboli. (Air, antifoam, foreign particles – calcium, etc., fibrin, spoliated plastic particles [16, 18, 27].

Thrombocyte aggregation [28]. The essential reaction in this circumstance appears to be as follows. Cell damage occurs as a result of cardiopulmonary bypass. This results in release of membrane arachidonic acid. Under the catalysis of cyclo-oxygenase (inhibited by aspirin), cyclic prostaglandin endoperoxides are formed, and these further react with cyclo-oxygenase and activated platelets. These activated platelets undergo complex reactions with adenosine diphosphate (ADP) and become alpha degranulated. This is associated with the release of measurable amounts of low affinity platelet factor 4 (LA-PF4 with anti-heparin effects). This reaction results in the creation of ecosanoids and two arms proceed. (1) Thromboxanes are released. Initially thromboxane A2 (half life of 30 seconds) is produced and rapidly converts into TXB2. The latter is stable and inactive and is produced in measurable quantities by cardiopulmonary bypass. This reaction is greater in nonpulsatile perfusion. TXA2 is a powerful platelet aggregant and a putative vasoconstrictor. It may result in cerebral subset veno-occlusive disease, due to platelet aggregation and deposition. (2) This arm is counterbalanced at least in part by the formation of prostacyclin. This has a half life of 5–10 min and is degraded into 6-keto-prostaglandin F_{1a}. The latter is measurable in the blood. This reaction is higher in pulsatile perfusion. This second arm (prostacyclin release), which may be overwhelmed by the thromboxane pathway especially in extensively utilized routine nonpulsatile perfusions, decreases platelet adhesiveness and is a potent vasodilator [29–33].

Stagnant capillary flow. (Intrinsic to nonpulsatile perfusion.)

Radioactive xenon studies indicate that there is a marked increase in cerebral blood flow during hypothermic cardiopulmonary bypass. During such bypass, brain metabolism is reduced and high brain blood flow must reflect uncoupling of flow and metabolism, and therefore, a state of luxury perfusion. This state of hypoperfusion could be a temporary diffuse microvascular blockade of at least moderate degree and related to extensive platelet consumption that occurs at the onset of bypass. Factors found to reduce hyperperfusion included reduced pCO_2 and a perfusion pressure less than 55 mm Hg. was associated with reduced cerebral blood flow, indicating that brain blood flow autoregulation was lost below this pressure.

Etiology

Central

Utilizing 2 MHz transcranial noninvasive Doppler studies focused on the middle cerebral artery during clinical bypass [18, 34], it has been shown that insertion of the aortic cannula was associated with a very high incidence of gaseous microemboli, that bubble oxygenators allowed frequent gaseous microemboli, and that this effect was fast flow dependent, but no such emboli were detected with membrane oxygenators [18, 35].

In patients with carotid artery disease undergoing cardiac surgery, the risk of central nervous system damage varies around 2 to 3%. The incidence of combined carotid and coronary atherosclerosis is reported to be as high as 49% [36]. Asymptomatic bruits may portend less risk than transient ischemic attacks or previous strokes, but there is no clear-cut relationship [37–40]. Recent evidence has demonstrated that clinical evaluation may overestimate the severity of carotid disease and duplex Doppler scanning may be the easiest noninvasive and most reliable method to evaluate the carotid disease [36].

Because of the lack of correlation of carotid disease and CNS events, some authors take the position that most of the CNS events are embolic, e.g., air and dislodgement of mural thrombus material [36].

Intracranial hemorrhages can also occur in association with cardiac surgery. These have a slightly higher incidence in children undergoing cardiac surgery. The more common hemorrhagic lesions encountered are epidural hematomas, but subdural hematomas, subarachnoid and intracerebral hemorrhages have also occurred. The pathogenesis is uncertain but anticoagulation, hypertonic intravenous solutions, e.g., bicarbonate, excessive diuresis, and venous (or arterial) hypertension have all been implicated.

Peripheral

In the circumstances of mononeuritis monoplex, suggested factors which promote its occurrence are prolonged malposition on the operating table with neuropraxia and axonotomesis due to compression, pre-existing diabetes mellitus, and atherosclerosis. Reported incidence is close to 0.1% [14, 41, 42]. The prognosis is good and complete resolution can be expected in the majority.

The ischemia may on occasion be due to diffuse inflammatory disease of the arteries, such as polyarteritis nodosa. In this instance, the arteries of the vasa nervorum produces the ischemic lesion [43].

Subacute bacterial endocarditis with friable lesions have been associated with both central and peripheral nerve tissue damage [44].

The effects of arterial filters and bubble oxygenators have been investigated and the possible role of gaseous microemboli in peripheral nerve lesions has been examined but so far these effects remain unconfirmed [14]

Reported syndromes include the following:

- Mononeuropathies of common peroneal nerve, saphenous nerve, and ulnar nerve.
- Brachial radiculoplexopathy.
- Singultus – following phrenic nerve injury, reported secondary to ice damage as well as division, etc. [45].
- Recurrent laryngeal injury
- Horner's syndrome
- Facial nerve neuropathy

The presumed causes include trauma associated with central venous cannulation, stretching of nerve roots due to retractors and prolonged malpositioning, cauterization or divisions, or direct nerve traction or pinching between forceps, etc.

Neurologic syndromes following open heart surgery

Two categories of acute nervous system syndromes occur:

(a) Transient
(b) Permanent

A. Transient syndromes

It is notable that these syndromes cannot be clearly correlated with the type or duration of cardiac surgery, nor with electrolyte or acid base balance. Microair embolism is a likely cause and recognition is difficult unless a transcranial Doppler velocimeter is scanning the middle cerebral artery [18]. The likely source of the air has been identified above. The brains of some patients who die for other reasons after cardiac surgery have been shown on occasions to have minute particles of plastic which has been spoliated from the Tygon (R) plastic pump head compression segments. These could be important causes for these syndromes. The neurologic deficits commonly last for only a few hours, and often are confined to the immediate postoperative period. Within a week or more that 60% can be expected to have resolved, and in general, recovery is rapid and complete. The reported incidence is approximately 25% [46]. The neurological deficits include the following:

Confusion and/or violent delirium. This may be associated with the so-called Anti-Cholinergic Brain Syndrome. This dramatic syndrome is associated with the preinduction and induction use of the acetyl cholinergic inhibitor (parasympathetic neuromuscular blocking – predominantly antimuscurinic) drugs such as scopolamine 1-hyoscine – Scope Reaction [47]. Postoperatively the patients may have both central and peripheral signs of toxicity. They appear drowsy and confused but with periods of alert orientation, in between episodes of disorientation, anxiety, hallucinations, and periodically seizures. The peripheral signs include tachycardia, hyperpyrexia, mydriasis, cycloplegia (loss of accommodation), vasodilation, urinary retention, gastric stasis, dry mouth and skin, and dry air passages.

Without warning, possibly as the result of release of a "cholinergic bomb" (building, due to the blocking effects of scopolamine), which suddenly hits disinhibited receptors and a large discharge occurs. This can result in an aggressive delirious attack on an unsuspecting nurse or physician, and injury can result. The patient frequently is crazed and hospital security may be needed to restrain the patient until the first dose of slow intravenous *Physostigmine* (Antilirium), a tertiary amine – reversible anticholinesterase which easily crosses the blood brain barrier, can be administered to settle the violent patient. This drug only lasts about 60 minutes and may need several administrations. The syndrome has the potential to recur several times. The best recommendation is to discontinue the use of scopolamine in these patients. Newer and less irritant anesthetics make this a reasonable approach.

An overdose of Antilirium can induce a Cholinergic Crisis, characterized by bradycardia, defecation, emesis, hypersalivation with respiratory insufficiency, and possible convulsions. Atropine is an antidote.

- Impaired consciousness.
- Memory defects.
- Visual hallucinations.

24

New positive archaic reflexes (lack of cortical and subcortical inhibition of brain stem reflexes), e.g., Palmomental reflex is considered a sign of subclinical cerebral impairment.

Impaired neuropsychologic evaluation (61% incidence in some series [48]. Wechsler Memory Scale and Adult Intelligence Scale).

The majority of these patients will be able to return to ordinary life once recovered from their cardiac surgery and they should be reassured that this syndrome is transient and related to extensive surgery.

An amnestic syndrome has been described in cardiac arrest patients which follows a brief period of postoperative confusion. It is not associated with coma. All patients show a bland and unconcerned affect and they will confabulate while amnestic. All patients are reported to have recovered within a month of surgery. The length of time required for complete recovery distinguishes this syndrome from transient global amnesia and the post-seizure state in which recovery is rapid and complete. CT scans and EEG studies fail to isolate a special lesion. This syndrome has been postulated to be due to reversible ischemic hypoxic stress to the hippocampi [49].

B. Permanent syndromes

Focal brain syndromes

Strokes varying from mild to severe may occur after profound or prolonged hypotension following particulate embolization, air embolization [50], cardiac arrest [12], and other less well-understood mechanisms.

A pre-existing carotid bruit should be carefully evaluated before such a patient is placed on cardiopulmonary bypass, and this patient may benefit from staged or simultaneous carotid endarterectomy [51, 52]. Patients who have such a stroke usually remain in coma for more than 12 hours after the insult.

As the patient wakens, system deficits and combinations such as hemiplegia, aphasia, visual field defects, bulbar palsy, nystagmus, quadriplegia, hemihypesthesia, cortical blindness due to disproportionate ischemia of both occipital lobes consequent upon their location in an arterial border zone, and bibrachial paresis, "man in the barrel," thought due to bilateral cerebral motor cortex infarction in the overlapping zone between the anterior and middle cerebral arteries [53], become apparent.

Recovery is commonly complete and is delayed over a time extending from weeks to months. Many patients will eventually resume an independent existence with limited residual neurologic deficits while others remain severely impaired and continue to be fully dependent.

Combined carotid and coronary disease and current strategies for management

Hemodynamically significant extracranial arterial stenosis is defined as carotid luminal reduction of 90% or a vascular diameter reduction of >70%. It can be expected in approximately 3% (1.3–16%) of patients presenting with coronary artery disease. A number of these patients will be asymptomatic while others will have histories of transient ischemic attacks (TIA), amaurosis fugax, or frank syncope. Some will have a history and perhaps evidence of an earlier stroke [54].

Patient screening, in addition to a careful history and physical, should include particular attention to neurologic and cerebrovascular symptoms. Both carotid arteries should undergo auscultation, and a duplex Doppler ultrascan should be organized. If the Doppler evaluation reveals a flow reduction of greater than 50%, then a digital subtraction angiogram, using intravenous contrast media, should be completed after discussion with the appropriate staff. Should the information be indeterminate (the real incidence of false negative and false positives is not known for this investigation), then selective carotid cineangiography should be performed, either synchronously or metachronously with the coronary artery cineangiogram.

A reduction of luminal diameter of ≥70%, intimal ulceration, or both, may be safely used as indications for carotid artery endarterectomy with or without symptoms provided the patient accepts the recommendations. Sometimes a second opinion should be advised. In general, about 67% of these patients will be asymptomatic, 26% will have a history of TIA's, and about 6% will have had a history of stroke. It is of interest to note that significant proximal brachiocephalic stenoses are only rarely associated with symptomatic coronary artery disease. There are no known reasons for this [40].

Strategies (>70% stenosis)

The most important point to recognize here is not to convert a stable clinical situation into an unstable one, resulting in both cerebral and myocardial infarction, or worse.

(1) Stable, chronic angina, "comfortable" left ventricular ejection fraction, absence of significant left main coronary artery stenosis. The risk of isolated carotid endarterectomy is low and the risk of cardiac decompensation is low; therefore, the most useful option is to complete the carotid surgery and then perform the cardiac surgery when recovered from the vascular procedure.

(2) Unstable cardiac situation

(a) Unilateral significant carotid artery stenosis. The author recommends a combined procedure with the carotid endarterectomy performed first. The option recommended by the author is as follows. The patient is skillfully anesthetized by an experienced anesthesia team with careful monitoring. If available, any of several cerebral function monitors may be useful adjuncts. Note: It should be mentioned that only unilateral signs should be considered significant, since anesthesia, brain temperature, etc., will produce global EEG alterations. The patient's sternum is opened, and the heart is cannulated after heparinization. The arterial cannula prior to insertion is cut and a T connector is placed in the line. The leg of the T is then connected to a Javid carotid shunt. The venous cannula is placed in the right atrium.

Attention is now turned to the carotid artery. The vessel is exposed and the Javid shunt is positioned distal to the obstruction. After carefully evacuating all air, the Javid clamp is removed but the clamp to the heart lung machine is left in place. The aortic line clamp is now removed and cerebral perfusion is completed by the aorta to carotid composite external shunt. Autoregulation will allow the correct amount of blood to enter the brain. The carotid endarterectomy is then proceeded with, with the security of the Jarvid shunt. Should the ECG change and cardiac status alter, then it is a simple matter to remove the line clamp to the heart lung machine and go on bypass and cool the patient. Both procedures can then be completed in the most stable of circumstances.

(b) Bilateral >70% and <70% carotid artery stenosis. The procedure is as described above. The carotid vessel chosen is the most stenotic. The contralateral carotid disease is repaired metachronously. The risk of stroke here is higher (8%) [54].

(3) Exigent cardiac disease with impending multiorgan failure. The risks of a stroke are explained to the sick patient or the relatives and a salvage operation is performed for the cardiac disease. The risk of stroke is outweighed by the risk of death. The patient may have a reasonable chance of not having a stroke and the carotid disease can be attended to following survival from the exigent cardiac disorder.

(4) Recent stroke. As long as the patient is stable defer the cardiac operation for six weeks.

(5) As more and more patients present for redo coronary revascularization and the patients move into an older age group, it is expected that there will be a slowly increasing number of patients who will need a reoperation event for both procedures. These will have to be individualized but in general the same principles as described above should apply.

An additional disorder that is being encountered follows the accidental puncturing of the carotid artery by the physician who is inserting the internal jugular line. The author's strategy in this situation is to some extent individualized. If only the needle has penetrated the artery and minimal bleeding/hematoma has formed, then simple pressure is acceptable and a delay of half an hour is recommended. Later, during the perfusion run and while heparinized, a frequent check to confirm no hematoma formation is imperative.

It is a different matter if an introducer sheath (9 Fr) has also been passed. This has occurred with more junior staff performing the stab, but can happen with any operator. The best policy here is to remove all equipment immediately and abandon the cardiac operation. There is a real chance that the patient may have a stroke and a cardiac problem. A very frank discussion with the relatives is recommended and careful hospital documents should be kept. If an extensive hematoma occurs exploration of the formerly normal carotid may become mandatory.

Spinal cord syndromes

The spinal cord appears in general to be more resistant to the damaging effects of transient hypotensive ischemic hypoxia when compared to the more rostral central nervous system components. Isolated complete necrosis of the central structures of the spinal cord has been reported [14, 41, 42, 55].

Since the cord has a radicular blood supply, the central sections will be more vulnerable to alterations in blood supply. In the cases reported all patients had flaccid paralysis of the lower limbs and urinary retention. Most patients had an upper sensory level in the thorax. Below this, fibers passing through the lateral spinothalamic tract (pain and temperature) which are rather equidistant to the posterolateral arterial trunk and the anterior spinal artery and therefore residing in the critical border zone area of the arteriae coronae, which unite the anterior and posterior spinal arteries around the periphery of the spinal cord, were more affected than either posterior column fibers (position sense), close to the posterior funicular artery or the ventral spinothalamic tract (light touch), close to the anterior sulcal artery [56].

Global cerebral damage syndromes

(A) Persistent vegetative state
(B) Neocortical brain death
(C) Total cerebral and brain stem death

This group of patients present as the result of resuscitation efforts of patients who have suffered widespread brain tissue destruction. Most remain in a vegetative state or die a brain death. Prognosis is bleak.

(A) Persistent vegetative state

Brain damaged patients who survive for more than one week sometimes revert from coma and regain small pupil, roving eye movements, sleep awake cycles and low level brain stem and spinal cord reflexes. Life support systems are not necessary for continued life. Encephalopathic response – any of the following: metabolic, hypoxic, ischemic, toxic, septic – can result in the encephalopathy. The prognosis is bleak.

(B) Neocortical brain death

In extreme cases of prolonged survival, the vegetative state is associated with an isoelectric EEG. Detailed neuropathologic examination has shown that the neocortex has been destroyed [57]. This particular syndrome had been reported occurring after cardiac arrest in a cerebral hypermetabolic state induced by generalized motor seizures.

(C) Total cerebral and brain stem death

This condition is incompatible with life and rapid death usually occurs without artificial life support measures. Usually all vegetative systems are unstable.

Miscellaneous neurologic syndromes:

Extrapyramidal tract dysfunction. This condition is quite similar to parkinsonism with tremor while awake, akinesia, and cogwheel rigidity. It may follow global ischemia.

Convulsions. These may be Jacksonian in nature, or generalized at commencement. They are controllable with anticonvulsants.

Myoclonic jerks. Synchronous, irregular, shock-like spasms of one or more limbs. They indicate diffuse damage, i.e., hemispheric, thalamic, brain stem, spinal cord, etc.

Action myoclonus syndrome. As above but they are reflex produced, e.g., light, sound, movement, etc. Some control of the intention myoclonus has been reported with various agents (58–61).

Guillain-barre. Acute polyradiculoneuropathy has followed cardiopulmonary bypass [61].

Neurologic injury in children presents with many of the same problems that plague adults, but there are some additional problems which are encountered.

The higher use of profound asanguinous circulatory arrest with a suggested "safe time" of 60 min has been incriminated as not being innocuous and that psychological developmental delays may occur [62]. This could result from ischemic encephalomalacia, and subsequent cerebral atrophy which may help to explain some of these findings [63].

The long-term neurologic sequelae of congenital heart disease and cardiac surgery have not been extensively studied, but clearly some infants and children with cardiac disease are "runts of the litter." They evidence failure to thrive, are often hypotonic and many exhibit delayed development of cerebration and motor skills prior to cardiac surgery, and those children who are cyanotic may be at greater risk for strokes (due to elevated hematocrits and a higher risk of cerebral thromboembolism) and intellectual and motor problems. But as cardiac repair is being done on younger babies, the effects of chronic hypoxia, pulmonary hypertension, and congestive heart failure are becoming less significant. The available literature would implicate the cardiac operation as being the most important event in the neurologic status of the young patient. Certain particular operations more commonly performed in children and babies deserve special mention for the particular risks they pose.

Coarctation. Requires aortic cross-clamping and therefore exposes the spinal cord to additional risks of paraplegia and spinal stroke.

Blalock-Taussig shunt. Performed for certain forms of cyanotic heart disease which have inadequate pulmonary blood flow, places the stellate ganglion at special risk and Horner's syndrome is well reported after this procedure.

The above operations also risk damage to the recurrent laryngeal nerve. This is particularly so in the circumstances of re-coarctation procedures.

Blalock-Hanlon Procedure has a significant potential to damage the right phrenic nerve and special attention should be paid to that nerve as the operation proceeds.

Communicating hydrocephalus has been reported in association with the Mustard Procedure for transposition. This is probably secondary to superior vena caval obstruction [64], and is due to baffle contraction along the superior limb of the intra-atrial repair. The clinical findings of the syndrome are typical [62].

Intraoperative cerebral monitoring is the same as in the adult patient and has consisted of EEG which is limited in deep hypothermia. The cerebral function monitor (computerized EEG) cannot differentiate between ischemia and hypothermic anesthesia. Transcranial Dopplers are being investigated as mentioned above. The use of SEP's – Somatosensory Evoked Potentials showing prolonged delays, indicating potential global brain injury may be useful in the future. However, this technology is influenced by alterations in pH, cardiopulmonary bypass, hypothermia, and anesthesia and these factors can produce interpretational difficulties.

The complexities of interpretation of the long-term sequelae of neurologic injury and cardiac surgery in children and babies are influenced by the following [65]:

- Small sample sizes.
- Varying socioeconomic levels.
- Pre-existing neurologic disorder.
- Preoperative cardiac failure and failure to thrive.
- The surgery – timing, complexity, duration, intraoperative problems, etc.
- Preoperative IQ.
- Perioperative cardiac arrest.
- Postoperative infection.
- Prolonged hospitalization and loss of parental bonding.
- Inappropriate tests on young children and babies.
- Prolonged absence from educational facilities depending upon age.

Follow-up findings

Long-term neurologic sequelae reported following cardiac surgery in babies and children include the following:

- Mental retardation.
- Cerebral palsy.
- Gait disorders.
- Seizure disorders.
- Deafness.
- Learning disorders.
- Memory and linguistic deficits.
- Poor academic achievement.

Diagnosis

Diagnostic examinations available at the bedside may assist in establishing the diagnosis. The most common occurrence being the nurse who reports that the patient is not moving some aspect of the body, or has inappropriate reflexes, e.g., nonreactive pupil, coma, hemiplegia, etc. A neurologic consult should be sent. The following tests are useful:

Physical examination

- Neurological examination (including funduscopy).
    Lumbar puncture (microscopy, chemistry, enzyme release and blood).
    Caloric testing.
    New archaic reflexes.
    Doll's eye test.
    EEG.
- CT scan.
- Radioisotopic tests – brain scan.
- Carotid angiography (delayed).

EEG: An abnormal EEG is a compelling indication to initiate anticonvulsant therapy regardless of how innocuous the patient's symptoms may appear. The EEG which is read as flat for two readings over 24 hours may be taken as legal evidence of brain death.

Lumbar puncture: This needs to be performed only in patients who are suspected of brain hemorrhage or infection. In patients who are anticoagulated, it is recommended that an experienced physician complete the procedure. This restriction should not defer a lumbar puncture when indicated.

Caloric response: Cold water instilled into the auditory canal results in contralateral horizontal nystagmus in the intact patient. A negative test usually indicates an unfavorable response.

Prognosis

Prognosis for patients in coma after a damaging cerebral event and cardiac surgery remains poor. More than half will die in coma, about 20% will remain functionally decorticate in a vegetative state, about 10% will remain severely disabled and will require extensive provider facilities, less than 5% will have only moderate disability, and about 8% can be expected to recover well [12].

Prognosticating factors are as follows:
- Brain stem involvement is unfavorable.
- Absent pupillary reflexes, corneal reflexes, motor response, or deep muscle tendon reflexes – imply a grave prognosis.

Absent doll's eyes sign and absent caloric response – predicts brain death or vegetative state, and a guarded prognosis at best (note this is not reliable in patients given ophthalmoplegic drugs such as Phenytoin [Dilantin]).

Pinpoint pupils are seen in association with pontine hemorrhages and should be considered unfavorable signs (note the effects of narcotic induced pupillary constriction).

Favorable prognoses are indicated by spontaneous roving eye movements appearing at less than 24 hours after the event. Thereafter it is noted in all patient groups and is nondiscriminant. Purposeful movements and withdrawal from noxious stimuli are favorable signs at all times. Speech and comprehension are favorable signs and identify patients with a good to moderate outcome.

The value of repeated assessments in the first 24 hours is obvious from the foregoing associations, and will assist in prognosis advice to relatives.

Treatment programs

Apart from the possible use of hyperbaric oxygen, the clinical management of comatose patients is both prophylatic and symptomatic and should be directed towards the prevention of further insults to the central nervous system, as well as the treatment of neurologic and cardiac complications should they occur, i.e., prevention of arrhythmias, hypotension, ischemia, hypoxia, cardiac arrest, postoperative low output syndrome, CSF hypertension with impending brain herniation, etc.

A ventilator is usually indicated until the patient stabilizes and spontaneous ventilation resumes. The use of brain resuscitation protocols and such agents as free radical scavengers (barbiturates and superoxide dismutase) and mannitol are still under evaluation.

It is advisable that the intracranial pressure be monitored with an intracranial screw, in certain patients undergoing brain resuscitation. This can be used as a monitor on patient progress. Should the ICP rise to high pressure, this might indicate the likelihood of "coning;" active deepening of a drug-induced coma could be indicated. Agents able to lower ICP may be indicated and might include barbiturates, mannitol, diamox, and muscle relaxants, etc., in seizure states [66].

Seizure prophylaxis should begin immediately upon determination that neurologic damage has been sustained. Dilantin 200 mg I.M. has been recommended, followed by 100 mg I.M. every eight hours in adult patients and in appropriate, weight-based doses in children. Barbiturates and other sedative agents should be used with caution until the level of consciousness is fully understood. Seizure control can be obtained with intravenous Valium or in status epilepticus with an intravenous infusion of barbiturate, e.g., sodium amytal. Muscle relaxants have a role to prevent the muscular contractions. Pavulon is commonly employed but this has a tendency to induce a tachycardia and other agents might be chosen. Sometimes a refractory seizure will respond to Mysoline suppositories.

Physiotherapy is indicated to reduce the tendency to contracture disorders, and to help mobilize the hemiplegic patients.

Reversibility

Beyond basic measures to restore hemostasis, no other measures have proved to reliably influence the outcome of the brain injured cardiac surgical patient. Attempts to control postischemic cerebral edema have met with limited success. Corticosteroids are commonly employed on an empirical basis, dehydrating agents, hypothermia and hyperventilation with lowering the pCO_2 and limiting cerebral blood flow in the swollen brain or hypoventilation and raising the pCO_2, inducing increased cerebral blood flow have not improved the outcome of such an injured patient.

Of more importance is the extent of the brain injury itself. Small damage will lead to limited swelling and the reverse is also true. Extensive loss of the neocortex will lead to massive swelling, and brain stem herniation is common, regardless of therapy.

Addendum

Very recently there has been a significant alteration in methodology in cardiac surgery at certain centers including our own practice which holds the possibility of lowering the rate of neurologic stroke injury. It may also result in improved myocardial protection and lower the overall risk of heart surgery.

Due to the imprecise technologies of the 1950 era it became accepted dictum (Bigalow *et al.*) that in order to protect both the brain and the heart, the two most critical organs in the human body, it was expedient to employ hypothermia both to the body and thus the brain, generally to 25–28°C and to the heart in particular, 14–20°C because of the ischemic insult that occurs when blood supply is interrupted to the heart for more than 3–4 min.

This fundamental hypothesis that cold cardiopulmonary bypass for heart surgery is safer for the patient has been seriously challenged for the first time in a scientific manner [67, 68].

The heart surgeons of the Western Heart and Lungs Surgeons, Ltd., have personally completed almost 100 consecutive open heart operations for coronary, valvular and congenital heart conditions and thus far there has not been a single major neurologic injury of any consequence. There have been five transient organic brain syndromes. These findings may be a result of warm heart surgery or they may be serendipidous. These patients are presently undergoing a careful review and will be compared to a recent group of similar population cold heart surgery patients with a focus on differences.

Initial impressions are as follows: The patients appear to wake up earlier, the neurologic injury rate appears diminished, the post operative cardiac performance appears improved, the need for warming devices in the postoperative period is obviated, there may be less postoperative bleeding due to the absence of cold repressed blood coagulation cascade autoregulation, cardiac reentry rates appear to be diminished, postoperative renal function appears less depressed. At present there is no evidence to suggest that ventilation requirements are diminished. Postoperative confusional states may be slightly diminished.

If it is subsequently demonstrated that there is a lowered rate of brain damage associated with normothermic cardiac surgery, then it follows that there must be a degree of damage occurring in the brain of an individual subjected to hypothermic cardiopulmonary bypass. It might further follow that this damage is due to preferential bypass routes that develop only under the conditions of hypothermia and dilution and thus allow peripheral or focal ischemic zones to occur. There has been no experimental data that the author knows of concerning cerebral monitoring devices employed under normothermic bypass.

Clearly warm heart surgery cannot realistically protect a patient from a particulate embolus. Its only benefit might be postulated in the prevention of preferred bypass routes that might occur only under cold conditions as mentioned above. This pathophysiologic cause of strokes in heart surgery patients may be more common than we have previously considered.

References

1. Budabin M. Neurologic complication of cardiac surgery: care of the cardiac surgical patient. In: Litwak R S, Jurado R A (eds). Appleton-Century-Crofts./Prentis Hall, Inc. 1982; p. 387.
2. Gilman S. Cerebral disorders after open heart surgery. N Egl J Med 1965; 272:489.
3. Javid H, Tufo H M, Najafi H, Dye W S, Hunter J A, Hulian O C. Neurologic abnormalities following open heart surgery. J Thorac Cardiovasc Surg. 1969; 58:502.
4. Tufo H M, Ostfeld A M, Shekelle R. Central nervous system dysfunction following open heart surgery. JAMA 1970; 212:1333.
5. Branthwaite M A. Neurologic damage related to open heart surgery. A clinical survey. Thorax 1972; 27:748.
6. Branthwaite M A. Prevention of neurologic damage during open heart surgery. Thorax 1975; 30:258.

34

7. Sotaniemi KA. Brain damage and neurological outcome after open heart surgery. J Neuro Neurosurg Psy 1980; 43:127.
8. Breuer AC, Furlan AJ, Hanson MR, Lederman RJ, Loop FD, Cosgrove DM, Greenstreet RL, Estafanous FG. Central nervous system complications of coronary artery bypass graft surgery: Prospective analysis of 421 patients. Stroke 1983; 5:682.
9. Furlan AJ, Breuer AC. Central nervous system complications of open heart surgery. Current concepts of cerebrovascular disease. Stroke 1984; 5:912.
10. McPherson RW. Intraoperative care of patients at risk of neurologic injury. Crit Care Clin Neurologic Intensive Care 1985; 1:355.
11. Kolkka R, Hilberman M. Neurologic dysfunction following cardiac operation with low flow, low pressure cardiopulmonary bypass. J Thorac Cardiovasc Surg 1980, 79:432.
12. Caronna JJ. Neurologic damage. Perioperative management in cardiothoracic surgery. Roe BB: Little Brown and Company, Boston 1st ed, 1981; p. 163.
13. Walsh JC. Mononeuritis monoplex complicating the post perfusion syndrome. Aust NZJ Med 1968; 17:327.
14. Keates JRW, Innocenti DM, Ross DN. Mononeuritis monoplex, a complication of open heart surgery. J Thorac Cardiovasc Surg 1975; 69:816.
15. Breuer AC, Furlan AJ, Hanson MR et al. Neurologic complications of open heart surgery. Cleveland Clinic 1981; 18:205.
16. Orenstein JM, Sato N, Aaron B et al. Microemboli observed in deaths following cardiopulmonary bypass surgery: Silicone antifoam agents and polyvinyl chloride tubing as sources of emboli. Human Pathology 1982; 13:1082.
17. Lieberman A, Kronzon I, Colvin S et al. Propranolol: An unrecognized cause of central nervous system dysfunction in patients undergoing cardiopulmonary bypass. Ann Thorac Surg 1980; 29:378.
18. Padayachee TS, Parsons F, Theobold R, Linley J, Gosling RG, Deverall PB. The detection of microemboli in the middle cerebral artery during cardiopulmonary bypass: A transcranial Doppler ultrasound investigation using membrane and bubble oxygenators. Ann Thorac Surg 1987; 44:298.
19. Henriksen L, Hjelms E, Lindeburgh T. Brain hypoperfusion during cardiac operations: Cerebral blood flow measured in man by intra-arterial injection of xenon 133: Evidence of intraoperative microembolism. J Thorac Cardiovasc Surg 1983; 86:202.
20. Bolsin SCN. Detection of neurological damage during cardiopulmonary bypass. Anesthesia 1986; 41:61.
21. Butler BD, Laine GA, Leiman BC, Warters D, Kurusz M, Sutton T, Katz J. Effect of the Trendelenberg position on the distribution of the arterial emboli in dogs. Ann Thorac Surg 1988; 45:198.
22. Murphy BP, Harford FJ, Glendall FS. Cerebral air embolism resulting from invasive medical procedures: Treatment with hyperbaric oxygen. Ann Surg 1985; 201:242.
23. Siesjo BK, Plum F. Pathophysiology of anoxic brain damage. Biology of brain dysfunction. Gaul GE (ed). Plenum New York 1972; 1:319.
24. Vaagenes P, Kjekshus J, Silvertsen E, Semb G. Temporal pattern enzyme changes in cerebrospinal fluid in patients with neurologic complications after open heart surgery. Crit Care Med 1978, 15:726.
25. Luft UC. Aviation physiology: The effects of altitude. Handbook of Physiology, Fenn WO, Rahl H (eds). Respiration, Washington, DC, American Physiology Society 1965; 2:1099.
26. Cohen MM. Clinical aspects of cerebral anoxia. In: Vinken PJ, Bruyn GW (eds) Handbook of Clinical Neurology. Amsterdam: North Holland Publishing Company 1976; 27:39.
27. Brierly JB. Neuropathological findings in patients dying after open heart surgery. Thorax 1963; 18:291.
28. Jenevein EP, Weiss DL. Platelet microemboli associated with massive transfusions. Am J Pathol 1964; 45:313.
29. Watkins DW, Peterson MB, Kong DL, Kono K, Buckley MJ, Levine FH, Philbin DM. Thromboxane and prostacyclin changes during cardiopulmonary bypass with and without pulsatile flow. J Thorac Cardiovasc Surg 1982; 84:250.

30. Addonizio V P, Smith J B, Strauss J F, Colman R W, Edmunds L H. Thromboxane synthesis and platelet secretion during cardiopulmonary bypass with bubble oxygenators. J Thorac Cardiovasc Surg 1980; 79:91.

31. Watkins D W, Peterson M B, Crone R B, Shannon D C, Levine L. Prostacyclin and prostaglandin E1 for severe idiopathic pulmonary artery hypertension. Lancet 1980; 1:1083.

32. D'Ambra M N, LaRaia P J, Philbin D M, Watkins D W, Hilgenberg A D, Buckley M J. Prostaglandin E1. A new therapy for refractory right heart failure and pulmonary hypertension after mitral value replacement. J Thorac Cardiovasc Surg 1985; 89:567.

33. Dewhurst W E. Prostaglandin E1 for refractory right heart failure after coronary artery bypass grafting. Case reports. J Cardiothorac Anesth 1988; 2:56.

34. Aaslid R, Markwalker T M. Nornes H. Noninvasive transcranial Doppler ultrasound recording of flow velocity in basal cerebral arteries. J Neurosurg 1982; 57:769.

35. Lundar T, Lindegaard K F, Froysaker T et al. Cerebral carbon dioxide reactivity during non-pulsatile cardiopulmonary bypass. Ann Thorac Surg 1986; 41:525.

36. Ennix E L, Lawrie G M, Morris G C et al. Improved results of carotid endarterectomy in patients with symptomatic coronary artery disease: An analysis of 1,546 consecutive carotid operations. Stroke 1979; 10:122.

37. Ropper A H, Wechsler L R, Wilson L S. Carotid bruit and the risk of elective surgery. N Engl J Med 1982; 307:1388.

38. Evans W E, Cooperman M. The significance of asymptomatic unilateral carotid bruits in preoperative patients. Surgery 1978; 83:521.

39. Turnipseed W D, Berkoff H A, Belzer F O. Postoperative stroke in cardiac and peripheral vascular disease. Ann Surg 1980; 192:365.

40. Jones E L, Guton R A, Michalik R A. Surgical treatment of combined carotid and coronary disease. In: Roberts A J (ed) Difficult Problems in Adult Cardiac Surgery. Year Book Medical Publishers, Inc. 1985; p. 117.

41. Parks B J. Postoperative peripheral neuropathies. Surgery 1983; 74:348.

42. Dhuner K C. Nerve injuries following operations: A survey of cases occurring during a six year period. Anesthesiol 1948; 11:289.

43. Braid Lord W J N. Brain's Diseases of the Nervous System, 7th edition. London: Oxford Univ. Press, 1969.

44. Royden J H, Siekert R G. Embolic mononeuropathy and bacterial endocarditis. Arch Neurol 1968; 19:535.

45. Lederman R J, Breuer A C, Hanson M R et al. Peripheral nervous system complications of coronary artery bypass graft surgery. Ann Neurol 1982; 12:297.

46. Mohr J P. Neurologic complications of cardiac valvular disease and cardiac surgery including systemic hypotension. In: Vinken P J, Bruyn G W (eds) Handbook of Clinical Neurology, Amsterdam: North Holland Publishing Company 1979; 38:143.

47. Weiner N. Atropine, scopolamine and related antimuscarinic drugs. In: Goodman and Gilman (eds) The Pharmacological Basis of Therapeutics, 7th ed. New York: Macmillan Publishing Company. Chapter 7, 1985; p. 130.

48. Aris A, Solanes H, Camara M L, Junque C, Escartin A, Caralps J M. Arterial line filtration during cardiopulmonary bypass: Neurologic, neuropsychologic, and hematologic studies. J Thorac Cardiovasc Surg 1986; 91:526.

49. Brierley J B. Pathology of cerebral ischemia. In: McDowell F H, Brennan R W (eds) Cerebral Vascular Disease. Eighth Princeton Conference. New York: Grune and Stratton 1980; p. 59.

50. Mills N L, Oschner J L. Massive air embolism during cardiopulmonary bypass: Causes, prevention and management. J Thorac Cardiovasc Surg 1980; 80:708.

51. Hertzer N R, Loop F D, Taylor P C, Beven E G. Staged and combined surgical approach to simultaneous carotid and coronary vascular disease. Surg 1978; 83:803.

52. Crawford E S, Palamara A E, Kasparian A S. Carotid and noncoronary operations. Simultaneous, staged and delayed. Surgery 1980; 87:1.

53. Mohr J P. Distal field infarction (abstract). Neurology 1969; 12:279.

54. Minami K, Sagoo K S, Breymann T, Fassbender D, Schwerdt M, Korfer R. Operative

36

strategy in combined coronary and carotid artery disease. J Thorac Cardiovasc Surg 1988; 95:303.

55. Richards RL. Ischemic lesions of peripheral nerves. A review. J Neurol Neurosurg Psych 1951; 19:76.

56. Chusid JG. Correlative neuroanatomy and functional neurology. Lange Medical Publications, 19th edition 1985; p. 87.

57. Brierley J B et al. Neocortical death after cardiac arrest. Lancet 1971; 2:560.

58. Van Woert M H et al. Long term therapy of myoclonus and other neurologic disorders with L-5-hydroxytryptophan and Carbidopa. N Engl J Med 1977; 296:70.

59. Goldberg MA, Dorman JD. Intention myoclonus: Successful treatment with Clonazepam. Neurology 1976; 26:24.

60. Fahn S. Post-anoxic action myoclonus: Improvement with Valproic Acid. N Engl J Med 1978; 299:313.

61. Constantino T, Weintraub A. The Guillian-Barre syndrome as a complication of the post-perfusion syndrome. Am Heart J 1972; 84:678.

62. Wells FC, Coghill S, Caplan HL et al. Duration of circulatory arrest does influence the psychological development of children after cardiac operations in early life. J Thorac Cardiovasc Surg 1983; 86:823.

63. Muraoka R, Yokota M, Aoshima M et al. Subclinical changes in brain morphology following cardiac oeprations as reflected by computed tomographic scans of the brain. J Thorac Cardiovasic Surg 1982; 81:364.

64. Markowicz RI, Kleinman CS, Hellenbrand WE et al. Communicating hydrocephalus secondary to superior vena caval obstruction. AJDC 1984; 138:638.

65. Ferry PC. Neurologic sequelae of cardiac surgery in children. AJDC 1987; 141:309.

66. Michenfelder JD, Lilde J H. Influence of anesthetics on metabolic, functional and pathological responses to regional cerebral ischemia. Stroke 1975; 6:405.

67. Lichtenstein S V, Ashe K A, Dalati H, Cusimano R J, Panos A, Slutsky A S. Warm heart surgery. J Thorac Cardiovasc Surg. 1991; 101:269.

68. Salerno T A, Christakis G R, Abel J, Houck J, Barrozo C A M, Fremes S E, Cusimano R J, Lichtenstein S V. Technique and pitfalls of retrograde continuous warm blood cardioplegia. Ann Thorac Surg 1991; 51:1023.

3. Prevalence and causes of cerebral complications in cardiac surgery

K. A. SOTANIEMI

Despite all the advances achieved during the past three decades of cardiac surgery, it remains clearly evident that the cardiac patient still faces the threat of cerebral complications in all the facets of the disease and its treatment. The outcome of the patient is essentially labelled by the vital interrelationship between the cardiac and cerebral functions. The cardiac disease itself carries a risk of cerebral disorders, mainly ischemic complications which, in turn, have been shown to impair the central nervous system's (CNS) ability to tolerate the numerous exceptionally strenuous conditions of the operative procedures. Also the necessary preoperative investigations expose the patient to cerebral consequences; their threat, however, being of minor importance when compared with the particular risks of cerebral embolism and hypoperfusion operant during and immediately after cardiopulmonary bypass. But the CNS risks of the cardiac patient are not limited to the pre- and intraorperative phases only. After operation, there remain a number of potential hazards for the CNS; e.g., those associated with the life-long anticoagulant treatment needed after valvular replacement and with embolism and infections related to the artificial value. On the other hand, it should not be forgotten, that cerebral disorders also carry a risk for cardiac dysfunction such as arrhythmias and ischemic cardiac damage which may lead to a vicious circle with the diseases of both the organs impairing the functions of each other. Thus, the cardiac and cerebral functions are closely inter-related determinants of the overall outcome of the cardiac surgery patient through the years achieved with surgical treatment.

Since the 1960s, a vast literature has accumulated devoted to the cerebral complications of cardiac surgery reporting disorders in virtually all the possible nervous system structures and functions. In the early years of cardiac surgery, severe CNS damage was not uncommon, resulting often in permanent deficits such as hemiplegia and even in cerebral death. Developments in surgical and anaesthesiological techniques and equipment have enormously diminished the occurrence of CNS disturbances and severe complications have become rare in modern heart surgery. On the other hand, the cerebral investigatory

37

methods have also improved at the same time, allowing the detection of more and more subtle dysfunction and even subclinical damage. It has become evident that cardiac surgery, particularly the procedure of cardiopulmonary bypass, almost always causes CNS dysfunction. Whether or not this dysfunction is detected, depends on the investigatory methods and criteria practised. In the 1980s, a relatively high level of cerebral safety has been achieved in both valvular and coronary artery bypass surgery (CABS) regarding severe CNS complications but, at the same time, such an advantageous development has not been gained in other important issues, such as neuropsychologic and psychiatric functions. Because these particular functions essentially determine the quality of life during the years achieved with surgical treatment, increasing attention has been devoted to these aspects of the outcome [1–9].

Preoperative factors of cerebral disorders have been dealt with in Meyendorf's chapter. This chapter reviews the features associated with the prevalence, determinants and detection of CNS dysfunction related to cardiac surgery.

Prevalence of postoperative cerebral damage

General considerations

Heterogeneity in the investigatory methods used and patient materials complicate the assessment of the prevalence of CNS disorders associated with cardiac surgery. The results are highly affected by the education of the authors, non-neurologists reporting substantially lower prevalence values than neurologists [10]. This is mainly due to the practice of the former of registering "obvious" or "clinically important" signs only, thus omitting findings that are less severe than frank paralyses while the latter investigators often include all the detectable abnormalities.

In addition to the criteria of CNS evaluation, the results vary according to the patient material. Neurologic complications have been reported to be much more common in valvular replacement surgery than in CABS but most common in heart transplantation operations [1–13]. Most valvular surgery reports date back to the 1960s and 1970s while the majority of the CABS studies have been published later which may overestimate the CNS complication prevalence associated with valvular surgery performed with modern techniques.

Further embarrassment in the evaluation of the cerebral complication rates is caused by the differences in the investigatory approaches and settings. As a rule, prospective studies [1–3, 11] have reported postoperative CNS complications to be very common and detectable in up to 80% of patients in contrast to considerably lower values of 1–6% reported in retrospective studies [14–16]. One comparison between prospective and retrospective evaluations has shown that while the former method revealed a prevalence value of postoperative neurologic complications of 37%, the latter method resulted in a value of only 6% which was two-thirds of the cases a neurologist would have discovered using inspection as the only investigation [10].

Prevalence of postoperative CNS damage in valvular surgery

In the early days of valvular replacement surgery, severe cerebral complications were not uncommon. In the 1960s, even 9–14% of the patients had fatal brain damage [17–19]. At the present, fatal damage has become rare, its prevalence having decreased to 0.5–2.6% [11, 14, 20]. The cause of severe brain damage is most commonly massive brain infarction or hemorrhage, multiple embolisation and/or extensive anoxic brain injury.

Almost all the possible kinds of neurologic disturbances have been encountered following cardiac surgery. Neurologic deficits, such as motor and/or sensory disorders of varying degree, primitive reflexes, visual field defects, cranial and peripheral neuropathy, spinal injury, as well as cognitive and psychiatric signs are among the most common abnormalities. The reported prevalence values of the somatic deficits have varied from 3% to 37% [11, 14, 20]. Most commonly, the clinical signs have been reported transient: by the time of discharge from the hospital most of the abnormalities have disappeared and persistent signs are encountered in only 2–3% of the survivors [2, 14, 20, 21].

As mentioned earlier, the neurologic outcome of the valvular replacement surgery patients have been given little attention recently, most of the studies being devoted to CABS patients. This should not be interpreted as reflecting that the risks of cerebral dysfunction have been eliminated in valvular surgery. In contrast, it is quite obvious that valvular replacement patients continue to be much more liable to cerebral consequences than CABS patients. This is due both to the differences between the diseases themselves (e.g., high embolisation rate in open-heart surgery) and to the more complicated procedures needed in valvular surgery when compared with CABS.

Most commonly, the postoperative neurologic follow-up has been limited to a few weeks or months. In one study [21], the follow-up was extended to five years. The prevalence of immediate postoperative neurologic signs was 49% but that of permanent abnormalities was 9%. Transient ischemic attacks occurred in five patients of 55. The rate of postoperative cerebral embolic events was 2.8 per 100 patient-years despite continuous and controlled anticoagulation therapy.

Postoperative disorders of the higher cerebral functions, psychiatric disturbances, and electrophysiological measures of valvular replacement surgery are dealt with in detail in other chapters.

Prevalence of postoperative cerebral damage in CABS

In coronary artery reconstructions, the available prospective studies report overall postoperative CNS complications in 17 to 64% and the prevalence of fatal cerebral damage as very low, 0–0.3% [1, 3, 22–24]. Stroke has been reported in about 5% of the patients [23–25]. In one study of 103 CABS patients [22], motor deficits were encountered in 1% while neuropsychologic disturbances were evident in 31% of the patients.

Two carefully conducted, prospective studies illustrate the present status of neurologic complications in CABS. In one study involving 421 patients [25], stroke occurred in 22 patients (5.2%), the prevalence of cases assessed as severe strokes being 2.0%, and postoperative encephalopathy was found in 49 patients (11.6%). Of the 22 strokes, 12 were hemispheral, five comprised of retinal or optic ischemia, and the remaining cases affecting the vertebro-basilar circulation. Full recovery was seen in six and partial recovery in nine stroke patients, six were disabled and one further stroke patient died. Of the 49 patients with prolonged encephalopathy, 39 recovered totally and the remaining 10 patients showed partial recovery at discharge. The potential cause of the brain damage could be demonstrated in half the cases with CNS complications but such determinants could be seen also in patients without any signs of brain damage.

In another study [3], the neurologic outcomes of 312 CABS patients and 50 patients undergoing major peripheral vascular surgery were compared. Postoperative neurologic abnormalities could be detected in 61% of the CABS patients and in 18% of the control patients. Neuropsychologic dysfunction was seen in 79% of the CABS patients and in 31% of the control patients. At discharge, 17% of the CABS patients had neurologic disability and 38% had neuropsychologic complications. The complications of the control group were mostly peripheral. Fifteen (5%) of the CABS patients suffered a stroke, four of them were severely incapacitated. In the CABS group, 39% of the patients developed primitive reflexes, ophthalmologic abnormalities were observed in 25%, peripheral nervous system complications in 12%, and postoperative psychosis was seen in 1% of the patients. Of the 191 patients with neurologic abnormalities, 48 had difficulties in their daily activities and four patients were severely disabled.

The prevalence values of CNS complications reported in retrospective studies have been, as expected, considerably lower than those mentioned above. In one study of 1427 patients [16], neurologic complications could be identified in only 18 cases (1.3%), cerebral infarction being found in 13 patients (0.9%). In another study, the prevalence of CNS damage was 3.8% (64 cases of 1669) [15]. Intraoperative stroke was seen in nine patients (0.5%), four of whom died. Four further patients developed stroke postoperatively. Altered mental state was registered in 57 patients (3.4%) and seizures in 5 patients (0.3%).

Comparisons between the prospective and retrospective studies clearly show the pitfalls of the latter. Identification of even major cerebral complications fails in the retrospective studies, which thus claim falsely optimistic prevalence values for cerebral disturbances.

Peripheral neurologic complications in cardiac surgery

As a reminder of the problems involved in differential diagnosis, there follows a brief review of peripheral nervous system complications. The prevalence of peripheral nerve injuries associated with cardiac operations has been of the magnitude of 12% in several prospective reports [3, 11, 26, 27]. Brachial plexopathy and phrenic nerve injury are the most common kinds of peripheral nerve damage [3, 27–30]. They are due to compression, traction or cold injury. Additionally, cranial neuropathy (e.g., facial palsy, extraocular muscle dysfunction, Horner's syndrome), radicular syndromes, peripheral mononeuropathy and multiple neuropathies have been reported [3, 11, 26, 37]. The peripheral injuries tend to resolve themselves within a few weeks or months suggesting conduction block to be the main pathophysiologic factor [26]. However, they may also entail severe complications, as in the case of phrenic nerve involvement [28–30]. Peripheral neurologic complications should not be overlooked: first, because they are frequent, cause considerable annoyance and may even be hazardous; second, because they are avoidable; and third, because they may be misdiagnosed as cerebral complications.

Causes of postoperative cerebral damage

Cerebral damage during heart surgery is well recognised but poorly understood. Sometimes specific causes as clear-cut infarctions due to demonstrable emboli, cerebral hemorrhages, and border-zone ischemia related to cerebral hypoperfusion can be identified [32–35]. However, it is often the case that either the cause of CNS damage remains inexplicable or else, because of the variety of concomitant harmful factors, it is impossible to pinpoint the actual exact cause of damage [1–3, 5, 8, 23]. Information concerning the determinants of intraoperative CNS damage is even more embarrassing than that concerning the occurrence of complications described previously in this chapter. This is obviously due not only to the differences in study designs, standards of pre-, intra- and postoperative care and surveillance, surgical and anaesthesiological skills, and to equipment and patient materials, but also quite evidently to the individual patients' particular abilities to tolerate the conditions operant during cardiopulmonary bypass (CPB). CPB, as well as the entire heart surgery procedure, expose the brain to a number of factors which all may result either in infarction due to embolisation or other causes, or in disturbed neuronal metabolism and transmission due to toxins or inadequate cerebral perfusion. Some of the most important mechanisms of cerebral injury are discussed below.

Embolism from the heart or the CPB apparatus is one of the most commonly suggested causes of cerebral damage and the most probable cause of severe stroke related to cardiac procedures. *Macroembolisation* may be caused by air or particulate matter (valve fragments, calcified debris, fat, mural thrombi) dislodged during manipulation of the heart or cross-clamping of the great vessels and embolising in the cerebral arteries [1, 15, 25, 36, 37]. Embolisation of calcium particles from the excised valves used to be very common in closed heart surgery but is rare in modern valvular replacements. Fat may be released during sternotomy or during excision of the mediastinal tissues, drain into the pericardial sac and then be sucked into the perfusion system. Fat emboli may also be formed when blood is exposed to a gas interface or when pooled blood contains free fat droplets [38]. Macroembolisation of air may occur when air is trapped in the heart or in the proximal parts of the great vessels is pushed forwards when the ventricles begin to eject [39–42]. Gaseous emboli may also be generated either from air suspended in stored cold blood, causing bubbles when the blood is rewarmed, or from foaming occurring in the CPB device, or by technical disturbances in the oxygenator.

Microemboli in the cerebral arteries may consist of aggregated blood elements, fibers from cotton gauzes or sponges, and small bubbles of air generated in the oxygenator. Normally, microemboli are trapped in the lungs but during CPB they are distributed throughout the arterial system. Aggregates of leucocytes, platelets, fibrin and denatured proteins may accumulate in stored blood, develop when blood is exposed to artificial surfaces, or form in blood vessels during episodes of hypotension and circulatory stress [44, 45]. Cotton fiber embolisation has been reported to be a rare cause of cerebral infarction. Microemboli or air, in turn, are considered to be the most common determinant of cerebral complications resulting in cerebral infarction or hypoperfusion [39–42, 45]. Oxygenation, particularly in bubble oxygenators, tends to produce bubbling and, as the available debubbling methods are still inadequate, large quantities of microbubbles can be detected in the carotid and cerebral arteries [40–42]. The amount of microemboli reaching the cerebral vessels can be diminished by developing more and more effective microfilters.

Membrane oxygenators produce considerably smaller quantities of microbubbles than the old bubble oxygenators. There is some evidence that postoperative CNS dysfunction, particularly neuropsychologic disorders, may be less frequent after membrane oxygenation than after bubble oxygenation [42, 46].

Cerebral hypoperfusion resulting in disturbed neuronal metabolism and transmission, may be caused by a number of things, of which embolisation, hypotension, low flow rate in CPB, malposition or obstruction of cannulae, and pre-existing carotid or cerebrovascular disease are among the most common [11, 15, 25, 36]. Cerebral blood flow falls markedly at various phases of the operative procedure, particularly at the onset of CPB, and the consequences in cerebral function are obvious, as reflected e.g. in the EEG [36, 47, 48].

Autoregulation of cerebral blood flow is greatly influenced by the acid-base balance. There are two main ways to control the carbon dioxide tension: the temperature-corrected regime (the so called pH-stat method) and the regimen in which temperature is not corrected (the alpha-stat method). The latter is shown to allow cerebral autoregulation to be maintained more effectively than the former [49–52]. There is some evidence that the alpha-stat method may be of benefit for postoperative outcome [53], but the question of the optimal way of protecting autoregulation of cerebral blood flow remains unsettled.

Also the type of blood flow during CPB may be important at the cerebral capillary bed level: pulsatile flow has been considered to provide a more adequate capillary perfusion than non-pulsatile flow [53], but the clinical significance of the question remains unsettled [54, 55].

The role of arterial blood pressure, perfusion pressure and *hypotension* during heart operations and particularly during CPB have remained controversial. Intraoperative hypotension has been considered one of the most important causes of cerebral complications by some investigators [1, 18, 19], but less important by others [11, 20, 22]. Although it is definitely clear that severe hypotension is disastrous to the brain, moderate hypotension seems to be tolerated, but no safe lower pressure limit can be stated and, after all, the cerebral perfusion rate is more important than the arterial blood pressure level itself.

The *duration of CPB* has been regarded as an overall index of the cumulative risks operant during perfusion. Several studies have shown a positive correlation between the prevalence and severity of postoperative clinical, neuropsychologic and electroencephalographic deterioration [1, 11, 23, 64] although this has not been the rule [25]. A critical time threshold of two hours has been stated in a number of reports. The influence of a long perfusion time has also been shown in long-term postoperative electroencephalographic follow-ups, revealing a less favourable five-year outcome in patients with long (>2 h) perfusion times than in patients with shorter perfusion times [21]. Correspondingly, follow-up of the neuropsychologic outcome showed that the scores of the long perfusion time group remained continuously lower than those of the short perfusion time group through the five-year follow-up period, despite equal preoperative values [2]. Furthermore, it was noted that the score difference between the two groups even became accentuated with time. This phenomenon could not be correlated to any neurologic or cardiologic cause. Thus, intraoperative conditions, of which perfusion time may be one example only, may entail consequences which are not apparent until long after operation.

In addition to the most common causes of cerebral dysfunction described above, there always remains a variety of other factors potentially harmful to the brain in such a complex procedure as heart surgery. Anaesthetics may cause disturbances in neurotransmission, there is a continuous threat of unexpected technical occurrences, toxins may be liberated or generated during the procedure, haematologic and immunologic disturbances may be generated, and even thus far unrecognised determinants of cerebral damage may be present. Furthermore, the patient's age, sex and cardiac measures may modify the influence of not only all the above mentioned potential single determinants of cerebral damage but also of their combinations. Study of the causes of CNS complications related to cardiac procedures has provided effective methods for both detecting and limiting, in some cases even eliminating, intraoperative cerebral damage. However, one should not forget that, apart from the intraoperative causes of brain dysfunction, the patient is also exposed to a variety of postoperative conditions, e.g., cardiogenic embolism and cardiac arrhythmias, through the years achieved with successful operative treatment.

Summary

The extensive literature devoted to the determinants of cerebral complications associated with cardiac surgery clearly shows the multiplicity of risk factors to which the patient is exposed in the various phases of both the disease itself and its treatment. Although the prevalence of severe cerebral damage has dramatically decreased during the past two decades, CNS disturbances still remain a major concern. Present technology and accumulated experience provide us with relatively reliable methods for the prevention of gross complications, but our knowledge of the subclinical level cerebral events associated with cardiac disease and surgery still seems to be far from perfect, as is reflected in recent neuropsychologic, neuroradiologic, neurochemical and neurophysiologic studies. Furthermore, the long-term effects of operative procedures are poorly defined and are only now in the process of receiving attention. All these aspects form a challenge for the multidisciplinary development of ever more safe and successful cardiac surgery and for effective multidimensional patient surveillance extended to all the phases of cardiac disease and its treatment.

References

1. Smith PLC, Newman SP, Ell PJ, Treasure T, Jospeh P, Schneidau A, Harrison MJG. Cerebral consequences of cardiopulmonary bypass. Lancet 1986; I:823.
2. Sotaniemi KA, Mononen H, Hokkanen TE. Long-term cerebral outcome after open-heart surgery. Stroke 1986; 17:410.
3. Shaw PJ, Bates D, Cartlidge NEF, French JM, Heaviside D, Julian DG, Shaw DA. Neurologic and neuropsychological morbidity following major surgery: comparison of coronary artery bypass and peripheral vascular surgery. Stroke 1987; 18:700.
4. Allen CMC. Cabbages and CABG. The risk of serious neurological damage from bypass operations is small. Br Med J 1988; 297:1485.
5. Folk DG, Freeman AM, Sokol RS, Reves JG, Baker DM. Cognitive dysfunction after coronary artery bypass surgery: a case-controlled study. South Med J 1988; 81:202.
6. Langeluddecks P, Fulcher G, Baird D, Hughes C, Tennant C. A prospective evaluation of the psychosocial effects of coronary artery bypass surgery. J. Psychosom Res 1989; 33:37.
7. Klonoff H, Clark C, Kavanagh-Gary D, Mizgala H, Munro I. Two-year follow-up study of coronary bypass surgery. Psychologic status, employment status, and quality of life. J Thorac Cardiovasc Surg 1989; 97:78.
8. Townes BD, Bashein G, Hornbein TF, Coppel DB, Davis KB, Nessly ML, Bledsoe SW, Veith RC, Ivey TD. Neurobehavioural outcomes in cardiac operations. A prospective controlled study. J Thorac Cardiovasc Surg 1989; 98:774.
9. Treasure T, Smith PL, Newman S, Schneidau A, Joseph P, Ell P, Harrison MJ. Impairment

of cerebral function following cardiac and other major surgery. Eur J Cardiothorac Surg 1989; 3:216.

10. Sotaniemi K A. Cerebral outcome after extracorporeal circulation. Comparison between prospective and retrospective evaluations. Arch Neurol 1983; 40:75.

11. Sotaniemi K A. Brain damage and neurological outcome after open-heart surgery. J. Neuro Neurosurg Psychiatry 1980; 43:127.

12. Hunt S A. Complications of heart transplantation. Heart Transplantation 1983; 3:70.

13. Montero C G, Martinez A J. Neuropathology of heart transplantation. Neurology 1986; 35:1149.

14. Branthwaite M A. Prevention of neurological damage during open-heart surgery. Thorax 1975; 30:258.

15. Coffey C E, Massey W M, Roberts K B, Curtis S, Jones R H, Pryor D B. Natural history of cerebral complications of coronary artery bypass graft surgery. Neurology 1983; 33:1416.

16. González-Scarano F, Hurtig H I. Neurologic complications of coronary artery bypass grafting: Case control study. Neurology 1981; 31:1032.

17. Gilman S. Cerebral disorders after open-heart operations. N Engl J Med 1965; 272:489.

18. Javid H, Tufo H M, Najafi H, Dye W S, Hunter J A, Julian O C. Neurological abnormalities following open-heart surgery. J Thorac Cardiovasc Surg 1969; 58:502.

19. Tufo H M, Ostfeld A M, Shekelle R. Central nervous system dysfunction following open-heart surgery. J Am Med Ass 1970; 212:1333.

20. Åberg T, Kihlgren M. Cerebral protection during open-heart surgery. Thorax 1977; 32–525.

21. Sotaniemi K A. Five-year neurological and EEG out-come after open-heart surgery. J Neurol Neurosurg Psychiatry 1985; 48:569.

22. Kolkka R, Hilberman M. Neurologic dysfunction following cardiac operations with low-flow, low-pressure cardiopulmonary bypass. J Thorac Cardiovasc Surg 1980; 79:432.

23. Shaw P J, Bates D, Cartlidge N E F, Heaviside D, Julian D G, Shaw D A. Early neurological complications of coronary artery bypass surgery. Br Med J 1985; 29:1384.

24. Carella F, Travaini G, Guzzetti S, Botta M, Pieri E, Mangoni A. Cerebral complications of coronary bypass surgery. A prospective study. Acta Neurol Scand 1988; 77:158.

25. Breuer A C, Furlan A J, Hanson M R, Lederman R J, Loop F D, Cosgrove D M, Greenstreet R L, Estafanous F G. Central nervous system complications of coronary artery bypass graft surgery: prospective analysis of 421 patients. Stroke 1983; 14:682.

26. Lederman R J, Breuer A C, Hanson M R, Furlan A J, Loop F D, Cosgrove D M, Estafanous F G, Greenstreet R L. Peripheral nervous system complications of coronary artery bypass graft surgery. Ann Neurol 1982; 12:297.

27. Sotaniemi K A. Branchial plexus lesion complicating sternotomy. J Neurol Neurosurg Psychiatry 1982; 45:568.

28. Watanabe T, Trusler G A, Williams W G, Edmonds J F, Coles J G, Hosokawa Y. Phrenic nerve paralysis after pediatric cardiac surgery. Retrospective study of 125 cases. J Thorac Cardiovasc Surg 1987; 94:383.

29. Abd A G, Braun N M, Baskin M I, O'Sullivan M M, Alkaitis D A. Diaphragmatic dysfunction after open heart surgery: treatment with a rocking bed. Ann Intern Med 1989; 111:881.

30. Curtis J J, Nawarawong W, Walls J T, Schmalz R A, Boley T, Madsen-Andersen S K. Elevated hemidiaphragm after cardiac operations: incidence, prognosis, and relationship to the use of topical ice slush. Ann Thorac Surg 1989; 48:764.

31. Keates J R W, Innocenti D M, Ross D N. Mononeuritis multiplex: a complication of open-heart surgery. J Thorac Cardiovasc Surg 1976; 69:816.

32. Brieley J B. Neuropathological findings in patients dying after open-heart surgery. Thorax 1963; 18:291.

33. Aguilar M J, Gerbode F, Hill J. Neuropathologic complications of cardiac surgery. J Thorac Cardiovasc Surg 1971; 61:676.

34. Humphreys R P, Hoffman H J, Mustard W T, Trusler G A. Cerebral hemorrhage following heart surgery. J Neurosurg 1975; 43:671.

35. Russell R W R, Bharucha N. The recognition and prevention of border zone cerebral ischaemia during cardiac surgery. 1978; 17:303.

46

36. Branthwaite, M A. Detection of neurological damage during open-heart surgery. Thorax 1973; 28:364.
37. Breuer A C, Franco I, Marzewski D, Soto-Velasco, J. Left ventricular thrombi are a significant risk factor for stroke in open-heart surgery. Ann Neurol 1981; 10:103.
38. Wright E S, Sarkozy E, Dobell A R C, Murphy D R. Fat globulemia in extracorporeal circulation. Surgery 1963; 53:500.
39. Mills N L, Ochsner J L. Massive air embolism during cardiopulmonary bypass. Causes, prevention, and management. J Thorac Cardiovasc Surg 1980; 80:708.
40. Deverall P B, Padayachee T S, Parsons S, Theobold R, Battistessa S A. Ultrasound detection of micro-emboli in the middle cerebral artery during cardiopulmonary bypass surgery. Eur J Cardiothorac Surg 1988; 2:256.
41. Blauth C I, Arnold J V, Schulenberg W E, McCartney A C, Taylor K M. Cerebral microembolism during cardiopulmonary bypass. Retinal microvascular studies in vivo with fluorescein angiography. J Thorac Cardiovasc Surg 1988; 95:668.
42. Blauth C, Smith P, Newman S, Arnold J, Siddons F, Harrison M J, Treasure T, Klinger L, Taylor K M. Retinal microembolism and neuropsychological deficit following clinical cardiopulmonary bypass: comparison of a membrane and a bubble oxygenator. A preliminary communication. Eur J Cardiothorac Surg 1989; 3:135.
43. Solis R T, Kennedy P S, Beall A C, Jr, Noon G P, DeBakey M E. Cardiopulmonary bypass. Microemboloization and platelet aggregation. Circulation 1975; 52:103.
44. Dimmick J E, Bove K E, McAdams A J, Benzing G. Fiber embolization – a hazard of cardiac surgery and catheterization. N Engl J Med 1975; 293:685.
45. von Reutern G-M, Hetzel A, Birnbaum D, Schloser V. Transcranial doppler ultrasonography during cardiopulmonary bypass in patients with severe carotid stenosis or ulceration. Stroke 1988; 19:674.
46. Pearson D T, Carter R F, Hammo M B, Waterhouse P S. Gaseous microemboli during open-heart surgery. In: Longmore D B (ed). Towards Safer Cardiac Surgery. Lancaster: MTP Press, 1981; p. 325.
47. Kritikou P E, Branthwaite M A. Significance of changes in cerebral electrical activity at onset of cardiopulmonary bypass. Thorax 1977; 32:534.
48. Arom K V, Cohen D E, and Strobl F T. Effect of intraoperative intervention on neurological outcome based on electroencephalographic monitoring during cardiopulmonary bypass. Ann Thorac Surg 1989; 48:476.
49. Murkin J M, Farrar J K, Tweed W A, McKenzie F N, Guiraudon G. Cerebral autoregulation and flow/metabolism coupling during cardiopulmonary bypass: The influence of PaO2. Anaesth Analog 1987; 66:825.
50. Nevin M, Colchester A C, Adams S, Pepper J R. Evidence of involvement of hypocapnia and hypoperfusion in aetiology of neurological deficit after cardioupulmonary bypass. Lancet 1987; 2:1493.
51. McNeill B R, Murkin J M, Farrar K K, Gelb A G. Autoregulation and the CO2 responsiveness of cerebral blood flow after cardiopulmonary bypass. Can J Anaesth 1990; 37:313.
52. Prough D S, Rogers A T, Stump D A, Gravlee G P, Taylor G. Hypercarbia depresses cerebral oxygen consumption during cardiopulmonary bypass. Stroke 1990; 21:1162.
53. Tranmer B I, Gross C E, Kindt G W, Adey G R. Pulsatile versus nonpulsatile blood flow ino the treatment of acute cerebral ischemia. Neurosurgery 1986; 19:724.
54. Brusino F G, Reves J G, Smith L R, Prough D S, Strump D A, McIntyre R W. The effect of age on cerebral blood flow during hypothermic cardiopulmonary bypass. J Thorac Cardiovasc Surg 1989; 97:541.
55. Henze T, Stephan H, Sonntag H. Cerebral dysfunction following extracorporeal circulation for aortocoronary bypass surgery: no differences in neuropsychological outcome after pulsatile versus nonpulsatile flow. Thorac Cardiovasc Surg 1990; 38:65.
56. Sotaniemi K A, Juolasmaa A, Hokkanen T E. Neuropsychological outcome after open-heart surgery. Arch Neurol 1984; 38:2.
57. Sotaniemi K A, Sulg I A, Hokkanen T E. Quantitative EEG as a measure of cerebral dysfunction betfore and after open-heart surgery. Electroenceph Clin Neurophysiol 1980; 50:81.

4. Perfusion related parameters affecting cerebral outcome after cardiac surgery

MARK KURUSZ

Introduction

The necessity to perform cardiopulmonary bypass (CPB) which permits open cardiac surgery has been considered one of the most significant medical developments of the 20th century. From animal laboratory experiments by physiologists more than 150 years ago to the clinical applications in the early 1950s, open-heart surgery with CPB has grown to the extent that more than 700 hospitals in the United States perform approximately 350,000 CPB procedures each year. Whereas congenital or valvular surgery predominated the early CPB experience, the advent of the coronary artery bypass graft (CABG) operation in the early 1970s has been largely responsible for the extraordinary growth in the number of cases. Despite a trend in recent years towards percutaneous transluminal coronary angioplasty (PTCA) procedures by cardiologists to treat coronary artery disease (which does not require use of CPB) the CABG operation remains the most frequent requirement for CPB today. The fact that many of these patients are middle-aged and actively employed further emphasizes the need for optimum cerebral protection during CPB.

Little is known about cerebral function and CPB in contrast to the considerable efforts that have been made to understand myocardial function associated with cardiac surgery. One reason is that studying the brain during and after CPB is often difficult when compared to the heart which is directly accessible and visible during the operation. Cardiac performance after CPB also is something of an all-or-none phenomenon: it either resumes effective pumping after the procedure or it does not. The brain, in contrast, is subject to anesthetic effects during the operation. Also, while cardiac pathology is often extensively studied and defined prior to the operation, few patients are subjected to extensive neurological examination before cardiac surgery, and even fewer have pre- and post-CPB neurologic or neuropsychological testing to gain insight as to the effects of CPB.

Controversy exists within the published literature regarding optimal cerebral protection during CPB. In fact, many fundamental studies were performed in the early decades (1950s and 1960s) when CPB was just beginning to be used at a limited number of larger medical centers. Much of our current practice in the 1990s can be traced to these earlier findings, and therefore many CPB concepts taught in perfusion schools today are dogmatic by nature.

The purpose of this chapter is to explain how CPB works, with an emphasis on perfusion techniques that are believed to enhance patients' cerebral outcome. It is acknowledged that variables beyond those attributable to CPB (namely, patient or operative) also can profoundly affect the brain during cardiac surgery.

It is the hope of all disciplines involved in open-heart surgery that we are on the threshold of answering several fundamental questions regarding optimum cerebral protection that have been posed since the inception of clinical application of CPB.

Cardiopulmonary bypass and cerebral physiology

Unlike other types of surgery, operations on the heart have special requirements due to the nature of the organ. That is, the heart is basically a two-chambered hollow muscle that pumps blood by rhythmically contracting, usually once every second. In this manner blood low in oxygen content (dark red in color) arrives at the right ventricle from veins where it is then ejected into the pulmonary arteries and passes through the lungs. The oxygen content is raised and carbon dioxide levels are lowered by diffusion gradients across multiple alveoli (membranes) in the lung. These alveoli contain air and oxygen. The now oxygen-rich blood (bright red in color) is then collected in the left ventricle which, upon contraction, ejects blood under pressure into the aorta, or main artery. After flowing through a series of multiple branching and progressively smaller vessels, blood cells (primarily red blood cells) are distributed to all tissues and organs (including the brain) for maintenance of normal cell metabolism. After perfusing these tissue beds, the once again oxygen-poor blood is drained into progressively larger and fewer veins that ultimately connect to the right ventricle, and the process begins all over again. It is a process that cannot be interrupted for longer than about five minutes in a human at normal temperature before cellular damage in the brain occurs. If perfusion is not maintained or restored after such brief interruptions, cells die, and the body is left injured or ceases to live.

The brain, under normal conditions, receives approximately 15% of the blood ejected from the left ventricle, despite representing only 2% of the total body mass [1]. The brain is supplied by two major arteries (right and left common carotids) that branch off the aortic arch. Both common carotids additionally branch into the external and internal carotid arteries on each side. A second set of two arteries, the vertebrals, also supply blood to the brain. The internal carotid arteries further branch into the smaller anterior cerebral and middle cerebral arteries, which are ultimately joined to the vertebrals by the circle of Willis. The anatomy of the circle of Willis provides some degree of protection of the brain by allowing for alternate blood flow should either an internal carotid or a vertebral artery become occluded [2]. Nearly all venous blood from the brain flows out through two internal jugular veins which join the superior vena cava via the right and left subclavian veins for transport of venous blood to the right ventricle.

The average cerebral blood flow in adults is approximately 50 cc/100 g of brain tissue, but nearly double this rate in children. Cerebral blood flow is remarkably constant, exhibiting autoregulation over a wide range of arterial blood pressure (50–150 mm Hg) under normal conditions. While on CPB, the range of autoregulation shifts downward to between 30 and 110 mm Hg [3]. Cerebral blood vessels dilate or constrict in response to arterial blood carbon dioxide levels (high levels > 45 mm Hg result in vasodilation and levels below 40 mm Hg cause vasoconstriction), which, other than total blood flow, is one of the few parameters that can be electively manipulated during CPB.

Cardiopulmonary bypass is used to provide the cardiac surgeon with a stiil, relatively dry operative field so delicate surgery can be performed on the normally beating heart. Patients are connected to CPB most often by insertion of two plastic tubes (called cannulae) placed in the right atrium/inferior vena cava or each vena cava for collection of venous blood, and, on the arterial side, in the ascending aorta. Blood in this manner is diverted away from the heart and lungs out of the patient's chest, which has been opened by median sternotomy, to the heart-lung machine.

The heart-lung machine in its simplest form consists of an artificial lung (called the oxygenator) and a pump which corresponds to the ventricle under normal conditions. With nearly all the systemic venous blood diverted to the CPB circuit, the heart is electively stopped by infusion of an ice cold solution that "arrests" the normal cardiac motion and metabolism and allows the heart to be functionally excluded from the circulation by placement of occlusive clamp on the ascending aorta. While technically the lungs do not have to be bypassed, they routinely are to avoid the necessity of placing additional cannulae which could obstruct the surgical field. When a patient is connected to the heart-lung machine (most often for about two hours), the surgeon is able to manipulate and open the heart and replace or repair defective valves, bypass blocked coronary arteries, or repair anatomic defects. For CABG operations, the ventricles are not opened, but small replacement grafts are sewn between the ascending aorta and coronary arteries to provide additional blood flow to the native coronary arteries which have become either partially or totally obstructed by vascular disease.

Perhaps the most important aspect of CPB from a cerebral outcome standpoint is that the entire perfusion of the brain is dependent on the heart-lung machine when the heart is arrested. Thus the quality and quantity of the blood (perfusate) exiting the arterial cannula in the ascending aorta will have a direct effect on maintenance of cerebral function during the open-heart operation. Factors that affect the quality of this perfusate are discussed shortly.

Two important adjuncts to conventional CPB are hypothermia and hemodilution, both of which have been shown to improve CPB perfusion and afford a degree of protection to all organs. The primary purpose of hypothermia, or lowering the body temperature, is to reduce oxygen demand which permits a lower blood flow. Lower blood flow decreases the degree of hemolysis (or blood damage) that inevitably occurs whenever blood is artificially pumped and oxygenated. A second benefit of hypothermia with reduced blood flow is to further limit the amount of blood that may be present at the operative site due to collateral circulation. A third benefit is to decrease the temperature gradient between the cold arrested heart and the warmer body, so as to delay the heart from rewarming when the aortic crossclamp is in place.

The body temperature during CPB is most often lowered to about 28°C (85°F), but, for more complex cases when extensive surgery is being performed, it is not unusual to lower the body temperature to 18 or 20°C (about 65°F). At these profoundly low temperatures, the circulation can be totally interrupted for short periods with no discernible ill effects. Total circulatory arrest is most often used on infants and only rarely on adults. Hypothermia also provides a margin of safety should there be a mechanical problem with the heart-lung machine necessitating temporarily stopping CPB until the problem is fixed. This also occurs only very rarely.

Hemodilution, or the purposeful lowering of the patient's hematocrit with crystalloid solution, was popularized in the early 1960s largely due to the burden open-heart surgery was making on blood banks. It was found later that because of the non-pulsatile nature of CPB blood flow, tissue and organ perfusion was actually improved with hemodilation despite the reduced oxygen-carrying capacity of blood with lower hematocrits. Typically, the hematocrit on CPB is approximately 20%, or about one-half that normally found in patients. It is not unusual now for most adult patients to have open-heart surgery without receiving any blood transfusion during their entire hospital stay, which has the added benefit of decreasing the risk to virtually zero of acquiring a blood-borne disease during their open-heart surgery.

In the late 1960s, it was found that blood transfusion carried with it the risk of microembolism [4]. Unlike a normal blood transfusion that is administered into a vein where the bank blood then passes through the lungs, blood transfusion during CPB entails transmission of microaggregates directly into the systemic arterial circulation, and the brain, instead of the lungs, is one of first recipient organs. Microemboli most often are composed of naturally-occurring blood products such as white blood cells and platelet aggregates which can block small arterial vessels, thus depriving tissues of nutrient blood flow.

Once the pathophysiology of microembolism was recognized, the solution to this problem was to develop filters to remove the microgaggregates before they were pumped out the CPB arterial line. Filters were first used on the venous side of the CPB circuit and then on the arterial. Filters used for the last decade most often consist of woven screen grids with pore sizes ranging between 20 and 40 microns. (Red blood cells are less than 10 microns, but blood microaggregates often exceed 50 microns and can be as large as 200–400 microns).

Besides the inherent risks of microembolism from blood bank transfusion into the CPB circuit, it was discovered that the CPB circuit itself could produce microaggregates. These microaggregates are caused by blood contact with the variety of foreign materials in the heart-lung machine (plastics, metals, and adhesives used in the fabrication of the oxygenator, reservoirs and circuitry). Unlike the normal vascular endothelium, these foreign surfaces alter blood in subtle ways still poorly understood [5].

Initiation of gross blood clotting during CPB, which normally occurs whenever blood leaves the normal vasculature, is prevented by administration of heparin, a potent anticoagulant. Regulation of heparin dosages prior to the mid 1970s was by protocol; that is, all patients were given a fixed dose based on their body weight with subsequent half-doses hourly when on CPB. In 1975 [6] it was found that individual patients' reactions to heparin could vary significantly, and the implication was that some patients were receiving too little anticoagulation leading to formation of small clots during CPB. These clots could circulate as microemboli and lodge in small vessels of organs perfused from the arterial line. A test called the activated clotting time (or ACT) was developed and used to more effectively regulate heparin anticoagulation during CPB [7]. By the early 1980s, virtually all open-heart teams in the USA were using ACTS, and this procedure along with arterial line filtration, which also was used by a majority of CPB teams, greatly decreased the incidence of emboli and coagulation abnormalities in patients undergoing open-heart surgery [8].

The most common manifestation of suboptimal heparin anticoagulation is development of abnormal bleeding as normal protein clotting factors and platelets in blood are consumed. The advantage of ACT measurements on brain protection is difficult to pinpoint, but minimizing the number of microaggregates and clots, at least from a theoretical viewpoint, has enhanced patients' cerebral outcome after CPB. The decreased incidence of abnormal bleeding after CPB now seen in patients is most likely due to better management of heparin anticoagulation with ACTS [9].

In addition, another type of microemboli formed during CPB consists of gas bubbles. Most often these were found to be bubbles of oxygen, particularly when a bubble oxygenator was used. Bubble oxygenators have been the preferred type for more than two decades, but within the last few years several models of membrane oxygenators have become available and are now being used with increasing frequency. Early criticisms of membrane oxygenators were: 1) limited gas transfer; 2) cost; and 3) complexity. These issues have largely disappeared with newer designs, and the primary added benefit is that membrane oxygenators produce negligible amounts of gaseous microemboli.

Current practice of CPB

Having described how CPB is used to substitute for normal circulation, the discussion now will focus on current CPB practices that are believed to favorably affect patients' cerebral outcome. It should be noted that every time a patient is connected to a heart-lung machine, all team members are acutely aware of the invasiveness of the procedure and utter dependence of the patient's life upon the CPB circuit and the skill of the team. Open-heart surgery, therefore, is approached with the seriousness and attention to detail commensurate with such an undertaking. Techniques and devices are gradually evolving and, for the most part improving, but the fundamental parameters of CPB practice are based on empiric knowledge gained through previous successful cases. If there was a way to do open-heart surgery without use of CPB, most cardiac surgeons would abandon CPB as we know it today, provided their patients could be kept alive with less morbidity and mortality as is currently experienced.

All blood-contacting components of conventional CPB circuits are disposable; that is, the oxygenators, reservoirs, filters, tubing, cannulae, and connectors are removed from sterile packaging, set up immediately prior to the beginning of surgery, used once, and then disposed of after the case. Of clear importance during this pre-CPB phase is the necessity to fully wet and debubble the blood-handling components of the circuit. This is described as "priming the pump." The various sterile components must be assembled together into a system by connecting them with tubing. This tubing, prior to adding priming solutions contains room air. As an aid to removing room air and debubbling the CPB circuit, filtered 100% carbon dioxide gas is flushed into the system. The rationale is that carbon dioxide is approximately 30 times more soluble in blood than room air which is four-fifths nitrogen. Nitrogen-containing bubbles are notoriously long-lived in solution [10]. After carbon dioxide flushing, balanced electrolyte solution and a plasma protein solution, most often human albumin, are added to the circuit. The volume required for adult CPB is approximately 2000 ml, which is about one-third the blood volume of the average-sized adult patient. Upon initiation of CPB this clear priming solution mixes with the patient's blood volume and the resulting patient/pump mixture has reduced hematocrit (to 20–25%), thus achieving the desired degree of hemodilution as discussed earlier.

Prior to CPB heparin is given according to protocol (usually 3–4 mg/kg), but its effect on blood coagulation is verified by measuring the ACT. A normal ACT is about 140 seconds; on CPB the minimum "safe" ACT is considered to be 400 seconds by most teams, and it is kept above this level by supplemental doses of heparin as needed and frequent ACT measurements to assess the effects.

The flow rates used during CPB are similarly calculated for each individual patient: larger patients require a higher total flow than smaller patients, but all patients are perfused according to well-established flow rates (50 to 60 ml/kg body weight or 2.2 to 2.4 L/min/m^2 body surface area). The flow rate used in children is slightly higher due to their higher metabolic demand. As discussed previously, the flow rate can be safely lowered after achieving hypothermia which decreases the oxygen (and therefore, blood flow) requirements.

However, in the absence of adequate total blood flow, regardless of the temperature, the brain will receive insufficient oxygen resulting in hypoperfusion which will deleteriously affect the cerebral outcome. Hence the importance of maintenance of CPB flows in the described "safe" ranges. Other causes of inadequate blood flow that occur infrequently are related to improper cannula placement in the ascending aorta. Equally important is the avoidance of venous cannula malposition, particularly if venous blood flow from the superior vena cava is obstructed. This can lead to elevated cerebral venous pressures which can quickly lead to cerebral edema, altered brain perfusion and injury.

In older patients who have known cerebrovascular disease (manifested by carotid bruits or a preoperative history of ischemic attacks or stroke) the flow rate and blood pressure on CPB are maintained slightly higher than normal to reasonably assure adequate cerebral perfusion. As noted earlier, cerebral perfusion is fairly constant over a wide range of arterial blood pressures, so in patients without cerebrovascular disease, the pressure is considered adequate so long as it remains above 40 mm Hg; in those patients with cerebrovascular disease it is kept above 70 mm Hg with the occasional administration of a vasoconstricting drug.

The characteristic of blood flow when patients are on CPB is mean (that is without the usual peaks and valleys called systolic and diastolic). Some studies have reported better organ perfusion, including that of the brain, with pulsatile flow which can be created by some pumps. However, the extensive literature devoted to examining this issue of mean versus pulsatile flow during CPB contains numerous contradictions, and no definitive studies have proven an overwhelming advantage to pulsatile flow for enhancing the cerebral outcome after CPB. It should be noted that for part of the time a patient is on CPB, flow is pulsatile during commencement and weaning when "partial CPB" is used. That is, the some flow originates from the heart-lung machine and some flow occurs naturally from left ventricular ejections.

In contrast, a number of studies have shown definite advantages when filtration is used on the CPB circuit. This includes prebypass filtration when priming to remove circuit debris or contaminants contained in priming fluids, filtration of many blood products administered through the heart-lung machine, cardiotomy (i.e., filtration of suctioned blood from the operative site), and finally, and perhaps most importantly, filtration of the arterial blood just prior to its reintroduction to the patient's aorta. While prebypass filtration for circuit debris is most usually down to a level of 0.2 to 5 microns, blood filtration for transfusion, cardiotomy, or arterial line is typically 20 to 40 microns. No convincing advantage is apparent for filtration at the lower end (i.e., 20 micron), and there are filter design and performance criterion that may make filtration with smaller pore-sized filters less forgiving than filters of 40 micron pore size. Likewise, there is a wide variety of current filter designs that promote separation and removal of gaseous microemboli prior to passage of the blood through the filter medium, but no obvious clinical advantage has been demonstrated to any particular filter brand, and a wide number are used by CPB teams today. The most recent purported design advantage of some arterial filters is the incorporation of either a heparin coating onto the filter medium or use of a chemically modified filter material that enhances its wettability. Both types of filters are easier to debubble when priming, and therefore, may offer some small advantage in terms of cerebral protection and outcome.

The other aspect of arterial filtration performance that can affect cerebral outcome is operation of the arterial filter with an active (i.e., open) purge line during CPB. In this manner, gaseous emboli (either micro or gross) will be shunted out of the filter instead of accumulating or possibly passing through the filter where they then could embolize to cerebral vessels. The amount of shunt created by an active purge line is insignificant (<5%) in relation to the total CPB blood flow.

The type of oxygenator used may have a direct bearing on cerebral outcome, but again a great number of papers in the literature provide contradictory information. What has become clearer in recent years, however, is that membrane-type oxygenators which have no direct blood/gas interface (in contrast to that found in bubble type) produce very few gaseous micro-emboli when primed and operated carefully. Therefore, it seems logical to assume better cerebral protection with use of membrane oxygenators, but definitive studies are sparse on this issue. A recent study [11] comparing a bubble to membrane oxygenator favored the membrane-type and was based on the observation of retinal microvascular occlusions during CPB and post-operative psychometric testing in patients. It may be coincidental that most CPB teams today use the membrane-type, primarily because manufacturers have provided devices that are cheaper and easier to use than those available 20 years ago.

As discussed previously, CPB must deliver adequate oxygen to and remove carbon dioxide from the tissues and organs perfused with blood. Thus besides providing blood flow, frequent monitoring of the levels of these gases in the blood exiting and entering the CPB circuit is one of the fundamental jobs of the perfusionist. Blood gases during CPB are altered from those seen in normal patients in the following way: the level of oxygen is elevated while the level of carbon dioxide is slightly lower. The primary reason for this is that maintaining the oxygen level somewhat higher is thought to provide a margin of safety under the altered physiology (e.g., mean flow) of CPB. Carbon dioxide levels are usually lower than normal primarily because of CPB hypothermia which decreases the production of carbon dioxide by the body. Carbon dioxide levels in arterial blood profoundly affect cerebral blood flow by causing vessels to dilate (with levels greater than 40 mm Hg) or conversely, constrict with lower levels.

The proper management of carbon dioxide levels during CPB is somewhat controversial. For many years it was thought to be advantageous to add carbon dioxide gas to the gas supplied to the oxygenator (termed pH-stat management) in the belief that this would ensure adequate cerebral perfusion by compensation for the lower levels caused by hypothermia and preventing vasoconstriction. However, about ten years ago persuasive evidence was put forth that suggested artificially elevating the carbon dioxide blood levels was, in fact, not the proper way to regulate blood gases on CPB. The new theory [12] has been to maintain the carbon dioxide content of the blood constant regardless of the temperature (termed alpha stat). In this way cerebral autoregulation of blood flow is maintained and the brain is neither over-perfused nor underperfused. The majority of CPB teams now use the alpha stat approach to blood gas management during CPB, despite few studies proving the superiority of this approach.

The induction and reversal (rewarming to normal temperature) of hypothermia during CPB can affect the cerebral outcome in patients. An impor-tant part of the oxygenator is a heat exchanger which circulates warm or cold water through it. By lowering the water temperature, the blood flowing through the oxygenator is cooled, as is subsequently the patient. Most current oxygenators contain efficient heat exchangers that are capable of either rapid cooling or rewarming the patient. A risk of rapid cooling and rewarming is the production of gaseous microemboli in the blood, so adherence to gradi-ents less than 10°C between the heat exchanger water and patient's temperature can protect the brain from gaseous microemboli.

Once the patient has been cooled to profoundly hypothermic levels, it may be technically necessary for the surgeon to employ a period of total circula-tory arrest with all blood flow from the CPB pump stopped. The period of "safe" circulatory arrest is generally thought to be less than 45 minutes, and in all cases, is kept as short as practically possible [13]. As mentioned earlier, this technique is used more often on infants or small children when the CPB cannulae are obstructing the operative site. The development of newer, thin-walled cannulae have enable many surgeons to avoid circulatory arrest because of its obvious potential for cerebral damage, and periods of low flow are preferred to total circulatory arrest.

An overriding concern with the practice of CPB is the avoidance of massive gas embolism which occurs in about one case out of every 8000 [14]. While a wide variety of mechanisms, as well as team members, have been shown to be responsible for massive gas embolism during CPB, the circuit should be equipped with at least two safety devices designed to prevent this cata-strophic accident. Many patients have died or been severely injured neurologically after massive gas embolism, and prevention of this complica-tion is a high priority whenever CPB is used.

Closing

In summary, much of the practice of CPB is empiric and most improvements over the last five decades have been subtle in nature. Many of the funda-mental questions regarding "proper" techniques and management of CPB were answered in the 1950s and 1960s. Most current CPB research is directed towards refinement or examination of subtle effects of CPB. Since the vast majority of patients make normal clinical recoveries after open-heart surgery,

56

little thought is given to their cerebral outcome, unless, of course, a major problem becomes apparent postoperatively. The growing body of literature examining the finer cerebral reactions to open-heart surgery may provide new information to teams as to the optimal techniques and devices to use. All involved in this remarkable technology hope we are on the threshold of obtaining such new information that will favorably alter the way CPB is currently practiced, so that the reported incidences of poor cerebral outcome attributed to CPB can be either eliminated or reduced to negligible levels.

References

1. Henry JP, Meehan JP. The Circulation. Chicago: Year Book Medical Publishers 1971; p. 133.
2. Reed C, Stafford TB. Cardiopulmonary Bypass, 2nd Edition. Houston: Texas Medical Press 1985; p. 27.
3. Sarnquist FH. Neurological outcome after "low flow, low pressure" cardiopulmonary bypass. In: Hilberman M (ed) Brain Injury and Protection during Heart Surgery, Boston: Martinus Nijhoff Publ, 1988; p. 13.
4. Hill JD, Aguilar MJ, Baranco A et al. Neuropathological manifestations of cardiac surgery. Ann Thorac Surg 1969; 7:409.
5. Royston D. Blood cell activation. Sem Thorac Cardiovasc Surg 1990; 2:341.
6. Bull BS, Korpman RA, Huse WM et al. Heparin therapy during extracorporeal circulation: I. Problems inherent in existing heparin protocols. J Thorac Cardiovasc Surg 1985; 69:674.
7. Bull BS, Huse WM, Brauer FS, et al. Heparin therapy during extracorporeal circulation: II. The use of a dose-response curve to individualize heparin and protamine dosage. J Thorac Cardiovasc Surg 1975; 69:685.
8. Kurusz M, Schneider B, Brown JP. Filtration during open-heart surgery: Devices, techniques, opinions and complications. Proc Am Acad Cardiovasc Surg 1983; 4:123.
9. Kurusz M, Conti VR, Arens JF et al. Perfusion accident survey. Proc Am Acad Cardiovasc Perfusion 1986; 7:57.
10. Butler DD. Biophysical aspects of gas bubbles in blood. Med Instrument 1985, 19:59.
11. Blauth CI, Smith PL, Arnold JV et al. Influence of oxygenator type on the prevalence and extent of microembolic retinal ischemia during cardiopulmonary bypass. Assessment by digital image analysis. J Thorac Cardiovasc Surg 1990; 99:61.
12. Swan H: The importance of acid-base management for cardiac and cerebral preservation during open-heart operations. Surg Gynecol Obstet 1984; 158:391.
13. Kirklin JW, Barratt-Boyes B. Hypothermia, circulatory arrest and cardiopulmonary bypass. In: Cardiac Surgery. New York: John Wiley, 1985; p. 29.
14. Kurusz M, Conti VR. Cerebral protection during cardiopulmonary bypass: Devices and techniques to prevent air embolism. In: Willner AE, Rodewald G (eds) Impact of Cardiac Surgery on the Quality of Life, Neurological and Psychological Aspects. New York: Plenum Press, 1990; p. 255.

5. The role of the surgical team in minimizing postoperative cerebral dysfunction

JONATHAN D. KATZ

Post-Cardiotomy Neurologic Dysfunction (PCND) is a descriptive term which encompasses a wide spectrum of neurologic complications. Depending upon the markers sought, complications in this family may range from minor transient neuropsychologic impairment to disabling stroke. Because of inconsistencies in definitions and research protocols, estimates of the frequency of PCND vary extensively, but it may occur in as many as 79% of patients subsequent to open heart surgery [1].

A number of circumstances and events during the peri-operative period are thought to contribute to this rather high occurrence of complication. Unfortunately, many of these risk factors are beyond the reach of the surgical team (see Table 1). For example, old age, aortic atherosclerosis, and a previous history of myocardial infarction place the patient at increased risk for PCND.

Table 1. Factors associated with post operative cerebral dysfunction-beyond control of the surgical team

Age
Previous neurologic disease
Presence of bruit
Brittle aorta
Left ventricular thrombus

On the other hand, as our understanding has deepened of the physiologic changes accompanying open heart surgery, we find that more of the damaging processes are accessible using contemporary technology (see Table 2). The purpose of this discussion is to review some pertinent elements of the clinical procedures of heart surgery with an emphasis on areas where interventions by the surgical team may potentially improve the neurologic outcome.

Pre-existing risk factors for post-cardiotomy neurologic injury

Factors in each stage of the peri-operative period influence the potential for

Table 2. Factors associated with post cerebral dysfunction-within the control of the surgical team

Surgical procedure
Choice of anesthetic agent
Oxygenator type
Use of filters
Duration of CPB
LV venting technique
Air removal technique
CPB flow
CPB pressure
Glucose management
Blood gas management

PCND. It is especially important to recognize that there is a substantial subset of cardiac surgery patients who evidence measurable neurologic abnormalities in the *preoperative period*, well before any surgical intervention. In studies by Breuer *et al.* [2], and Shaw *et al.* [3], close to 35% of *preoperative* patients had demonstrable neurologic disease. This observation serves as a significant reminder as to the vital importance of a thorough neurologic examination to establish the patient's preoperative baseline.

There is evidence to suggest a higher incidence of new post-operative neurologic disease in those who enter the operating room with pre-existing neurologic impairment. This is especially so among those patients with prior neurologic symptoms related to vascular insufficiency (stroke, TIA) [4].

More controversial is whether the presence of *asymptomatic* cerebrovascular disease places the patient at increased risk for PCND. Conflicting results have appeared in the literature, depending upon a number of variables in study design, most notably the nature of the evaluation for cerebrovascular disease and the reportable complication (i.e., stroke, neuropsychological deficit). The majority of studies indicate that the presence of pre-operative bruits is not associated with a higher incidence of post-operative strokes [5]. And Harrison *et al.* reported no increase in neuropsychological deficit in patients with carotid artery disease as demonstrated by angiography [6]. On the other hand, Reed *et al.* demonstrated a significant increase in risk of stroke after coronary bypass surgery in patients with carotid bruits [7].

With no clear-cut conclusion as to whether or not asymptomatic carotid disease is a risk factor, it is extremely debatable if prophylactic carotid endarterectomy is indicated. A key question is whether the risk of stroke subsequent to cardiac surgery exceeds that of the prophylactic carotid artery surgery. The reports by Barnes [8] and by Turnipseed [9] concluded that prophylactic carotid endarterectomy in otherwise asymptomatic patients was not indicated.

Pre-operative medication may play a role in PCND. It is standard practice to utilize a potent pre-operative medication regimen in order to minimize the stress of the immediate pre-operative events (transport to the operating room, placement of invasive monitors). Potent sedatives such as scopolamine and the potent long acting benzodiazepines may have prolonged effects, especially in critically ill patients, and may contribute to coma or delirium in the early post-operative period.

Intraoperative events associated with PCND

Intraoperative events play a dominant role in the appearance of postoperative cerebral injury. It is estimated that some 70% of the peri-operative neurologic injuries occur during the operative period [10].

One frequently overlooked intervention that may contribute to PCND is the placement of intravascular monitors. Usually placed in the operating room immediately prior to anesthetic induction, these monitors usually include; a central venous catheter - placed via the subclavian or internal jugular vein, a pulmonary artery catheter - via the subclavian or internal jugular vein, and an intra-arterial catheter - via the radial or femoral artery.

In the case of the central venous and the pulmonary artery catheters, the complications of immediate concern during placement are subclavian or carotid artery puncture, arrythmia, and air embolism. Each of these events hold the potential for compromising cerebral circulation.

Intra-arterial catheter placement carries with it the risk of air or thrombus embolization. This potential for retrograde embolization to the central circulation was well demonstrated in a study by Lownstein who showed retrograde flow with as little as a 3 ml flush of the radial arterial catheter [11]. Additionally, in those patients in whom the distance from catheter site to the central circulation is shortened (i.e. children, temporal artery catheters) the risk is heightened [12].

Events during the induction of anesthesia have been implicated in the appearance of PCND. One period of special vulnerability occurs during the anesthetic induction when it is not unusual for there to be sudden and extreme variations in blood pressure in patients with known cardiovascular disease, and even more so when the cardiovascular disease is inadequately controlled.

There have been suggestions that the choice of anesthetic may influence the outcome in patients at risk for PCND. Much attention has been directed to the possible role of various anesthetic agents in offering cerebral protection when there is heightened risk of hypoxemic injury. Barbiturates have been most thoroughly studied, with inconsistent findings. Nussmeier et al. used a thiopental infusion titrated to maintain EEG burst-suppression in patients who were undergoing open-chamber (intracardiac) surgery [13]. They found a beneficial influence on the incidence and severity of neurologic complications. Unfortunately, this was not accomplished without a cost. The patients who received the thiopental treatment were more hemodynamically unstable, and required more inotropic support than the controls. The thiopental group also required prolonged mechanical ventilation. On the other hand, in a more recent study evaluating patients undergoing CABG procedures, Zaidan et al.

failed to demonstrate any beneficial brain protection from high dose thiopental [14]. They also reported some degree of morbidity associated with administration of the drug.

Other anesthetic agents have been promoted as potentially beneficial in brain protection. Isoflurane has been shown to produce a dose-dependent decrease in $CMRO_2$ and suppression of cortical electrical activity [15]. The cerebral energy state is also preserved when challenged with hypotension [16]. Additionally, it has been suggested that isoflurane protects cerebral autoregulation during CPB [17]. Unfortunately, isoflurane has other properties, such as direct cerebral vasodilation which may produce a "steal" phenomenon, that counteract the beneficial reduction in $CMRO_2$ and negates the theoretical ability to provide cerebral protection [18].

Events during Cardiopulmonary bypass (CPB) clearly play a dominant role in the development of PCND [4]. A large number of studies have reported that duration of CPB bears a direct relationship with the incidence of neurologic injury [19]. Less clear are the exact events during the CPB which expose the individual patient to increased risk.

Inadequate cerebral perfusion to meet cerebral metabolic demand during CPB is generally acknowledged to be among the primary causative events for PCND. The etiology for the presumed hypoperfusion is much more controversial. Earlier reports warned about the dangers of hypotension during CPB [20, 21]. The specific concern expressed by these authors was that autoregulation of the cerebral circulation would not be adequate to maintain cerebral blood flow when systemic blood pressure was permitted to drop below a certain minimum level - i.e. 50 mm Hg. More recent evidence has demonstrated that there is no known absolute minimum safe arterial blood pressure because of the interactions with a number of other factors; hematocrit, blood viscosity, temperature, pH and pCO_2 management, flow rate and type, age and preexisting condition of patient, to mention just a few. In the study by Murkin *et al.*, there was no decrement in cerebral blood flow with blood pressures as low as 25 mm Hg, utilizing the alpha stat (see below) method of pH management [22]. Even more to the point, Slogoff *et al.* failed to demonstrate a relationship between neurologic outcome and perfusion pressure [23].

There are circumstances under which autoregulation during CPB is not maintained. This may occur during profound hypothermia, in patients with diabetes mellitus, uncontrolled hypertension, and certain neurologic diseases. It has been suggested that autoregulation can be compromised in the presence of certain inhalation anesthetics, especially the halogenated hydrocarbons. And finally, pH-stat blood gas management has been shown to obliterate cerebral autoregulation [24].

It has been proposed that loss of pulsatile flow during CPB is another mechanism producing inadequate cerebral perfusion. This argument suggests that non-pulsatile flow transmits less energy into the central circulation which results in compensatory vasoconstriction and insufficient perfusion. Several studies have documented physiologic changes affecting the cerebral microcirculation as a result of nonpulsatile flow [25]. On the other hand, there has been no documentation that neurologic outcome is improved when pulsatile perfusion is utilized.

And finally, hypoperfusion may result from faults in surgical technique. Aortotomy and cardiotomy may produce showers of gaseous, atheromatous or thrombotic emboli [26]. Inappropriate use of the cardiotomy suction may be a major contributor of embolic debris [27]. Additionally, incorrect placement of the arterial perfusion cannula can result in aortic dissection and impeded or channeled flow through the aorta.

Micro- (<150 µm in diameter) and macroemboli are thought by other authors to be the primary causal agent for PCND [28]. Gaseous (air, N_2O) and particulate (fat, fibers, plastic chips, aggregates of platelets, leukocytes, atherosclerotic debris and fibrin) embolization have all been shown to occur. In a study utilizing M-mode echocardiography, Oka et al. showed that intracardiac and aortic microbubbles were present in 79% of patients during open cardiac procedures and 11% during closed cardiac procedures [29]. Using transcranial Doppler, Von Reutern et al. demonstrated gaseous microemboli in the middle cerebral artery of as many as 50% of patients during CPB [30]. Of concern to the anesthesiologist is the suggestion that the presence of N_2O may enlarge the gaseous emboli and exacerbate the neurologic injury associated with CPB [31].

It is important to recognize that there is no clear understanding of the exact relationship between entrapped air in the circulation and CNS dysfunction. A recent report by Moody et al. identified in brain specimens what they claim is the anatomical correlate of the neurological deficits resulting from CPB [32]. These "SCADs" (small capillary and arteriolar dilatations) are thought by the authors to represent the anatomic sites of fat and air emboli.

Solid microscopic debris is also embolized in great volume during CPB. A number of types of emboli have been demonstrated including atheromatous and thrombotic debris, aggregates of fibrin, leukocytes and platelets and even plastic chips. Modification of surgical techniques, especially avoiding excessive aortic manipulation, can play a major role in minimizing the amount of atheromatous and calcific emboli [33]. Special attention must also be given to maintaining adequate anticoagulation to minimize the volume of fibrin and platelet aggregates.

A recent report by Nakajima et al. has focused on the rewarming period following hypothermic CPB as a potential vulnerable period for neurologic damage [34]. Using an oximeter catheter to measure jugular venous oxygenation, they were able to demonstrate reduced saturation during the rewarming period. This was interpreted as representing inadequate cerebral perfusion during an interval of rapidly increasing cerebral metabolic demand resulting from the increasing brain temperature. Neurologic outcomes in this small clinical study were not reported.

A number of modifications in CPB protocol have been introduced in an attempt to limit the quantity of emboli and the potential for cerebral injury. For example, it has been shown that the number of microscopic gas emboli is diminished when membrane oxygenators are substituted for bubble oxygenators [35]. Similarly, the introduction of arterial and cardiotomy suction filters diminish the number of microparticles larger than 20 μm in diameter that can embolize to the general circulation [36].

Unfortunately, the desired outcome, i.e. the demonstration of improved neurologic outcome has not been forthcoming. Clinical studies looking for improved neuropsychologic outcome have failed to conclusively demonstrate protection from arterial filtration or from use of membrane oxygenators and have been, at best, contradictory [37]. In fact, it appears that one period of enhanced jeopardy occurs at a moment when neither of these interventions would be effective - during aortic cannulation and the initiation of CPB [38].

A second area of controversy exists regarding the correct management of arterial blood gases during CPB. The crux of the argument centers about whether it is desirable to maintain normal pH and pCO_2 as measured at 37° (alpha stat) or as corrected to body temperature (pH stat). The theoretical advantage of alpha stat management is that cerebral autoregulation is maintained even at low flows and blood pressures. The theoretical advantage of pH stat management is that, although autoregulation is abolished, overall CBF is higher and cerebral venous oxygen saturation is maintained higher than with alpha-stat. There are persuasive arguments to support both methods of management during routine cases. However a recent study found no difference in neuropsychologic outcome as a result of differences in CO_2 management [39].

A number of other interventions have been proposed to reduce the incidence and severity of PCND. Moderate hypothermia and hemodilution are routinely employed during CPB. Hypothermia provides decreased cerebral requirements for oxygen and glucose. Hemodilution is employed to reverse the increase in blood viscosity resulting from hypothermia and low flow states. The beneficial influence of hypothermia varies depending upon the nature and duration of the insult and the brain region affected. In general, hypothermia seems to confer greater protection for global than for focal ischemia [40]. Hemodilution provides protection only to the point where the increased oxygen delivery compensates for the decreased oxygen content. The lower limit of hemodilution is not well delineated but it appears that this limit probably is represented by hematocrits in the low 20's. In Shaw's report, neuropsychological outcome was worse in patients with the greatest reductions in hemoglobin [4].

The pharmacologic control of blood glucose during CPB is another area of controversy. Laboratory models of focal [41] and global [42] cerebral ischemia indicate a worse neurologic outcome in the face of hyperglycemia. On the other hand, clinical studies have not implicated hyperglycemia during CPB as a factor in poor neurologic outcome [43]. And, from the vantage point of other outcome parameters, hyperglycemia appears to offer some beneficial properties [44]. In the face of these conflicting findings, the current recommendation is to attempt to maintain euglycemia.

The potential role of anesthetic agents in protection from the neuroendocrine stress response secondary to cardiac surgery and CPB is a relatively unexplored area. During, or after CPB, a large number of vasoactive markers of the stress response have been identified. These include; cortisol, epinephrine and nor-epinephrine, thromboxane, leukotrienses, prostaglandins, and complement. Each of these exert their own, characteristic pathophysiologic effect on the microcirculation. It is likely that these contribute to the potential for PCND [45]. It has been documented that various anesthetics can blunt these hormonal stress responses [46] and that the depth of anesthesia influences this response [47]. Unfortunately, no studies to date have demonstrated a relationship between specific type or depth of anesthesia, mediators of stress, and neuro-logic outcome.

Calcium channel blockers have been advanced as possible agents for cerebral protection. The basic theory is that ischemia results in increased intra-cellular calcium which appears to be a key component of many terminal chain reactions [48]. Calcium channel blockers inhibit calcium influx, and should attenuate the neurologic injury from ischemia. Unfortunately, calcium channel blocker pharmacology is extremely complex, and they are associ-ated with a host of activities, including interactions with excitatory neurotransmitter and impairment of autoregulatory vasoconstriction. In select situations, calcium channel blockers may produce beneficial effects, but a different blocker, or slightly altered conditions may yield the opposite result. In general, there is no good evidence to support the use of calcium channel blockers in the expectation of cerebral protection.

Post operative events associated with PCND

Often overlooked are the contributions of the post-operative period to the emergence of neurologic injury. Approximately 30% of strokes occur in the post-operative period, frequently appearing as late as the second post-opera-tive day [10].

A number of events in the post- operative period might contribute to this complication. In the study by Breuer et al. it was pointed out that the use of vasopressors and the need for an intra-aortic balloon assist device were associated with a higher incidence of post-operative encephalopathy [2]. Similarly, Slogoff et al. reported that cardiovascular failure in the recovery period requiring cardiopulmonary resuscitation was one of the major risk factors for PCND [23].

Monitoring for cerebral injury

Controversy exists on the utility and validity of the various available tools for monitoring cerebral function during cardiac surgery and CPB. It was expected that intraoperative electroencephalography (EEG) would serve as a predictor of post-operative neurologic dysfunction [49]. Potentially dangerous intraoperative events such as gaseous or particulate embolism, hypoxia, aortic dissection, impaired venous drainage all produce easily recognizable EEG changes. Unfortunately, these changes may be camouflaged by the alterations produced by a number of other more innocuous influences. For example the anesthetics in use may produce EEG changes that could be mistaken for those of hypoxemia. The commonly used synthetic opiods such as fentanyl or sufentanyl cause a suppression of high frequency beta, alpha and delta waves and the superimposition of lower frequency delta waves. EEG changes associated with hypothermia also resemble those of ischemia and add further to the difficulty in accurate EEG diagnosis. And the presence of an enormous amount of extraneous electrical "noise" in the operating room makes interpretation of intraoperative EEG very difficult.

Because of these and other limitations, the EEG has not proven to be a reliable predictor of postoperative PND. In a re-analysis of data from a previously published prospective study, Bashein calculated a 60% false positive and a 75% false negative fraction for intraoperative EEG abnormalities and ultimate outcome [50]. The main problem with single or dual lead or processed EEG is that it can help to detect the (rare) episodes of global cerebral hypoperfusion but does not reliably detect the (more common-place) episodes of focal neurologic injury.

Some improvement in yield from intraoperative EEG monitoring has resulted from the introduction of computer- assisted analysis. However, as is the case with raw data EEG, these types of monitors are extremely vulnerable to artifactual competition, such as from effects of the anesthetic regimen and from other electrical "noise" in the operating room environment.

As a result of the above-mentioned limitations, the intraoperative EEG has not become a routine monitor of cerebral perfusion during cardiac surgery. However, in certain specific situations, EEG analysis can play a vital role. If it is considered important to administer barbiturate or isoflurane in an attempt to provide cerebral protection, the obligatory endpoint is EEG burst suppression. The EEG may also provide important information to avoid instances of awareness during pure narcotic anesthesia. And finally, the EEG can be a valuable tool in those patients at risk for global or hemispheric ischemia; i.e. patients with severe carotid stenosis or occlusion.

More recently, investigators have reported on other monitors as predictors of PND. These include Doppler and (other) measures of CBF, and evoked potential. Other chapters in this volume deal with this topic more extensively.

Summary

It is apparent that the risk of Post-Cardiotomy Neurologic Dysfunction is multifactorial. Injury results from the interaction of a large number of circumstances and events. Cerebral ischemia and infarction represents a spectrum of injury and is not an all-or-none phenomenon. To further complicate any study of this subject, cerebral injury produces an assortment of symptoms, ranging from subtle neuropsychologic dysfunction to overt neurologic deficit such as stroke. As we have discussed, a large number of factors have all been proposed as the culprits in the appearance of PCND. And for each of the potential offenders a number of remedies have been offered. However, it is apparent that there is no simple panacea for this serious complication. This is well illustrated in a comparative analysis of data derived from 2 separate institutions where diametrically opposite techniques for surgical and CPB management were employed [51]. In this report, the severity of postoperative neuropsychological dysfunction was similar, despite these large differences in technique. The authors concluded that, at least when considering subtle cognitive deficits after CPB, all of the individual factors which have been proposed as causative agents have been "overemphasized" and the precise etiology remains undetermined.

References

1. Shaw PJ, Bates D, Cartlidge NEF et al. Neurologic and neuropsychological morbidity following major surgery: Comparison of coronary artery bypass and peripheral vascular surgery. Stroke 1987; 18:700.
2. Breuer AC, Furlan AJ, Hanson MR et al. Central nervous system complications of coronary bypass surgery: Prospective analysis of 421 patients. Stroke 1983; 14:682.
3. Shaw PJ, Bates D, Cartlidge NEF et al. Early neurologic complications of coronary artery bypass graft surgery. Brit Med J 1985; 291:1384.
4. Shaw PJ, Bates D, Cartlidge NEF et al. An analysis of factors predisposing to neurological injury in patients undergoing coronary bypass operations. Quart J Med 1989; 72:633.
5. Ivey TD, Strandness DE, Williams DB et al. Management of patients with carotid bruit undergoing cardiopulmonary bypass. J Thorac Cardiovasc Surg 1984; 87:183.
6. Harrison MJG, Schneidau A, Ho R et al. Cerebrovascular disease and functional outcome after coronary artery bypass surgery. Stroke 1989; 20:235.
7. Reed GL III, Singer DE, Picard EH, DeSanctis RW. Stroke following coronary bypass surgery: A case-control estimate of the risk from carotid bruits. New Engl J Med 1988; 319:1246.
8. Barnes RW, Liebman PR, Marszalek PB et al. The natural history of asymptomatic carotid disease in patients undergoing cardiovascular surgery. Surgery 1981; 90:1075.
9. Turnipseed WD, Berkoff HA, Belzer FO. Postoperative stroke in cardiac and peripheral vascular disease. Ann Surg 1980; 192:365.
10. Coffey CE, Massey EW, Roberts KB et al. Natural history of cerebral complications of coronary bypass surgery. Neurology 1983; 33:1416.
11. Lowenstein E, Little JW, Lo HH. Prevention of cerebral embolization from flushing radial artery cannulae. New Engl J Med 1971; 285:1414.
12. Prian GW, Wright GB, Rumack CM et al. Apparent cerebral embolization after temporal artery cannulation. J Pediatr 1978; 93:115.
13. Nussmeier NA, Arlund C, Slogoff S. Neuropsychiatric complications after cardiolpulmonary bypass: Cerebral protection by a barbiturate. Anesth 1986; 64:165.
14. Zaiden JR, Klochany A, Martin WM et al. Effect of thiopental on neurologic outcome following coronary bypass grafting. Anesth 1991; 74:406.
15. Newberg LA, Milde JH, Michenfelder JD. The cerebral metabolic effects of isoflurane at and above concentrations that suppress cortical electrical activity. Anesth 1983; 59:23.
16. Newberg LA, Michenfelder JD. Cerebral protection by isoflurane during hypoxemia or ischemia. Anesth 1983; 59:29.

66

17. Aladj LJ, Croughwell N, Smith LR, Reves JG. Cerebral blood flow autoregulation is preserved during cardiopulmonary bypass in isoflurane-anesthetized patients. Anesth Analg 1991; 72:48.
18. Nehls DG, Todd MM, Spetzler RF et al. A copmparison of the protective effects of isoflurane and barbiturates during temporary focal ischemia in primates. Anesth 1987; 66:453.
19. Sotaniemi KA, Mononen H, Hokkanen TE. Long-term cerebral outcome after open-heart surgery. Stroke 1986; 17:410.
20. Stockard, JJ, Bickford RG, Schauble JF. Pressure-dependent cerebral ischemia during cardiopulmonary bypass. Neurology 1973; 23:521.
21. Branthwaite MA. Prevention of neurologic damage during open-heart surgery. Thorax 1975; 30:258.
22. Murkin JL et al. Cerebral auto regulation and flow/metabolism coupling during cardiopulmonary bypass: Influence of PaCO2. Anesth Analg 1987; 66:825.
23. Slogoff S, Reul GJ, Keats AS. Role of perfusion pressure and flow in major organ dysfunction after cardiopulmonary bypass. Ann Thorac Surg 1990; 50:911.
24. Henriksen L, Hjelms E, Lindeburgh T. Brain hyperperfusion during cardiac operations. J Thorac Cardiovasc Surg 1983; 86:202.
25. Sanderson JM, Wright G, Sims FW. Brain damage in dogs immediately following pulsatile and non-pulsatile blood flows in extracorporeal circulation. Thorax 1972; 27:275.
26. Gallagher EG, Pearson DT. Ultrasonic identification of sources of gaseous microemboli during open heart surgery. Thorax 1973; 28:295.
27. Solis RT, Kennedy PS, Beall AC et al. Cardiolpulmonary bypass: Microembolization and platelet aggregation. Circulation 1975; 52:103.
28. Newman M, Frasco P, Kern F et al. Central nervous system dysfunction after cardiac surgery. Adv Cardiovasc Surg 1992; 3:243.
29. Oka Y, Moriwaka KM, Hong Y et al. Detection of air emboli in the left heart by M-mode transesophageal echocardiography following cardiopulmonary bypass. Anesth 1985; 63:109.
30. Von Reutern GM, Hetzel A, Birnbaum D, Schlosser V. Transcranial Doppler ultrasonography during cardiopulmonary bypass in patients with severe carotid stenosis or occlusion. Stroke 1988; 19:674.
31. Wells DG, Podolakin W, Mohr M et al. Nitrous oxide and cerebrospinal fluid markers of ischaemia following cardiopulmonary bypass. Anaesth Intensive Care 1987; 15:431.
32. Moody DM, Bell MA, Challa VR et al. Brain microemboli during cardiac surgery or aortography. Annals Neurol. 1990; 28:477.
33. Van Der Linden J, Casimir-Ahn H. When do cerebral emboli appear during open heart operations? A transcranial Doppler study. Ann Thorac Surg 1991; 51:237.
34. Nakajima T, Masakazu K, Hayashi Y et al. Clinical evaluation of cerebral oxygen balance during cardiopulmonary bypass: On-line continuous monitoring of jugular venous oxyhemoglobin saturation. Anesth Analg 1992; 74:630.
35. Padayachee TS, Parsons S, Theobold R et al. The detection of microemboli in the middle cerebral artery during cardiopulmonary bypass: A transcranial Doppler ultrasound investigation using membrane and bubble oxygenators. Ann Thorac Surg 1987; 44:298.
36. Padayachee TS, Parsons S, Theobold R et al. The effect of arterial filtration on reduction of gaseous microemboli in the middle cerebral artery during cardiopulmonary bypass. Ann Thorac Surg 1988; 45:647.
37. Blauth CI et al. Influence of oxygenator type on the prevalence and extent of microembolic retinal ischemia during cardiopulmonary bypass. Assessment by digital image analysis. J Thorac Cardiovasc Surg 1990; 99:61.
38. Pugsley W et al. Microemboli and cerebral impairment during cardiac surgery. Vasc Surg 1990; 24:34.
39. Bashein G et al. A randomized study of carbon dioxide management during hypothermic cardiopulmonary bypass. Anesth 1990; 72:7.

40. Michenfelder JD, Milde JH. Failure of prolonged hypocapnia, hypothermia, or hypertension to favorably alter acute stroke in primates. Stroke 1977; 8:87.
41. Nedergaard M. Transient focal ischemia in hyperglycemic rats is associated with increased cerebral infarction. Brain Res 1987; 408:79.
42. Lanier WL, Strangland KJ, Scheithauer BW et al. The effects of dextrose infusion and head position on neurologic outcome after complete cerebral ischemia in primates: examination of a model. Anesth 1987; 66:39.
43. Frasco P, Croughwell N, Blumenthal J et al. Association between blood glucose level during cardiopulmonary bypass and neuropsychiatric outcome. Anesth 1991; 75:A55.
44. Metz S, Keats AS: Benefits of a glucose-containing priming solution for cardiopulmonary bypass. Anesth Analg 1991; 72:428.
45. Reves JG. Anesthesia and cardiopulmonary bypass. International Anesthesia Research Society; 1991 Review Course Lectures 1991; p. 93.
46. Samuelson PN, Reves JG, Kirklin JK et al. Comparison of sufentanil and enflurane-nitrous oxide anesthesia for myocardial revascularization. Anesth Analg 1986; 65:217.
47. Flezzani P, Croughwell N, Mcintyre RW, Reves JG. Isoflurane decreases the cortisol response to cardiopulmonary bypass. Anesth Analg 1986; 65:1117.
48. White BC, Winegar CD, Wilson RF et al. Possible role of calcium blockers in cerebral resuscitation: A review of the literature and synthesis for future studies. Crit Care Med 1983; 11:202.
49. Arom KV, Cohen DE, Strobl FT. Effect of intraoperative intervention on neurological outcome based on electroencephalographic monitoring during cardiopulmonary bypass. Ann Thorac Surg 1989; 48:476.
50. Bashein G, Blesdoe SW, Townes BD, Coppel DB: Tools for assessing central nervous injury in the cardiac surgery patient. In: Hilberman M (ed) Brain Injury and Protection During Heart Surgery. Boston: Martinus Nijhoff, 1988; p. 109.
51. Nussmeier NA, Fish KJ. Neuropsychological dysfunction after cardiopulmonary bypass: A comparison of two institutions. J Cardioth & Vasc Anesth 1991; 5:584.

6. The causes of postoperative cerebral damage

PETER L. C. SMITH and STANTON P. NEWMAN

The consequences of cerebral damage which occurs as a result of surgery may be considered as presenting at three major levels of clinical disability. The first, which follows overwhelming cerebral insult, leads to the patient's death or severe coma. The second level concerns focal neurological deficit or 'stroke'. This usually manifests either in hemiplegia or a retinal field defect but may selectively influence other higher cortical functions. The deficits are clearly evident on clinical neurological examination and will also be demonstrable on neuropsychological assessment. The third is a more subtle level of disability where the patient shows neuropsychological deterioration in the absence of clear neurological changes. Concomitant emotional changes are frequently reported postoperatively in major surgery patients. The aetiology of these emotional changes are difficult to discern and although they may on occasion be associated with a cerebral injury this is not necessarily the case [1]. In the case of cardiac surgery the mood changes observed in patients appear not be associated with cerebral injury [2].

All forms of surgery may be associated with cerebral morbidity but certain types, particularly cardiac surgery with cardiopulmonary bypass and neurosurgery are particularly liable to major cerebral complications. We do not propose, in this chapter, to discuss the specialized problem of cerebral complications following neurosurgery but intend to confine our observations to the cerebral morbidity associated with major general surgery and cardiac surgery with cardiopulmonary bypass. In the process of describing the impact of surgery on cerebral functioning we will discuss a study we have performed.

Subjects and methods in study

We carried out a prospective study of 79 coronary artery bypass surgery (CABS) patients and 30 comparison major vascular and thoracic non-cardiopulmonary bypass patients to determine the incidence of post-operative cerebral complications and the major factors associated with this cerebral morbidity. In the non-cardiac surgery group 25 patients had major vascular surgery 3, patients had a lung resection and 2 patients had closed cardiac surgery. Surgery in the cardiac group was rigidly standardised both in terms of technique and anaesthesia. Similarly in the comparative group, though technique was more heterogeneous by the group's nature, anaesthesia was standardised. All patients underwent preoperatively, at 8 days, 8 weeks and one year postoperatively detailed neurological, neuropsychological and psychiatric examinations. An additional neurological examination was carried out at 24 hours postoperatively. The neuropsychological test battery consisted of ten tests, some computer administered, especially chosen to be sensitive to diffuse cortical damage and resistant to practice effect. The neuropsychological tests used were as follows:

1) Two computer administered, non-verbal recognition tests (Figure 1).
2) Computer administered, two-choice reaction time test.
3) Computer administered symbol digit replacement test (Figure 2).
4) Trail Making Tests A & B.
5) Purdue Pegboard test for each and both hands.
6) Block design subtest from the Weschler Adult Intelligence Scale (WAIS).
7) Letter cancellation task.
8) The Rey Auditory Verbal Learning Test (verbal memory).

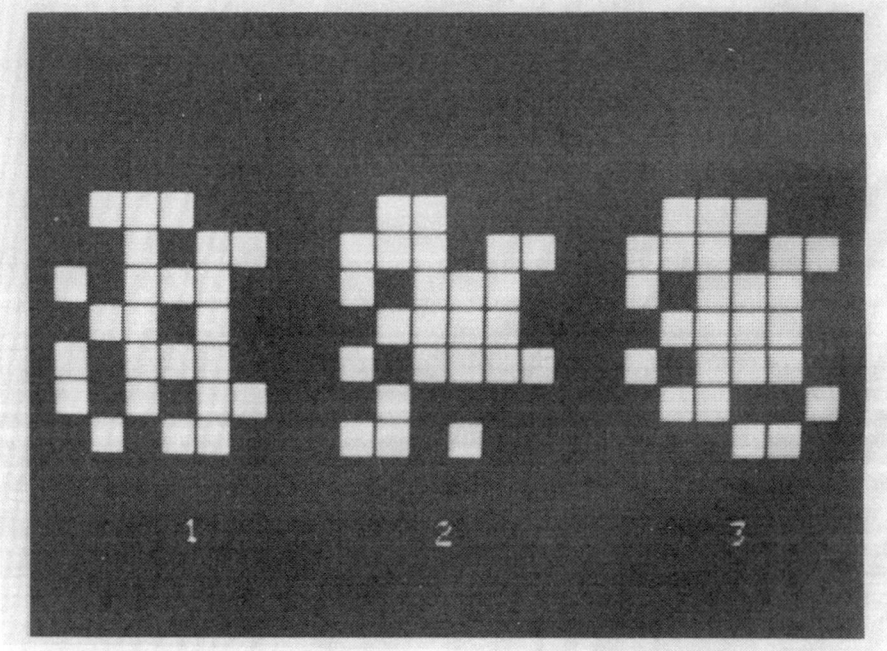

Fig. 1. A photograph showing the type of patterns used in the non-verbal memory test on the Apple microcomputer.

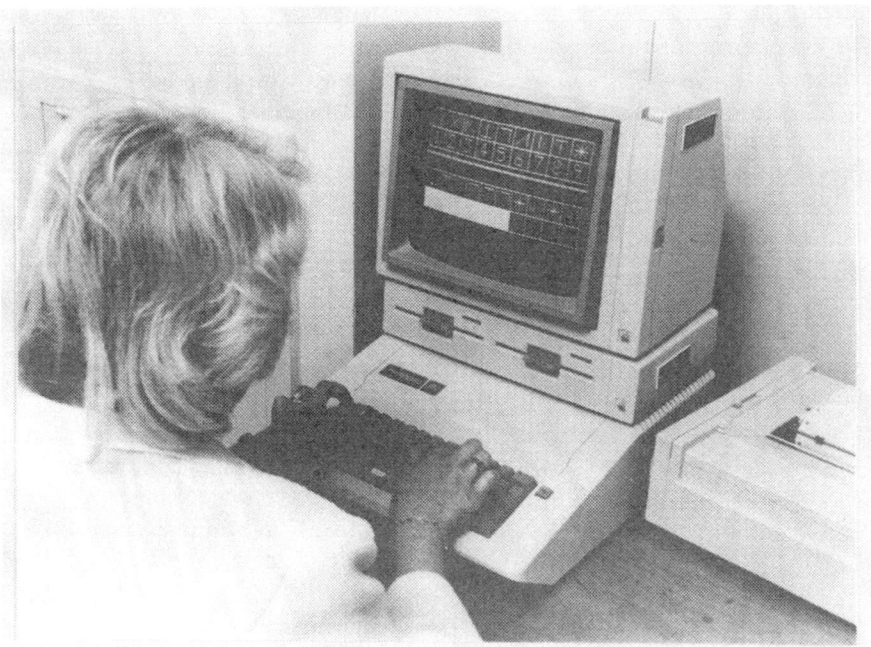

Fig. 2. The symbol digit replacement test being carried out by a patient in the study using an Apple microcomputer.

Neuropsychological performance was considered in relation to the standard deviation of all preoperative scores on each test. An individual was considered to have produced a 'significantly deteriorated performance' in a test if they exhibited a drop from their pre-operative performance of greater than the standard deviation observed in all preoperative performances. A 'significant neuropsychological deficit' was considered to have occured if an individual produced a 'significantly deteriorated performance' in two or more tests.

All drugs given with dosage during the operative stay in hospital were recorded. In addition, physiological observation during operation and immediately postoperatively was extensive including recording of mean arterial pressure, blood gases and temperature.

The extent of cerebral morbidity found following surgery

Overwhelming cerebral insult leading to death is rare following general surgery and unusual following cardiac surgery with cardiopulmonary bypass. On the occasions it has been reported in general surgical patients, it has often been associated with unexpected preoperative predisposition such as cerebrovascular disease. Other factors associated with massive cerebral insult may be severe haemorrhage, myocardial infarction or hypoxia. In cardiac surgery patients its occurrence is probably more common than in general surgical

72

patients. This is because of the particular problems of cardiopulmonary bypass and the opening of the chambers of the heart leading to, on very rare occasions, massive embolism of air or interruption of the circulation. Through improvement of techniques, there has been a steady reduction in mortality rates following cardiopulmonary bypass. In our study of 79 patients no instance of overwhelming cerebral insult occurred.

A number of studies have examined the incidence of stroke in CABS. Many of these are retrospective studies and, as such, appear to understimate the true incidence of stroke. Two recent prospective studies have been performed. Breuer in his prospective study of 421 such patients showed an incidence of stroke of 5% [3] and Shaw studying 320 coronary artery bypass surgery patients showed an incidence of stroke of 4.8% [4]. In our study six patients presented with focal neurological signs when they were assessed at 24 hours after coronary artery bypass surgery (7%). By 8 weeks only one patient still exhibited focal neurological deficit (2%). This finding emphasises the importance of the time chosen postoperatively to assess focal neurological change. An additional important finding in our study was that none of the general surgical patients exhibited focal neurological signs 24 hours after surgery.

Given the relative infrequency of major cerebral insults, there have been an increasing number of studies directed towards a more subtle analysis of the possible cerebral consequences of CABS. Neuropsychological assessment provides a sensitive tool for considering these subtle changes. In our study we found a relatively large frequency of neuropsychological deficits following CABS. Significant neuropsychological deficit was found in 73% of coronary artery surgery patients 8 days after surgery, 37% 8 weeks after surgery and 35% one year after surgery [5–7] (Figure 3). A relatively similar incidence has been reported by Shaw in her studies of 312 coronary artery surgery patients. Shaw found neuropsychological deficit in 79% of 259 patients at 7 days and 57% at six months following surgery [8, 9].

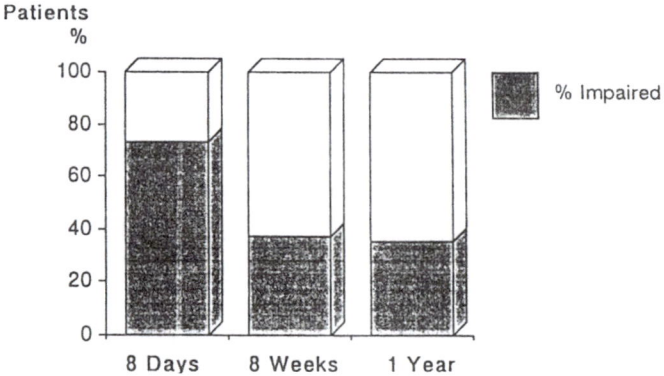

Fig. 3. Significant neuropsychological deficit 8 days, 8 weeks and 1 year after surgery expressed as a percentage (n=67), in the coronary artery bypass surgery group.

We were surprised to find that our small comparison group also showed significant neuropsychological deficit 8 days, 8 weeks and 1 year after surgery (Figure 4).

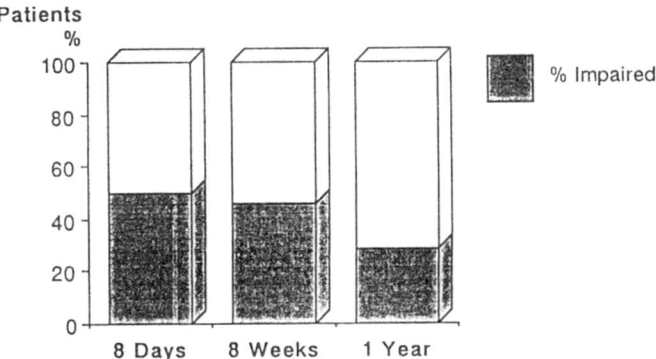

Fig. 4. Significant neuropsychological deficit 8 days, 8 weeks and 1 year after surgery expressed as a percentage (n=24), in the non-cardiopulmonary bypass comparative group.

This finding contrasts with Åberg who found that none of 46 general surgical patients tested with a detailed neuropsychological test battery had a significant neuropsychological deficit following surgery [10], confirming the results previously reported by Gruvstadt [11]. In Åberg's study, however, the general surgical cases studied involved relatively simple surgery, while in our study the patients received more complicated procedures. Other studies which have used relatively detailed neuropsychological procedures have also found a proportion of surgical patients suffering from postoperative neuropsychological deficits. Shaw has recently reported the findings from a group of 50 major vascular surgery patients who underwent an extensive neuropsychological test battery preoperatively and at approximatly one week postoperatively. She found that 15 of 48 patients (31%) had deteriorated in one or more test scores at the postoperative examination compared with the preoperative scores. No patient however showed severe deficit defined as being a significant deficit in 3 or more tests [12]. Rollason investigated 27 patients undergoing retropubic prostatectomy with spinal anaesthesia, with a neuropsychological test battery preoperatively and at 5 days and 6 weeks postoperatively. Reduced intellectual performance was shown to be present at 5 days postoperatively but at 6 weeks postoperatively performance was, in fact, increased probably due to practice effect [13].

Further examination of our small comparison group suggests not only that they were in poorer health than other general surgical groups studied, but also perhaps marginally older, with unusual numbers staying in the Intensive Care Unit or being metabolically disturbed following surgery. The conclusion that we have tentatively drawn from the findings on this small group is that significant neuropsychological deficit does occur following major general surgical procedures but we consider that the pattern of deficits and recovery may indicate that the aetiology of the changes differs from that observed in CABS' patients [7].

The causes of postoperative cerebral damage after major surgery

We showed a degree of neuropsychological impairment in patients following major general surgery. Though we could not show any specific aetiological factors to be important, speculation would suggest that several might be involved.

Peroperative stroke may potentially occur in any form of major surgery particularly if the patient is older with preoperative hypertension and carotid artery disease. The stroke may be due to cerebral embolus of haemorrhage. Less severe changes following general surgery have been demonstrated by Bedford [14] who showed that general surgery in the elderly often leads to noticeable diminution in mental faculties following the procedure. Many subsequent studies have confirmed this [15]. It has been speculated that the increasing atherosclerotic disease found in the cerebral circulation of the elderly might be aetiologically implicated.

Several factors may lead to critical cerebral hypoperfusion peroperatively leading to a postoperative cerebral deficit. Sudden profound hypotension can result from torrential uncontrolled haemorrhage or from sudden left ventricular failure notably due to peroperative myocardial infarction. Peroperative dysrhythmias of the heart can lead to hypotension if uncontrolled, and cardiac arrest, that is not promptly reversed, may lead to a grossly brain damaged patient on eventual resuscitation.

Though Sorenson [16] concluded that a properly administered anaesthetic did not cause subsequent changes in brain function measured by neuropsychological testing, many anaesthetic agents have, more recently, been shown to lead to a deficit in intellectual performance postoperatively eg. Halothane and nitrous oxide at a few hours postoperatively [17] or cyclopropane at 6 days following surgery [18]. Drummond [19] felt that not only may the change in intellectual performance be due to the anaesthetic agent but also that the anaesthetic agent may produce changes in brain physiology. Jouvet [20] considered that changes in the level of neurohumoral and transmitter substances was produced by anaesthetic agents for a period of time following their administration.

Other factors implicated as being of aetiological importance in the genesis of postoperative intellectual deficit are reductions of cerebral blood flow during surgery either due to inadvertent or purposely induced hypotension; hypocarbia and hypoxia. Evidence both for and against these assertions exist. Gruvstadt [11] and Echenhof [21] felt that hypotension was not a significant factor but Harp [22] has suggested that it is very significant if combined with a degree of hypoxia. Wollman [23] showed that a PCO_2 of less than 24 mms of Hg inspired for a period of time was followed by a significant increase in reaction time but Blenkarn [24] found no difference between hypocarbic and normo-carbic anaesthetic techniques.

Metabolic disturbance, usually renal or hepatic in origin, is also occasionally encountered following major surgery leading to possible encephalopathic states.

Sleep deprivation and abnormal sensory stimulation, as experienced by the surgical patient in the intensive care unit or the recovery room, has been shown to lead to subsequent poor performance in neuropsychological testing. As has the anxiety and emotional response that is an inevitable concomitant for the patient undergoing surgery [25, 26]. The manifestation or presentation of cerebral damage incurred at surgery may be profoundly effected by the psychological response of the patient to his illness and its management.

Sometimes microemboli occur in the bloodstream during general surgical procedures. Cerebral atheromatous emboli have been found in the post-mortem brains of patients who have had a major vascular surgical operation without cardiopulmonary bypass or indeed without intracardiac mixing of the circulations through an abnormal connection and it is well known that unfiltered blood transfusion can lead to mircoemboli in the circulation of the patient.

A review of the literature appertaining to intellectual performance following general surgical procedures leads to three particular conclusions. The first being that the timing of the postoperative neuropsychological examination is of great importance in determining the amount of intellectual deficit found. In particular early assessments may indicate a transient disturbance which does not reflect any permanent damage to the brain. The second is that much argument exists as to whether a particular intellectual deficit is of significance to the patients everyday functioning. This is likely to be dependent upon the relative demands that the individual experiences in their lives and the extent to which they may make adjustments to their activities following major surgery. The third conclusion is the increasing evidence of the importance of age in the aetiology of postoperative intellectual deficit following general surgery.

The causes of postoperative cerebral damage after cardiac surgery with cardiopulmonary bypass

Stroke, presenting in the early postoperative period following cardiac surgery is likely to be due to a major cerebral embolic event. Large particles may be introduced into the circulation during aortic cannulation from dislodged atheromatous plaques or from dislodged clots from the mural surface of the left ventricle [27]. Massive air embolism could occur through the aortic cannulation site, cardioplegia needle site, or if the left ventricle was vented, through the left ventricle vent site [28]. In addition, malfunction within the cardiopulmonary bypass circuit has also been implicated in massive air embolus, particularly if the cardiotomy reservoir blood level is allowed to become dangerously low.

The causes of neuropsychological deficit following cardiac surgery with cardiopulmonary bypass are probably similar to those observed in stroke but lesser in magnitude and extent. It is probable for a proportion of patients, that during the period on cardiopulmonary bypass, a degree of diffuse cortical damage takes place which can later manifest itself in measurable neuropsychological impairment. The diffuse cortical damage is probably an expression of cerebral microemboli generated during the bypass and/or by relative cerebral hypoperfusion occuring at the same time. Pathological findings offer us some evidence regarding the mechanism producing the deficit. Aguilar in 1971 reported the pathological findings of the brains of 206 patients who had died following cardiac surgery at the Pacific Medical Center in San Francisco. Eighty five percent of the patients showed either fibrin-platelet, crystalline or fat emboli, acute petechial, perivascular or focal subarachnoid haemorrhages or acute ischaemic neuronal damage [29].

The microemboli are largely generated in the cardiopulmonary bypass circuit [30], and may consist of air, platelet aggregates, fibrin or silicone [31–34]. Many authorities have stressed the importance of fat as a cerebral micro-embolus [35, 36]. However fibrin platelet aggregates are of equal or greater importance [37]. Microemboli have been measured with a transcranial doppler [38] and directly visualised from the retina during cardiopulmonary bypass by the use of retinal fluorescein angiography [39–41] (Figures 5 and 6).

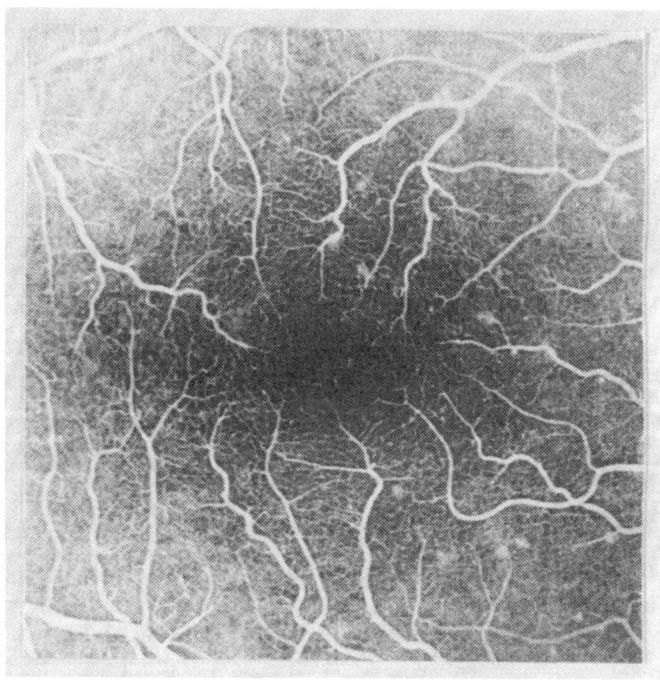

Fig. 5. A normal retinal fluorescein angiogram in an operative coronary artery bypass surgery patient.

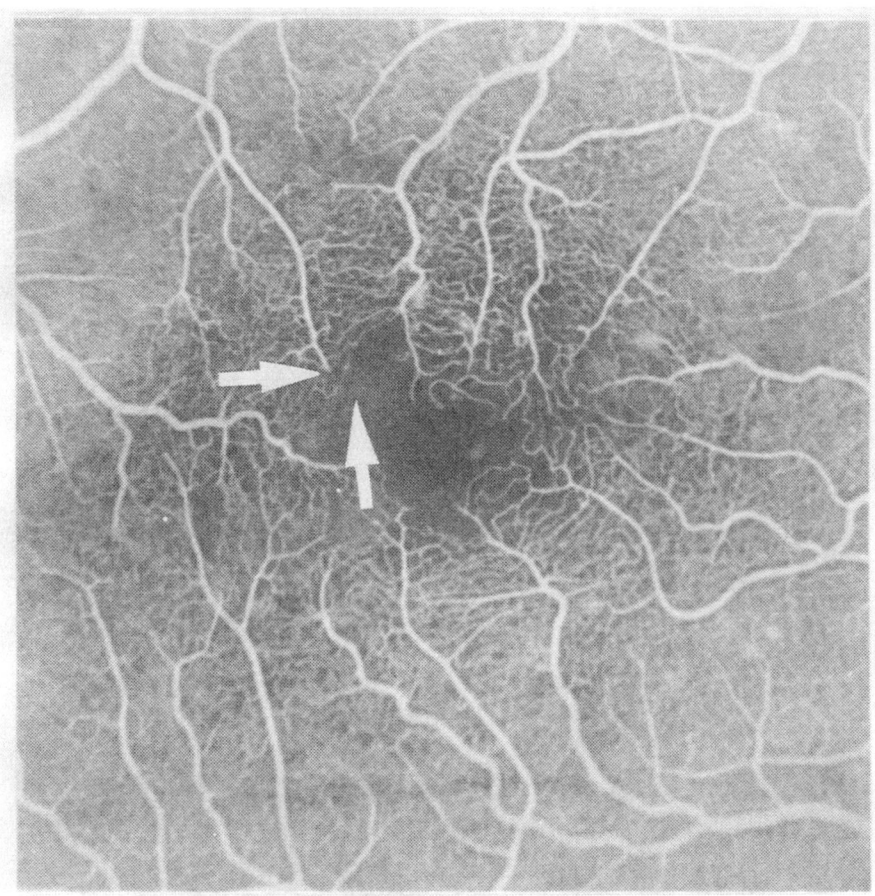

Fig. 6. An abnormal retinal fluorescein angiogram taken five minutes before the end of car-diopulmonary bypass. The arrows indicate a truncated arteriole thought to be indicative of microembolisation and an adjacent area of retinal non-perfusion.

The mechanism whereby fibrin-platelet aggregates cause cerebral damage is probably both direct and indirect. Patterson showed the presence of microvas-cular blockade with microparticles following cardiopulmonary bypass in dogs. This was transient in nature and he speculated that this form of damage might be the reason for the transient encephalopathy seen in patients after cardiac surgery with cardiopulmonary bypass [42]. Taylor, however, feels that the mechanism producing cerebral damage is not just simple obstruction to flow but may be alteration in the clotting-lysis cascade with platelet activation at the site of the blockade and release of damaging vasoactive substances and free radicals [43]. The dynamic balance between thromboxane and prostacy-clin present in the normal circulation has been shown to orientate towards thromboxane during cardiopulmonary bypass [44]. Cerebral microembolic insult undoubtedly occurs during cardiopulmonary bypass and many authorities would now consider it the major aetiological factor causing cerebral damage during cardiac surgery [45].

An alternative or additional aetiological factor is poor cerebral perfusion associated with low cerebral blood flow occuring during cardiopulmonary bypass. However, several workers have shown that permanent cerebral damage is unlikely at normothermia unless cerebral blood flow is less than 10 ml/100 g/min [46]. It is very rare for this to happen during routine cardiopulmonary bypass. Theoretically if low perfusion had caused cerebral damage then it should appear maximally in the so called "water shed" areas of the brain. These are boundary zones between areas of distribution of different cerebral arteries [47]. There is little convincing evidence that this occurs.

It is likely that PCO_2 management during cardiopulmonary bypass is of importance in the degree of cerebral injury which takes place [48]. Nevin has shown a relationship between PCO_2 management and the extent of early postoperative neuropsychological deficit found in a study of 65 patients who had undergone coronary artery bypass graft surgery [49]. PCO_2 management may be either pH-stat, using temperature corrected data, with the addition of PCO_2 to the oxygenator to maintain a $PaCO_2$ of near 40 mm Hg with a pH of approximately 7.4, or alpha-stat, using temperature uncorrected data, with the result that $PaCO_2$ falls, reducing cerebral blood flow. It can be argued, that alpha-stat PCO_2 management is more physiological, matching cerebral blood flow to demand which is desireable when trying to minimize microembolic mediated cerebral damage.

A scrutiny of recent papers considering predictors of neuropsychological deficit following cardiac surgery presents evidence that increasing age of the patient at operation and increasing bypass time are the two major predictors of an increased neuropsychological deficit following surgery [50–52].

Smith has also shown that low mean arterial pressure on cardiopulmonary bypass maybe implicated in the genesis of postoperative neuropsychological deficit [6].

There is a risk of peroperative cerebral damage with all major surgery but especially with cardiac surgery utilising cardiopulmonary bypass. The risk of subtle diffuse neuropsychological deficit after the latter is probably substantial. Because of this many cardiac surgery units are endeavoring to minimize this risk using 40 micron main arterial line filters, membrane oxygenators, minimal suction of shed blood, alpha-stat PCO_2 management and possibly in the future covering the operations with the new groups of cerebroprotective drugs that are being developed.

Acknowledgements

The authhours would like to acknowledge the support of the Medical Research Council, the British Heart Foundation and the Jules Thorn Trust.

References

1. Newman S. Anxiety, Surgery & Hospitalisation. In: Fitzpatrick R, Hinton J, Newman S, Scambler G, Thompson J (eds). The Experience of Illness. Tavistock Press, Ch. 7, 1984; p. 133.
2. Newman S, Klinger L, Venn G, Smith P, Harrison M, Treasure T. Subjective reports of cognition in relation to assessed cognitive performance following coronary artery bypass surgery. J Psychosomatic Res 1988; 33:227.
3. Breuer A C, Furlan A J, Hanson M R, Lederman R J, Loop F D, Cosgrove D M, Estafanous G. Central nervous system complications of coronary artery bypass graft surgery. Stroke 1983; 14:682.
4. Shaw PJ, Bates D, Cartildge N E F, Heaviside D, Julian D G, Shaw D A. Early neurological complications of coronary artery bypass surgery. Br Med J 1985; 291:1384.
5. Smith P L C. Treasure T, Newman S P, Joseph P, Ell P J, Schneidau A, Harrison M J G. Cerebral consequences of cardiopulmonary bypass. Lancet 1986; ii:823.
6. Smith P L C. The cerebral complications of coronary artery bypass surgery. Ann Roy Coll Surg of Engl 1988; 70:212.
7. Newman S, Smith P, Treasure T, Joseph P, Ell P, Harrison M. Acute neuropsychological and regional cerebral blood flow consequences of coronary artery bypass surgery. Contempor Psychol Res Rev 1987; 6:115.
8. Shaw PJ, Bates D, Cartlidge N E F, French J M, Heaviside D, Julian D G, Shaw D A. Early intellectual dysfunction following coronary bypass surgery. Quart J Med 1986; 58:59.
9. Shaw PJ, Bates D, Cartlidge N E F, French J M, Heaviside D, Julian D G, Shaw D A. Long term intellectual dysfunction following coronary artery bypass surgery: a six-month follow-up study. Quart J Med 1987; 62:259.
10. Åberg T. Effect of open heart surgery on intellectual function. Scand J Thorac Cardiovasc Surg 1984; 15 (Suppl):1.
11. Gruvstad M, Kebbon L, Lof B A. Changes in mental function after induced hypotension. Acta Psychiatr Scand 1962; 37 (Suppl):163.
12. Shaw PJ, Bates D, Cartlidge N E F, Heaviside D, French J M, Julian D G, Shaw D A. Neurologic and neuropsychological morbidity following major surgery: comparison of coronary artery bypass and peripheral vascular surgery. Stroke 1987; 18:700.
13. Rollason W N, Robertson G S, Cordiner C M, Hall D J. A comparison of mental function in relation to hypotensive and normotensive anaesthesia in the elderly. Br J Anaesth 1971; 43:561.
14. Bedford P O, Leeds M D. Adverse effects of anaesthesia on old people. Lancet 1985; i:259.
15. Simpson B R, Williams M, Scott J F, Smith A C. The effects of anaesthesia and elective surgery on old people. Lancet 1961; ii:887.
16. Sorenson H R, Lindeberg, J. Cerebral injury and cerebral function following anaesthesia. Acta Chir Scand 1950; 99:40.
17. Bruce D L, Arbit J. Trace anaesthetic effects on perceptual, cognitive and motor skills. Anesthesiology 1974; 40:453.
18. James F M. The effects of cyclopropane anaesthesia without surgical operation on mental functions of normal man. Anesthesiology 1969; 30:264.
19. Drummond C B. The assessment of post operative mental function. Br J Anaesth 1975; 47:130.
20. Jouvet M. Biogenic amines and the states of sleep. Science 1969; 163:32.
21. Eckenhoff J E, Compton J R, Larson A, Davies P M. Assessment of cerebral effects of deliberate hypotension by psychological measurement. Lancet 1964; ii:711.
22. Harp J R, Wollman H. Cerebral metabolic effects of hyperventilation and deliberate hypotension. Br J Anaesth 1973; 45:256.
23. Wollman S B, Orkin L R. Post operative human reaction time and hypocarbia during anaesthesia. Br J Anaesth 1968; 40:920.

24. Blenkarn GD, Briggs G, Bell J, Sugioka K. Cognitive function after hypocapnic hyperventilation. Anesthesiology 1972; 37:381.
25. Sveinsson IS. Post operative psychosis after open heart surgery. J Thorac Cardiovasc Surg 1975; 70:717.
26. Orr WC, Stahl ML. Sleep disturbance after open heart surgery. Am J Cardiol 1977; 39:196.
27. Breuer AC, Franco I, Marzewski D, Soto-Velasco J. Left ventricular thrombi seen by ventriculography are a significant risk factor for stroke in open-heart surgery. Ann Neurol 1981; 10:103.
28. Utley JR, Stephens DB. Prevention of major perioperative neurological dysfunction: a personal perspective. Perfusion 1986; 1:135.
29. Aguilar MG, Gerbode F, Hill JD. Neuropathologic complications of cardiac surgery. J Thorac Cardiovasc Surg 1971; 61(5):676.
30. Kessler J, Patterson RH. The production of microemboli by various blood oxygenators. Ann Thorac Surg 1970; 9:221.
31. Lindeberg DAB, Lucas FV, Sheagren J, Malm JR. Silicone embolisation during clinical and experimental heart surgery employing a bubble oxygenator. Am J Pathol 1961;39: 129.
32. Pearson DT, Carter RF, Hammo MB, Waterhouse PS, Gaseous microemboli during open heart surgery. In: Longmore DB (ed). *Towards Safer Cardiac Surgery*. Lancaster: MTP Press, 1981; p. 327.
33. Orenstein JM, Noriko S, Aaron B, Buchholz B, Bloom S. Microemboli observed in deaths following cardiopulmonary bypass surgery: silicone antifoam agents and polyvinyl chloride tubing as sources of emboli. Hum Pathol 1982; 13:1082.
34. Solis RT, Kennedy PS, Beall AC Jr, Debakey ME. Cardiopulmonary bypass. Microembolization and platelet aggregation. Circulation 1975; 52:103.
35. Miller JA, Fonkalsrud EW, Latta HL, Maroney JV. Fat embolism associated with extracorporeal circulation and blood transfusion. Surgery 1962; 51:448.
36. Caguin F, Carter MG. Fat embolism with cardiotomy with the use of cardiopulmonary bypass. J Thorac Cardiovasc Surg 1963; 46:665.
37. Dutton RC, Edmunds LH Jr, Hutchinson JC, Roe BB. Platelet aggregate emboli produced in patients during cardiopulmonary bypass with membrane and bubble filters. J Thorac Cardiovasc Surg 1874; 67:258.
38. Deverall PB, Padayachee TS, Parsons S, Theobald R, Battistessa SA. Ultrasound detection of microemboli in the middle cerebral artery during cardiopulmonary bypass surgery. Eur J Cardiothorac Surg 1988; 2:256.
39. Williams IM. Intravascular changes in the retina during open heart surgery. Lancet 1971; ii:688.
40. Blauth C, Arnold J, Kohner EM, Taylor KM. Retinal microembolism during cardiopulmonary bypass demonstrated by fluorescein angiography. Lancet 1986; ii:837.
41. Blauth C, Arnold J, Schulenberg WE, McCartney A. Taylor KM. Cerebral microembolism during cardiopulmonary bypass. Retinal microvascular studies in vivo with fluorescein angiography. J Thorac Cardiovasc Surg 1988; 95:668.
42. Patterson RH, Rosenfeld L, Porro RS. Transitory cerebral microvascular blockade after cardiopulmonary bypass. Thorax 1976; 31:736.
43. Taylor KM. Pathophysiology of brain damage during open heart surgery. Texas Heart Instit J 1986; 13:91.
44. Watkins WD, Peterson MD, Kong DL, Kono K, Buckley MJ, Levine FH, Philbin DM. Thromboxane and prostacyclin changes during cardiopulmonary bypass with and without pulsatile flow. J Thorac Cardiovasc Surg 1982; 84:250.
45. Taylor KM. (Editorial) Brain damage after open heart surgery. Lancet 1986; ii:1161.
46. Astrup J, Symon L, Branston MN, Lassen NA. Cortisol evoked potential and intracellular K+ and H+ at critical levels of brain ischaemia. Stroke 1977; 8:51.
47. Ross-Russel RW, Bharucha N. The recognition and prevention of border zone cerebral ischaemia during cardiac surgery. Quart J Med 1978; 187:303.

48. Swan H. The importance of acid-base management for cardiac and cerebral preservation during open heart operations. Surg Gynecol Obstet 1904; 158:391.

49. Nevin M, Adams S, Colchester ACF, Pepper JR. Evidence for involvement of hypocapnia and hypotension in aetiology of neurological deficit after cardiopulmonary bypass. Lancet 1988; ii:1943.

50. Savageau JA, Stanton BA, Jenkins CD, Klein MD. Neuropsychological dysfunction following elective cardiac operation. I. Early assessment. J Thorac Cardiovasc Surg 1982; 84:585.

51. Savageau JA, Stanton BA, Jenkins CD, Frater RWM. Neuropsychological dysfunction following elective cardiac operation. II. A six-month reassessment. J Thorac Cardiovasc Surg 1982; 84:595.

52. Newman SP. The incidence and nature of neuropsychological morbidity following cardiac surgery. Perfusion 1989 (In press).

7. Central nervous risk factors in cardiac surgery*

†G. RODEWALD, B. DAHME, TH. EMSKÖTTER, P. GÖTZE,
L. LACHENMEYER, U. LAMPARTER, P. KALMAR,
H-J. KREBBER, H-J. MEFFERT and H. POKAR

Summary

Serious complications involving the central nervous system in the course of
cardiac surgical procedures have become rare. Nevertheless, CNS dysfunctions
are still observed in a considerable number of patients, exceeding by far the
number of those at risk from preoperative neurological hazards. The influence of extracorporeal circulation performed and of hypothermia on the
physiology of cerebral autoregulation, as well as micro-embolization occurrences seem to be crucial factors in this context. The resulting regional or global
posthypoxic changes in brain metabolism may lead to the manifestation of
various neurological and psychiatric disorders in the postoperative course.
These often minor disturbances of CNS function can only be detected
regularly and diagnosed correctly in a prospective way by consulting specialists
in neurology, psychiatry and psychology, as has been the practice at the
Department of Thoracic and Cardiovascular Surgery in the University Hospital
in Hamburg since 1974, and currently in an international multi-centre study.
We found postoperative neurological abnormalities in more than 50% of our
patients. While irreversible brain damage occurred in only 0.5% of cases, about
two-thirds exhibited transient symptoms that were no longer apparent after
eight to ten days postoperatively. Obvious psychopathological symptoms were
noted in 10% of cases after surgery and minor, likewise transient, psychiatric disturbances were seen in up to 50% of patients; 20% suffered from
long-lasting psychic problems. Subjective complaints in these cases exceeded
the numbers derived from objective assessments to a remarkable extent.
The discussion focuses on a critical assessment of clinical and supple-
mentary examination techniques and on the potential pathophysiological
mechanisms induced by extracorporeal circulation.
In conclusion, the disorders of CNS function still encountered today in open-

†Deceased.
*Based on a lecture delivered at the 56th Annual Congress of the German Society for Cardiac
and Circulatory Research in Mannheim, Germany, on 20–22 April, 1990.

heart surgery do not on the whole challenge the success of cardiac-ECC operations and the requirement for these, but clearly emphasize the need for an improvement in patient information and concomitant treatment.

Introduction

For a start, some preliminary remarks:

1. Along with Lehmann and his colleagues, back in 1962 we were already addressing the problems which risk factors in the CNS presented for cardiac surgery [1]. In constant cooperation with colleagues from the neurology, psychiatry and psychology departments, appropriate research has been conducted in Hamburg since the Seventies [2, 3]. That applied especially during the years 1974–1980 for a research project supported by the German government and conducted under the supervision of H. Speidel [4], and still does to a study being carried out internationally at nine centres in North and South America, as well as Europe [5]. In Germany, units at Bad Krozingen, Hamburg and Kiel are participating.
2. By definition the CNS consists of the brain and the spinal chord. The comments below relate only to the brain in adult patients.
3. The problem is that while CNS risk factors exist for cardiac patients, far more disturbances to the CNS are evident in connection with open heart surgery that bear no relation to risk factors discerned preoperatively. Extracorporeal circulation is largely responsible.

Following the downturn in hospital mortality and morbidity, such disturbances are attracting more attention in cardiac surgery, although it must also be said that the frequency of severe dysfunctions of the CNS have also declined.

We intend to discuss some physiological parameters and the changes in these caused by extracorporeal circulation, and then the pathogenetic factors, research procedures, and the frequency and severity of neurological and psychological-psychiatric dysfunctions.

Physiological parameters

The brain amounts to 2% of the body weight, and under resting conditions it requires 13% of cardiac output and 20% of total oxygen consumption. Perfusion and oxygen uptake differ greatly between the regions. Areas of higher oxygen consumption show a greater density of mitochondria and are particularly sensitive to hypoxia.

Blood supply occurs via four main arteries. The cerebral arterioles are terminal branches. In other words, in the event of an occlusion, sufficient collateral circulation cannot be maintained by precapillary inter-arteriolar anastomoses. The arteriolar tonus is mainly conditioned by biochemical factors of blood and tissues, while vasomotor nervous regulation plays only a minor role.

Extracorporeal circulation

As the simplified example of perfusion in hypothermia of 27°C in a patient weighing 70 kg with a body surface area of 1.8 m² demonstrates, extracorporeal circulation makes for a substantial intervention in normal conditions (see Table 1):

Table 1. Alterations in some physiological parameters during extracorporeal circulation (ECC) – Body-weight: 70 kg, BSA: 1.8 m²

		Normal	ECC
t°C		37	37
Blood pressure	(mm Hg)	120/80	≥ 50
cardiac output	(l/min)	5.0	3.24
Vb brain	(ml/min)	750	?
V_{02} brain	(ml/min)	48	?
Hematocrit	(%)	40	20–30
PO_2a	(mm Hg)	90	> 90
PCO_2a	(mm Hg)	40	25–55
ph	(mm Hg)	7.42	7.2–7.55

During extracorporeal circulation, the median blood pressure is lower than normal, as a rule the flow is not pulsatile, and total output is lower. Depending on hypothermia, blood circulation can be increased, normalized or reduced, whilst oxygen consumption can be reduced in accordance with the degree of hypothermia, or also be reduced more steeply. Hematocrit is lowered by hemodilution. Arterial oxygen pressure is generally higher than normal. A special problem, to be covered below, is the question of adequate values for pCO and pH under hypothermic conditions.

In the past, perfusion was done at normal temperatures and with total blood. The changes shown here have become essential for extracorporeal circulation:

With hemodilution and auto-transfusion, the homologous blood syndrome is avoided and blood viscosity is influenced, among other considerations. Hypothermia reduces the oxygen needed and thus extends the revival period; compensates for the reduced 0_2 capacity caused by blood thinning, and renders diminished perfusion through the heart-lung machine possible.

With a Q_{10} of 2.8 [6], the survival time of the brain is increased from 22 to 28 minutes at 27°C. Except in the case of operations affecting planned interruption of the circulation, and of rare incidents, tolerance for total ischemia is barely required at all in cardiac surgery. Postoperative findings in the central nervous system are the consequence of local occurrences induced by the vascular bed. The mediator in these is regional hypoxia.

In these circumstances, glycolysis and lactateacidosis occur, leading to functional disturbances which can extend as far as paralysis. Should the period necessary for maintenance or revival of the structure be exceeded, then irreversible damage ensues. Also contributing to tissue damage is the occurrence of cytotoxic edema involving swelling of the astrocytes, which can in turn cause malfunction of the circulation. The sensitivity of the brain to lack of oxygen is at its greatest in the neocortex, then in the basal ganglia, the hippocampus and cerebellum, in that order.

Pathogenetic factors

Table 2 illustrates the reasons for hypoxia and ischemia. The *heart-lung machine system* can of itself cause micro-embolism: Gas emboli and particle emboli from accumulations of blood or particles, in the form of fat or discarded fragments of plastic [7–20] and complement activation have been described [21, 22]. An important role is played by autoregulation of vascularization of the brain during hypothermia and perfusion, and this depends primarily on the pCO_2 and pH content. In blood gas analysis, a distinction is made between what is known as the pH-stat procedure and the alpha-stat procedure. During hypothermia, the first causes acidosis, in that the pCO_2 is kept constant, whilst the CO_2 content (cCO_2) is progressively increased, whilst in the alpha-stat procedure the cCO_2 is kept constant by reducing the pCO_2. The pH content of the blood thus increases in parallel to the shift in water's assay point at 27°C, e.g., from 7.40 to 7.55 [23, 24].

Table 2. Possible causes of CNS dysfunctions

ECC	Micro-emboli	
		Gas bubbles
		Particles
		Complement
		activation
	Autoregulation	
Operation	Emboli	Atheroma
		Thromboses
		Calcification
		"Surgical air"
Patient	Arterio-sclerosis	
	Hypertension	
	Prior CNS dysfunctions	
	Age	

Autoregulation renders the brain's blood supply independent of pressure in a range from 50 to 130 mm Hg. The pH-stat procedure, i.e., local acidosis, leads to a de-coupling of cerebral blood supply and metabolism in the sense of a hyper-perfusion and a far-reaching loss of autoregulation. By contrast, the alpha-stat procedure maintains autoregulation as far down as a median arterial pressure of approx. 50 mm Hg.

There is sufficient evidence to show that disruption of autoregulation (caused by abnormal pCO_2, pH and possibly also pO_2 ratings) can cause dysfunction of the brain [10, 23, 25, 26].

Embolisms as a result of surgery and due to various causes are also possible. A specially dreaded part here is played by what is known as "surgical air" following closure of a heart after an open-heart procedure.

The patient may also harbour such risk factors as the repercussions of arteriosclerosis, previous CNS impairments, hypertension, cardiac insufficiency, age, etc.

Investigative procedures

As reported in the literature, the frequency of neurological dysfunction varies from 3 to 60%. This is not primarily due to varying perfusion techniques, but is primarily a matter of the type and timing of investigations. Retrospective surveys indicate fewer losses than prospective investigations by specialists.

For our own patients, our findings were as follows:

Of 1,873 patients operated on between 1987 and 1989, 3.4% showed neurological dysfunction whilst in the intensive care unit. These figures include 120 patients in a simultaneously conducted prospective study, of whom 50% showed neurological changes. This discrepancy confirms the theory that we can only find what we seek.

The findings in the 3.4% of the cases in the intensive care unit indicated serious changes of a kind which as a rule necessitated a consult, whilst the findings in the prospective survey were preponderantly based on minor symptoms.

Similar considerations apply to *Psychological-psychiatric disorders*, which after purely clinical observation, have been included under the heading of organic (brain) psycho-syndromes. These manifested themselves in very different ways, however, extending from frequently observed disturbances in attention and orientation, to rarely present delusions, illusions and hallucinations.

Basing themselves on the system developed by the Working Group for Methods and Documentation in Psychiatry (AMDP) [27], Götze and Dahme developed the Hamburg Rating Scale for Psychiatric Disorders (HRDP) [28], containing 36 items instead of the AMDP's 116. This reduction permits application of the scale to cardiac surgery cases in the intensive care unit.

The 36 characteristics were used to form eight symptom groupings:

  I.   Disorientation
  II. Impaired concentration and thinking
  III. Paranoid-hallucinatory symptoms

IV.   Anxiety symptoms
V.   Sullen inadequacy (restrained depression)
VI.   Hostility
VII.   Loss of control
VIII.   Giving up

In each of these groups, the 36 symptoms were weighted in four degrees of intensity. Six groups or clusters were formed on that basis, ranging from those with inconspicuous to paranoid-hallucinatory and delirious characteristics.

Neuro-psychological test procedures are used to examine cognitive functions involving the cortex. Attention, alertness, visualization of three-dimensional space, memory, recall and the ability to reach logical conclusions are among the abilities which can be tested in this way, with preoperative and postoperative findings being compared (Trail making test, WAIS Block Design, WAIS Digit Symbol, Figure Rotation test [29], Bethune and Williams Delayed Recall test, [30], CLAT-test [31]). All the same, anxiety, depression and fatigue can also impair cognitive functions.

The great advantage of clinical test procedures lies in the fact that they enable cross-sectional pictures to be recorded of preoperative and postoperative changes.

The critical objection, whether dysfunctions of the central nervous system are not better captured by using objective research methods, needs to be treated with caution.

Within the range of definition available, such *neuro-radiological procedures* as DSA, 133-Xenon scintography [32–37] and computer and MRI tomography [38] demonstrate larger structural lesions in the vascular system within the cerebral parenchyma. CT and MRI, for example, show the consequences of a stroke or larger lacunar infarcts. That also applies to the use of PET and SPECT. The preponderant element of neurological impairment is of a transitory and functional nature and occurs in an area in which the extent of definition available through these methods is inadequate.

EEG monitoring may be used for the non-specific recording of functional impairments [11, 39–42]. Continuous trans-cranial Doppler ultrasonography can be used to record changes in the brain's global circulation [9, 12, 17, 19, 43, 44]. *Doppler sonography* of the carotid arteries can show the existence of micro-embolisms. Åberg is the only person to have *determined the content of adenyline kinase in cerebro-spinal fluid in human beings* [45], but in animals the same has been done by Taylor so as to measure CRK and CKBB [46]. *Fluorescein retinoscopy* has also been conducted immediately following perfusion [47].

The upshot is that for the early detection and continuous observation of transient symptoms, clinical-neurological examinations are currently far superior to procedures using apparatus.

Findings

The literature puts the frequency of *irreversible brain damage* as the cause of death in cardiac surgery at 0.3–2% [48]. In our hospital, of over 5,000 patients undergoing operations, 245 died. 27 of these, representing 0.52% of those operated and 11% of all deaths, suffered irreversible brain damage. Preponderantly caused by embolisms, 0.2% of these cases were directly related to the operation. Causes indirectly related to the operation consisted mainly of inadequate revival procedures and post-operative brain hemorrhages [49].

Stroke is the main cause of more prolonged neurological complications. The literature puts the frequency of these at 2–5% [50, 51]. Larger embolisms, as well as inadequate blood flow during perfusions, are regarded as the causes.

One risk factor for a stroke related to surgery is atheroma of the large blood vessels in the neck. This cannot be attributed solely to carotid stenosis, since a number of other factors related to extracorporeal circulation could have contributed. At all events, it has hitherto been impossible – with the exception of one preoperative stroke [51] – to establish any significant link between pre-, intra- and post-operative variables.

The question of whether surgery on a stenosis of the carotid vessel should be conducted preoperatively or simultaneously with the operation is a matter of controversy among cardiac surgeons [26, 52–59]. Surgical removal of a severe asymptomatic stenosis of the carotid is conducted in some centres prior to cardiac surgery, the objective being to eliminate the risk of inadequate ipsilateral blood supply during perfusion. Research by the Freiburg working party using intraoperative trans-cranial Doppler sonography has demonstrated that even in cases of severe asymptomatic stenosis of the carotid artery, the blood circulation of the brain is not diminished in the course of extracorporeal circulation [44]. In the authors' view, the only indication for a two-step procedure is provided by transitory ischemic attacks and strokes in the patient's previous history. Simultaneous surgery should be confined to those cases where the coronary illness represents an enhanced risk for carotid reconstruction conducted in advance, or the cardiac operation brooks no delay.

Given that the frequency of carotid murmur among patients with coronary disease can reach 20%, this indicator symptom deserves special attention. Transitory ischemic attacks or strokes are important occurrences in the patient's past history, but can be either incorrectly represented or even, where they had occurred some time ago, entirely forgotten by a patient.

Most other postoperative neurological findings are a matter of minor symptoms. For some patients, neurological occurrences are indicated by their anamnesis or form part of pre-operative findings, so that a distinction needs to be made post-operatively between the continuance or the worsening of existing symptoms, or the occurrence of new ones.

In 52 of 100 patients, Götze described occurrences in the anamnesis and pre-operative findings [60]. In 42 of 67 patients, we ourselves found neurological occurrences in the previous history. At the pre-operative stage, 28 of these showed neurological symptoms which were mainly a matter of the areas supplied by the vertebro-basilar circulation system or by the posterior cerebral artery. With one exception, these symptoms were also present post-operatively [49].

It is worth mentioning that not infrequently, the related details in the documentation of patients transferred to us were incomplete. Occurrences in the anamnesis or forming part of the preoperative findings are of significance, not only for scientific purposes but in certain circumstances for establishing legal liability.

A summary of the literature and of our own findings is supplied by Table 3. Postoperative neurological incidents have been listed in the approximate order of frequency. Here again, most of these disturbances can be attributed to the areas supplied by the vertebro-basilar circulation and the posterior cerebral artery and, in very rare cases, the arteria cerebri media.

Table 3. Postoperative neurological findings listed in approximate order of frequency*

Nystagmus
Anisocoria
Vertigo
Primitive reflexes
Double images
Central facial paralysis
Interferences to visual field
Other motor failures
Retinal defects

*According to the literature and our own findings.

The frequency of neurological dysfunctions reported in prospective studies is up to 60% in the literature [9, 41, 51, 61], but 39% with Götze [60], for example, and 51% with us [49].

The significance of this large total diminishes if one calls to mind that the first four symptoms barely affect the patient beyond causing dizziness, and that two-thirds of them are no longer in evidence by the eighth to the tenth day after the operation. All the same, the last four, far rarer symptoms can persist for some time, with the exception of double vision. Except for central facial paralysis and motor dysfunctions, scarcely any of these consequences are detected in retrospective studies based on the documentation.

In connection with any visual dysfunctions, fluorescein angiograms of the retina can prove revealing. Blauth and his team examined 40 patients with coronary disease five minutes before the end of perfusion, finding micro-embolic occlusions of the vessels of the retina affecting between 0.02 and 2.5% of the surface of the visible retina. The use of membrane oxygenators produced less failures than was the case with bubble oxygenators. Similar changes must be assumed to take place within the cerebral microcirculation [47].

Psychological-psychiatric complications have been described since the beginnings of cardiac surgery, but also previously in patients with heart disease generally, and also in connection with closed commissurotomy of mitral stenosis [62, 63]. The frequencies varied between 5 and 40%. Once again, these were caused by differences in methods of examinations and in classification.

We shall now confine ourselves to the findings derived with the aid of the HPRD. Table 4 shows that on the basis of the cluster formation described above, 60 of 99 patients displayed no symptoms from the first to the fourth postoperative days, and that 23 others revealed minimal psycho-organic symptoms. Several dysfunctions were found in 16 patients. Here it needs to be said that paranoid-hallucinatory symptoms appeared mainly on the third and fourth days after the operation. These symptoms were found in 99 patients in 1978, who had had 57 valve replacement and 23 bypass operations and other heart surgery [28].

Table 4. Six clusters demonstrating the severity of psychological dysfunctions on the first to the fourth postoperative days. From [28]

Cluster	Degree of dysfunction	n	n
1	Unremarkable	28	
2	Almost unremarkable	32	83
3	Mild psycho-organic symptoms	23	
4	Severe psychological syndrome	4	
5	Hostility, paranoid-hallucinatory	8	16
6	Delirious symptoms	4	
		99	99

Figure 1 below illustrates the frequency of the eight symptom groups in 67 patients operated for coronary heart disease in 1987/88. The symptoms have not been weighted here in accordance with severity, in the same way as would be required for forming clusters. Three strips show the number of patients noticeable at the anamnesis state, preoperatively, on the first to the third postoperative days, and between the fifth and the seventh. Whereas few patients indicated dysfunctions at the anamnesis stage, dysfunctions of concentration and thought processes were evident in one-third of them immediately prior to the operation, along with anxiety in two-thirds of them and depression in 28 of the 67 patients. These symptoms were evident again after the operation. Here four-fifths of the patients were affected by impairments of concentration, and almost three-quarters by anxiety and depression, and these were still persisting on the seventh postoperative day. It should be noted that one-fifth of the patients were hostile both preoperatively and postoperatively [49].

Between three and five years after the operation, Annegret Boll found 20% of patients displaying moderate to severe symptoms. Yet these were irrespective of dysfunctions soon after the operation, and were related mainly to the operation itself and coronary disease, to physical and mental abilities, and to the social environment.

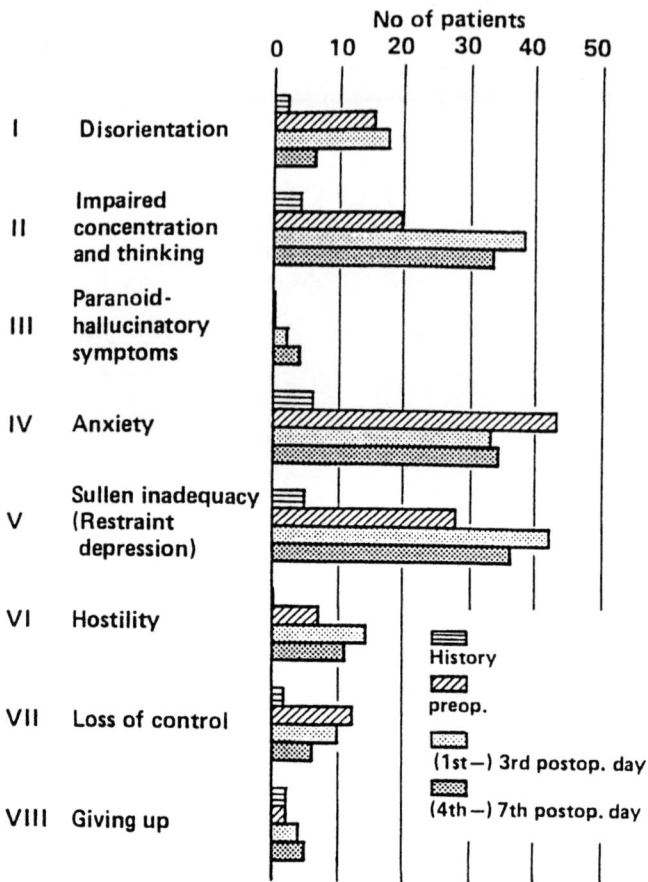

Fig 1. Frequency of the 8 HRPD-symptom groups before and after open-heart surgery.

One interesting point here was a frequent discrepancy between these findings and physical condition [64]. These patients often regarded the operation as the cause of their problems. As with accident surgery, one could speak here of a one-time subjective, determinant deterioration in the sense of a causal attribution of problems and dysphoric moods derived from quite different "real" but not realized causes.

The literature puts the frequency of *impairments of the cognitive functions* immediately after the operation at between 12.5 and 79% [65]. Many authors have tried to relate these findings to the parameters imposed on the operation and extracorporeal circulation as well as the risk factors affecting the patients. Whether in terms of the duration of the operation and extracorporeal circulation, intra-operative hypotension, brain perfusion or the degree of hypothermia, the results are contradictory. The majority of the authors do find a link between postoperative impairment of cognitive functions and age above 60 or 70.

Yet cognitive dysfunctions come to be of more importance later on. After between two and six months, the frequency of these can reach 35% [65]. This may be partly due to the fact that most studies pay insufficient attention to anxiety and depression, which are well known to have the effect of impairing functions.

Sotaniemi examined 44 patients five years after valve replacement surgery. Twenty three of these who had showed no signs of neurological dysfunction immediately after surgery achieved significantly better results than 21 with postoperative neurological symptoms [41, 66].

A survey by Newman and his team is of special interest in this context [67]. They questioned 62 coronary patients about one year after their operations about their subjective estimate of their cognitive functions. More than one-quarter complained of memory impairment, for example, and about one-sixth of impairments of thinking, the proportion of impairments of concentration t ing about the same. A comparison of the findings of objective tests on thet ⸗ patients and on those who did not mention any dysfunctions indicated tha⸗ performance in the two groups was more or less normal, and that no significant differences existed between them. By contrast, there was a marked difference between the two collectives in the intensity of anxiety and depression. Here again, there is much to suggest that subjective complaints of impairments ⸗ᶜ memory, concentration and thinking are not a result of the operation, but are instead an expression of unconscious anxiety and depression.

Discussion

The question whether the disturbances of the central nervous system described here are specifically consequences of cardiac surgery requires comparable research into patients undergoing other surgery of special interest. Unfortunately very little material is available.

Treasure [35] and Pamela Shaw [68] found a considerably greater frequency of neurological symptoms among cardiac patients than among those primarily undergoing vascular surgery. In the two collectives operated with the assistance of extracorporeal circulation, postoperative frequency of these was 59% and 60% respectively, whereas for those undergoing vascular surgery it was 20 and 4%, respectively. Shaw's findings in respect to cognitive functions were very similar. The 20 patients operated on without extracorporeal circulation by Treasure included a similar proportion with impairments of cognitive functions, which were still to be observed after eight weeks and, for him, were explained by the greater age and poorer state of health of this group. Treasure noted psychic disturbances to much the same extent in the cardiac and vascular patients alike.

In 87 cardiac patients, finally, Åberg found a significant rise in adenyline kinase in the cerebrospinal fluid, whereas the content was normal in eight patients after lung surgery. A significant correlation existed between the increase in adenyline kinase and the deterioration in results in cognitive tests [45].

Even if one agrees with Woody Allen that the brain is our second most essential organ, these findings leave no room for doubt that with regard to cardiac surgery, it is probably the most sensitive one.

As indicated at the outset, far more dysfunctions of the central nervous system are found postoperatively than could be explained by the preoperative risk factors. These latter are limited to greater age, advanced arteriosclerosis, and carotid complaints involving such symptoms as ischemic attacks and strokes in the anamnesis; the type and severity of heart disease, hypertension, diabetes, etc., play little or no part. These factors can entail a greater risk, yet this is almost impossible to predict in the individual case, as clinical experience shows. By contrast, factors determined by the operation are of greater significance. The use of arterial filters, the improvement of oxygenation, improvement of the conduct of extracorporeal circulation itself [16, 69–73] and operating techniques which have become increasingly discriminating have led to a considerable reduction of apparent complications down the years. Too much weight should not be attached to the frequency of minor symptoms established in prospective neurological examinations, still less give grounds for reluctance to indicate a cardiac operation when this has proven advantageous over traditional treatment or a procedure involving invasive cardiology. Yet the consequences of such operations for the central nervous system cannot be overlooked for two reasons:

1. However minimal this may be, the frequency of lasting cerebral dysfunctions must be mentioned to the patient in an appropriate manner prior to the operation. It should also perhaps be pointed out that where results are otherwise positive, later postoperative dysfunctions are demonstrably not linked with early postoperative dysfunctions, but can be caused by the psychic state of the patient.
2. Quite irrespective of the minimal clinical importance of most dysfunctions, prospective examinations, in an attempt to further explain the causes of these, are absolutely indispensable. That this is within the realms of the possible has been illustrated by the improvements evident since the beginning of open-heart surgery.

As Taylor said, one can view these problems in the manner adopted by some surgeons, with Nelson's blind eye, as it were, and say: "None of my patients has ever suffered brain damage". On the other hand, one can take an electron microscope to this one aspect of all the problems involved, and arrive at an over-estimate of its importance for cardiac surgery [74].

References

1. Lehman HJ, Grahmann H, Hauss K, Rodewald GW, Schmitz Th. Akute organische Psychosyndrome nach Herzoperationen. Der Nervenarzt 1968; 39:529.

2. Becker R, Katz J, Polonius MJ, Speidel H (eds). Psychological and Neurological Dysfunctions Following Open Heart Surgery. Berlin, Heidelberg, New York, Springer, 1982.
3. Speidel H, Rodewald G (eds). Psychic and Neurological Dysfunctions After Open Heart Surgery. Thieme, Stuttgart, New York, 1980.
4. Speidel H. Analyse von Bedingunsfaktoren der postoperativen psychopathologischen und neurologischen Auffälligkeiten bei Herzoperierten mit extrakorporaler Zirkulation. SFB 115, Projekt A 3/A 20, Hamburg. Bericht an die Deutsche Forschungsgemeinschaft, 1981.
5. Willner A E, Rodewald G (eds). The Impact of Cardiac Surgery on the Quality of Life: Neurological and Psychological Aspects. Plenum Publ. Corp., New York, 1990.
6. Kent B, Peirce E C. Oxygen consumption during cardiopulmonary bypass in the uniformly cooled dog. J Appl Physiol 1974; 37:917.
7. Ärztezeitung 2.3.89. Materialabrieb von Rollenpumpen – eine Zeitbombe im Kreislauf?
8. Branthwaite M A. Prevention of neurological damage during open-heart surgery. Thorax 1975; 30:258.
9. Deverall P B, Padayachee T S, Parsons S, Theobold R, Battistessa S A. Ultrasound detection of micro-emboli in the middle cerebral artery during cardiopulmonary bypass surgery. Eur J Cardiothorac Surg 1988; 2:256.
10. Henriksen L, Hjelms E, Lindeburgh Th. Brain hyperperfusion during cardiac operations. J Thorac Cardiovasc Surg 1983; 86:202.
11. John E R, Prichep L S, Chabot R J, Isom W O. Monitoring brain function during cardiovascular surgery: hypoperfusion vs. microembolism as the major cause of neurological damage during cardiopulmonary bypass. In: Refsum H, Sulg I A, Rasmussen K (eds). Heart and Brain Berlin, Heidelberg, Springer, 1989; p. 405.
12. Grefe C, Krebber H J, Ayisi K. Emission of micro-bubbles in bubble (BO) and membrane-oxygenators (MO); A comparative investigation. In: Willner A E, Rodewald G (eds). The Impact of Cardiac Surgery on the Quality of Life: Neurological and Psychological Aspects. New York, Plenum Publ. Corp., 1990; p. 273.
13. Landew M, Bowles L Th, Gelman S, Lowenfels A B, Tepper R, Lord J W Jr. Effects of intra-arterial microbubbles. Am J Physiol 1960; 199:485.
14. Pearson D T. Microemboli: Gaseous and particulate. In: Taylor K M (ed). Cardiopulmonary Bypass, Principles and Management. London Chapmann and Hall, 1986; p. 313.
15. Pearson D T. Assessing cerebral damage. Perfusion 1989; 4:101.
16. Pearson D T. Blood gas control during cardiopulmonary bypass. Perfusion 1988; 3:113.
17. Pedersen T, Hatteland K, Karlsen H, Semb G. An in vivo investigation of the creation and transportation of free gas bubbles in the extracorporeal circulation system by means of a doppler ultrasound system. In: Hagl S, Klövekorn W P, Mayr N, Sebening F. (eds). Thirty Years of Extracorporeal Circulation. Deutsches Herzzsentrum München 1984; p. 511.
18. Schaldach M. New aspects of biomaterial research for extracorporeal circulation. In: Hagl S, Klövekorn W P, Mayr N, Sebening F. (eds). Thirty Years of Extracorporeal Circulation. Deutsches Herzzentrum München 1984; p. 407.
19. Semb B K H, Pedersen T, Hatteland K, Storstein L, Lillcaasen P. Doppler ultrasound estimation of bubble removal by various arterial line filters during extracorporeal circulation. Scand J Thor Cardiovasc Surg 1982; 16:55.
20. Wozniak G, Dapper F, Strube I, Thiel A, Kasseckert S, Hehrlein F W. Nachweis zerbraler Mikroembolisationen während extrakorporaler Zirkulation im pulsatilen Betrieb mittels transkraniellem Doppler-Monitoring. ECC International 1990; 1:64.
21. Salama A, Hugo F, Heinrich D, Höge R, Müller R, Kiefel V, Müller-Eckhardt Ch, Bhakdi S. Deposition of terminal C5b-9 complement complexes on erythrocytes and leukocytes during cardiopulmonary bypass. New Engl J Med 1988; 318:408.
22. Wastaby S, Kirklin J K, Blackstone E H, Kirklin J W, Chenoweth D E, Pacifico A D. Complement activation and morbidity after cardiopulmonary bypass. In: Hagl S, Klövekorn W P, Mayr N, Sebening F (eds). Thirty Years of Extracorporeal Circulation. Deutsches Herzzentrum München 1984; p. 389.
23. Hazel J R, Garlick W S, Seelner P A. The effects of assay temperature upon the pH optima of enzymes from poikilotherms: a test of the imidazole alphastat hypothesis. J Comp Physiol 1978; 123:97.

96

24. White FM. A comparative physiological approach to hypothermia. J Thorac Cardiovasc Surg 1981; 82:821.
25. Lundar T, Lindegaard KF, Froysaker T, Aaslid R, Grip A, Nornes H. Dissociation between cerebral autoregulation and carbon dioxide reactivity during nonpulsatile cardiopulmonary bypass. Ann Thorac Surg 1985; 40:582.
26. Turnipseed WD, Berkoff HA, Belzer FO. Postoperative stroke in cardiac and peripheral vascular disease. Ann Surg 1980; 192:365.
27. Angst J, Battegay R, Bente D, Berner P, Brocren W, Cornu F, Dick P, Engelemeier P, Heimann H, Heinrich K, Helmenhen H, Hippius H, Pöldinger W, Schmidlin P, Schmitt W, Weiss P. Das Dokumentationssystem der Arbeitsgemeinschaft für Methodik und Documentation in der Psychiatric (AMDP). Arzneim Forsch 1969; 19:399.
28. Götze P, Dahme B, Wessel W. Die Hamburger Schätzskala für psychische Störungen nach Herzoperationen (HRPD). Eur Arch Psychiatr Neurol Sci 1985; 234:308.
29. Sweetland RC, Keyser DJ. Tests. A Comprehensive Reference For Assessments in Psychology, Education And Business. Test Corporation of America, Kansas City, 1986.
30. Bethune DW. Test of delayed memory recall suitable for assessing postoperative amnesia. Anaesthesia 1981; 36:942.
31. Willner AE, Rabiner CJ, Wisoff RG, Hartstein M, Struve FA, Klein DF. Analogical reasoning and postoperative outcome. Arch Gen Psychiatry 1976; 33:255.
32. Henriksen L. Cerebral blood flow during cardiopulmonary bypass. In: Refsum H, Sulg IA, Rasmussen K (eds). Heart and Brain. Berlin, Heidelberg, Springer, 1989; p. 422.
33. Medinews. Hirndurchblutung und zerebrovaskuläre Reservekapazität. Messmethoden und klinische Bedeutung. Wiss Symp 9–10.6.1989, Med Hochschule Hannover. München: Publimed Verlag, 1989.
34. Prough DS, Stump DA, Roy RC, Gravlee GP, Williams Th, Mills SA, Hinshelwood L, Howard G. Response of cerebral blood flow to changes in carbon dioxide tension during hypothermic cardiopulmonary bypass. Anesthesiology 1986; 64:576.
35. Treasure T, Smith PLC, Newman S, Schneidau A, Joseph P, Ell P, Harrison MJG. Impairment of cerebral function following cardiac and other major surgery. Eur J Cardiothorac Surg 1989; 3:216.
36. Venn GE, Sherry K, Klinger L, Newman S, Treasure T, Harrison M, Ell PJ. Cerebral blood flow during cardiopulmonary bypass. Eur J Cardiothorac Surg 1988; 2:360.
37. Venn GE. Cerebral vascular autoregulation during cardiopulmonary bypass. Perfusion 1989; 4:105.
38. McConnnell IR, Fleming WH, Sarcafian LB. Magnetic resonance imaging of the brain in infants and children before and after cardiac surgery: A prospective study. In: Willner AE, Rodewald G (eds). The Impact of Cardiac Surgery on the Quality of Life: Neurological and Psychological Aspects. New York, Plenum Publ. Corp., 1990; p. 121.
39. Boezeman EHJF, Simons AIR. Automatic EEG monitoring in cardiac surgery. In: Willner AE, Rodewald G (eds). The Impact of Cardiac Surgery on the Quality of Life: Neurological and Psychological Aspects. New York, Plenum Publ. Corp., 1990; p. 111.
40. Sotaniemi KA, Juolasmaa A, Hokkanen TE. Neuropsychologic outcome after open-heart surgery. Arch Neurol 1981; 38:2.
41. Sotaniemi KA, Mononen H, Hokkanen TE. Long-term cerebral outcome after open-heart surgery. A five year neuropsychological follow-up study. Stroke 1986; 17:410.
42. Strobl FT, Arom KV, Chohen DE. EEG monitoring during cardiopulmonary bypass procedure. In: Willner AE, Rodewald G (eds). The Impact of Cardiac Surgery on the Quality of Life: Neurological and Psychological Aspects. New York, Plenum Publ. Corp., 1990; p. 343.
43. Lundar T. Cerebral hemodynamics during nonpulsatile cardiopulmonary bypass. In: Refsum H, Sulg IA, Rasmussen K. (eds). Heart and Brain. Berlin, Heidelberg, Springer, 1989; p. 432.
44. Reutern G von, Hetzel A, Birnbaum D, Schlosser V. Transcranial doppler ultrasonography during cardiopulmonary bypass in patients with servere carotid stenosis or occlusion. Stroke 1988; 19:674.

45. Åberg T, Ronquist G, Tyden H, Brunnkvist S, Hultman J, Bergström K, Lilja A. Adverse effects on the brain in cardiac operations as assessed by biochemical, psychometric, and radiologic methods. Thorac Cardiovasc Surg 1984; 87:99.

46. Taylor KM, Devlin BJ, Mittra SM, Gillan JG, Brannen JJ, McKenna JM. Assessment of cerebral damage during open-heart surgery. A new experimental model. Scand J Thor Cardiovasc Surg 1980; 14:197.

47. Blauth C, Smith P, Newman S, Arnold J, Siddons F, Harrison MJ, Treasure T, Klinger L, Taylor KM. Retinal microembolism and neuropsychological deficit following clinical cardiopulmonary bypass: Comparison of a membrane and a bubble oxygenator. Eur J Cardiothorac Surg 1989; 3:135.

48. Shaw PJ. The incidence and nature of neurological morbidity following cardiac surgery: A review. Perfusion 1989; 4:83.

49. Rodewald G, Meffert HJ, Emskötter T, Götze P, Lachenmayer L, Lamparter U, Krebber HJ, Kalmar P, Pokar H. Head and heart – neurological and psychological reactions to open-heart surgery. Thorac Cardiovasc Surg 1988; 36:254.

50. Breuer AC, Furlan AJ, Hanson MR, Lederman RJ, Loop FD, Cosgrove DM, Greenstreet R, Estafanous FG. Central nervous system complications of coronary artery bypass graft surgery: prospective analysis of 421 patients. Stroke 1983; 14:682.

51. Furlan AJ, Jones SC. Central nervous system complications related to open-heart surgery. In: Furlan AJ (ed). The Heart and Stroke. Berlin, Springer, 1987; p. 287.

52. Barnes RW, Marszalek PB. Asymptomatic carotid disease in the cardiovascular surgical patient: Is prophylactic endarterectomy necessary? Stroke 1981; 12:497.

53. Barnes RW, Liebmann PR, Marszalek PB, Kirk CL, Goldman MH. The natural history of asymptomatic carotid disease in patients undergoing cardiovascular surgery. Surg. 1981; 90:1075.

54. Barnes RW, Archie JP, Batson RC. Advocates in vascular controversies. Surg 1984; 95:339.

55. Breslau PJ, Fell G, Ivey TD, Bailey WW, Miller DW, Strandness DE. Carotid arterial disease in patients undergoing coronary artery bypass operations. J Thorac Cardiovasc Surg 1981; 82:765.

56. Easton JD, Hart RG. Asymptomatic carotid artery disease in patients undergoing open-heart surgery: A neurologic viewpoint. In: Furlan AJ (ed). The Heart and Stroke. Berlin, Springer, 1987; p. 319.

57. Evans WE, Cooperman M. The significance of asymptomatic unilateral carotid bruits in preoperative patients. Surg 1978; 521.

58. Hertzer NR, Loop FD, Beven EG. Management of coexistent carotid and coronary artery disease: A surgical viewpoint. In: Furlan AJ (ed). The Heart and Stroke. Berlin, Springer, 1987; p. 305.

59. Ivey TD, Strandness E, Williams DB, Langlois Y, Misbach GA, Kruse AP. Management of patients with carotid bruit undergoing cardiopulmonary bypass. J Thorac Cardiovasc Surg 1984; 87:183.

60. Götze P. Psychopathologie der Herzoperierten. Enke, Stuttgart 1980.

61. Tufo HM, Ostfeld AM, Shekelle R. Central nervous system dysfunction following open-heart surgery. JAMA 1970; 25:1333.

62. Capon D. Psychologic prognostication for mitral valvoplasty. Section of Res in Psychodynamics, Dept. of Psychiatry, University of Toronto, 1959.

63. Meyendorf R. Psychopathology in heart disease aside from cardiac surgery. A historical perspective of cardiac psychosis. In: Speidel H, Rodewald G (eds). Psychic and Neurological Dysfunctions After Open-heart Surgery. New York, Thieme, 1980; p. 14.

64. Boll A. Längerfristige psychische Anpassung Herzoperierter. Dissertation, Universität Hamburg 1986.

65. Newman S. The incidence and nature of neuropsychological morbidity following cardiac surgery. Perfusion 1989; 4:93.

66. Sotaniemi KA. Cerebral outcome after open-heart surgery: A long-term multidimensional follow-up of valvular replacement patients. In: Refsum H, Sulg IA, Rasmussen K (eds). Heart and Brain. Berlin, Heidelberg, Springer, 1989; p. 440.

67. Newman S, Klinger L, Venn G, Smith P, Harrison M, Treasure T. Subjective reports of cognition in relation to assessed cognitive performance following coronary artery bypass surgery. J Psychosom Res 1988; 33:227.
68. Shaw PJ, Bates D, Cartlidge NEF, French JM, Heaviside D, Julian DG, Shaw DA. Neurologic and neuropsychological morbidity following major surgery: Comparison of coronary artery bypass and peripheral vascular surgery. Stroke 1987; 18:700.
69. Kurusz M. Cerebral protection and cardiopulmonary bypass: A review. Proc Am Acad Cardiovasc Perf 1986; 7:115.
70. Kurusz M. Perfusion safety. Perfusion 1988; 3:97.
71. Marshall L. Filtration in cardiopulmonary bypass: past, present and future. Perfusion 1988; 3:135.
72. Tanzeem A, Vahl C, Schäfer H, Hagl S. Success of the low flow – low pressure perfusion in reducing postoperative psychological disturbances. In: Willner AE, Rodewald G (eds). The Impact of Cardiac Surgery on the Quality of Life: Neurological and Psychological Aspects. New York, Plenum Publ. Corp., 1990; p. 353.
73. Taylor KM. Cardiopulmonary Bypass. Principals and Management. London: Chapmann and Hall, 1986.
74. Taylor KM. The cerebral consequences of cardiac surgery. Perfusion 1989; 4:Editorial.

PART TWO

Techniques for assessing cerebral damage

8. Neuropsychological methods for evaluating regional brain dysfunction

As in any scientific discipline, progress in the behavioral neurosciences is constrained by the availability of techniques to probe its subject matter. Understanding of how human behavior is regulated by the brain has been particularly slow to advance because until recently there were relatively few techniques or controlled experimental procedures that can be applied to live humans. Inferences have been drawn from animal data, but much of the insight came from clinical observations of patients with brain damage. A number of rather ingenious means that can be used in normal subjects have been devised for examining hypotheses on hemispheric asymmetry of brain function. The latter have included the tachistoscopic, dichotic listening and dichaptic techniques in which stimuli are presented to the left or right sensory fields, and inferences on hemispheric asymmetry of function are made from differences in performance *see other articles in this issue*. Electroencephalography (EEG) used to be the only method for measuring regional brain activity, and it can also be used to examine intra-hemispheric effects. However, its spatial resolution is poor and the relationship between patterns of electric activity and the underlying rate of neural activity is still being debated.

In recent years, a number of techniques have been developed for measuring parameters of regional brain physiology. These techniques make use of the fact that active neurons have metabolic needs for oxygen and glucose, and that cerebral blood flow rates change in response to these needs. Such measures can help identify regions of abnormal physiologic activation associated with behavioral deficits. Furthermore, such measures obtained during the performance of cognitive tasks could help delineate brain regions necessary for regulating cognitive processes. These techniques will be described briefly, and some initial data will be presented.

In 1948, Kety and Schmidt [1] described a technique for measuring brain metabolism and blood flow. The technique used nitrous oxide and measurement of arterial-venous differences in concentration yielded accurate and reproducible data. However, this technique is limited to providing whole-brain values and could not be used widely because of its invasiveness. Regional measurements were first made possible by the introduction of the 133-Xenon

101

clearance techniques for measuring regional cerebral blood flow (rCBF), and more recently by the development of position emission tomography (PET), which enables the application of different isotopes for measuring a diverse range of physiologic parameters including glucose and oxygen metabolism as well as blood flow.

The highly diffusable 133-Xenon can be administered as gas mixed in air or in saline. Its clearance from the brain can be measured by scintillation detectors, and from the rate of clearance it is possible to quantify with considerable accuracy rCBF in the fast clearing gray matter compartment, as well as mean flow of gray and white matter. Initial applications used carotid injections [2], which only enabled measurements in one hemisphere at a time and invasively. In 1975, Obrist and colleagues have reported the 133-Xenon inhalation technique [3], and presented models for quantifying rCBF with this noninvasive technique. The technique permits simultaneous measurements from both hemispheres, and the number of brain regions that can be measured depends on the number of detectors. Initial studies were performed with up to 16 detectors, 8 over each hemisphere, but there are now commercially available systems with 32 detectors and recently a system has been introduced that enables the placement of up to 254 detectors. Figure 1 shows a topographic display of rCBF obtained with such a system. The main limitation of the technique is that it measures rCBF from cortical areas only.

PET has made it possible to measure in vivo biochemical and physiological processes in the human brain, with three dimensional resolution. Initial

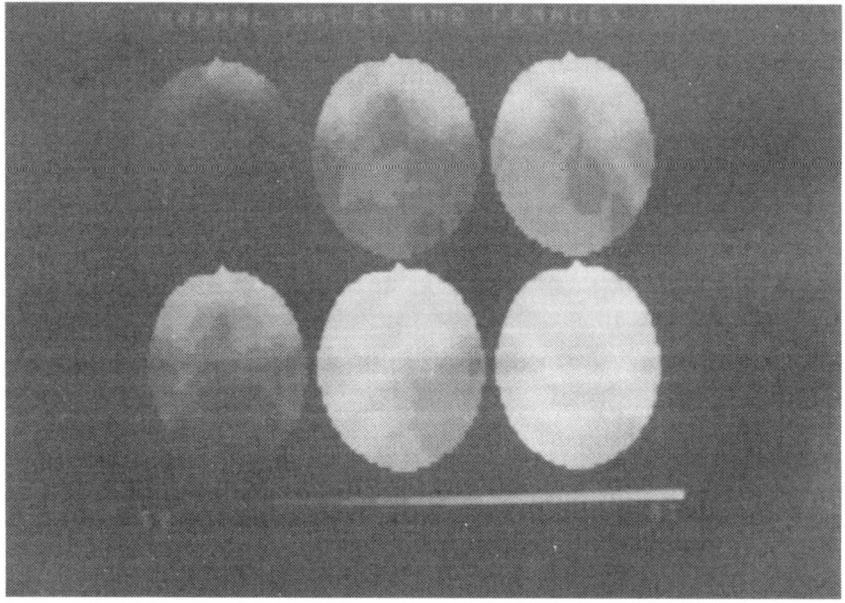

Fig. 1. A topographic display of rCBF in a group of normal males (upper row) and females (lower row) during rest (1st column), a verbal analogies task (middle column), and a spatial line orientation task (last column). NOTE the hyperfrontal pattern at rest, the higher CBF in females and the increased CBF in the left for the verbal and the right for the spatial task.

work with animals used selectively labeled chemical compounds, called radio-isotopes, to measure the rate of the chemical process. This has been extended to humans by principles of computed tomography [4], and now the technique has been adapted to use with various radionuclides (such as carbon-11, nitrogen-13, oxygen-15 and fluorine-18) that decay through the emission of positrons. Subjects are administered radionuclides that are unstable because their nuclei have an excess positive charge. The radionuclides are usually given intravenously, and are taken up by tissue. Through the emission of a positron they get rid of their energy and undergo the process of annihilation where the positron interacts with a negatively charged electron. The two photons emitted travel in opposite directions and the energy generated is detected and measured by PET devices which consist of detector arrays. By computed tomography principles, the coincidental counts are used to generate images reflecting the regional rate of radionuclide uptake. This information enables the calculation, depending on the specific radionuclide, of such varied physiologic parameters as oxygen and glucose metabolism, blood flow, or receptor density of neurotransmitters. In order to relate this physiologic information to anatomic regions of interest (ROI), an atlas of brain anatomy is required. These can be based on computerized images of sliced brains, or on X-ray CT scans. Multiple brain "slices" can be obtained with PET. Figure 2 illustrates the principles and setting of PET.

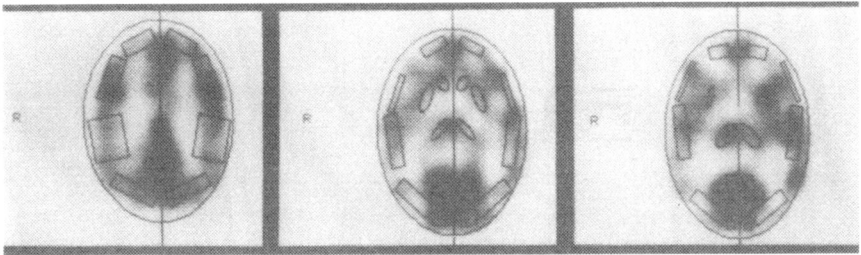

Fig. 2. Placement of regions of interest. (Figure 2 appears in Gur *et al,* Regional brain function in schizophrenia. I. A positron emission tomography study. *Archives of General Psychiatry* 1987; 44:119. Copyright 1987 by the AMA).

Another technique recently introduced for three dimensional imaging of rCBF is single photon emission tomography (SPECT). The technique enables three-dimensional imaging of CBF using radionuclides which, unlike positron emitters, do not require the availability of a dedicated cyclotron for their production. However, at present, reliable quantitation of rCBF with available radionuclides that can be safely administered is still very problematic, and much more work is required to make it applicable in systematic neurobehavioral research.

Finally, an old technique for measuring regional brain activity is now being adapted for imaging. Techniques have been developed for representing computer EEG parameters, reflecting neural electric activity, as topographic displays such as the one shown in Figure 3.

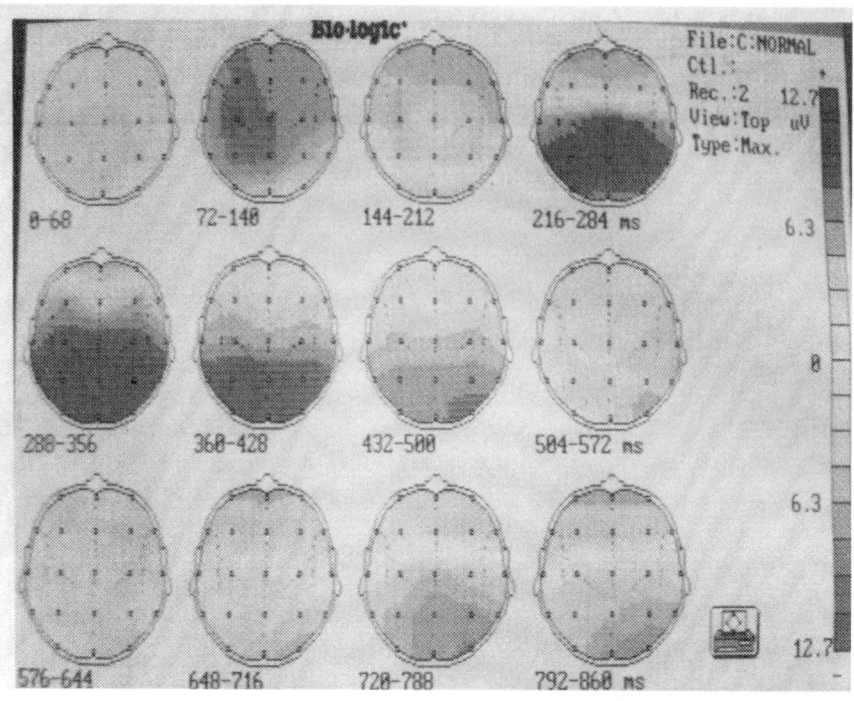

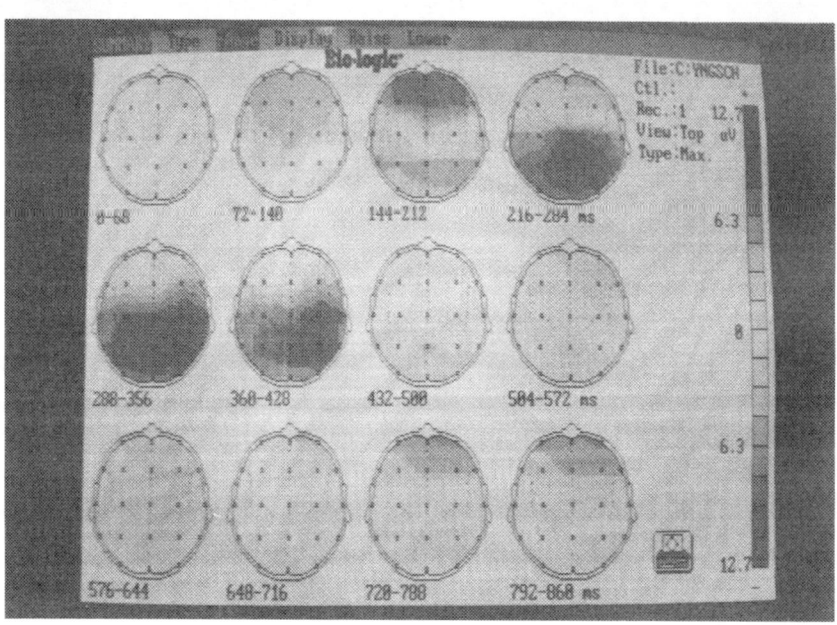

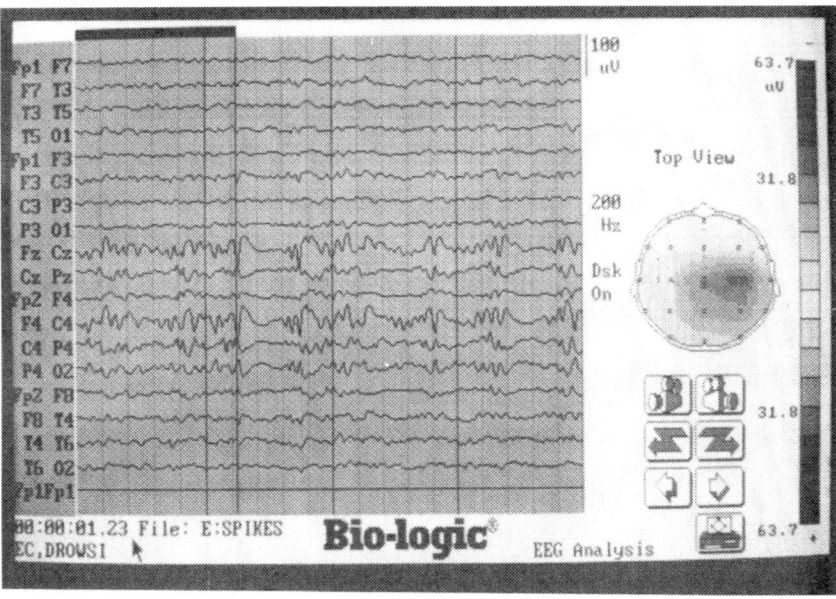

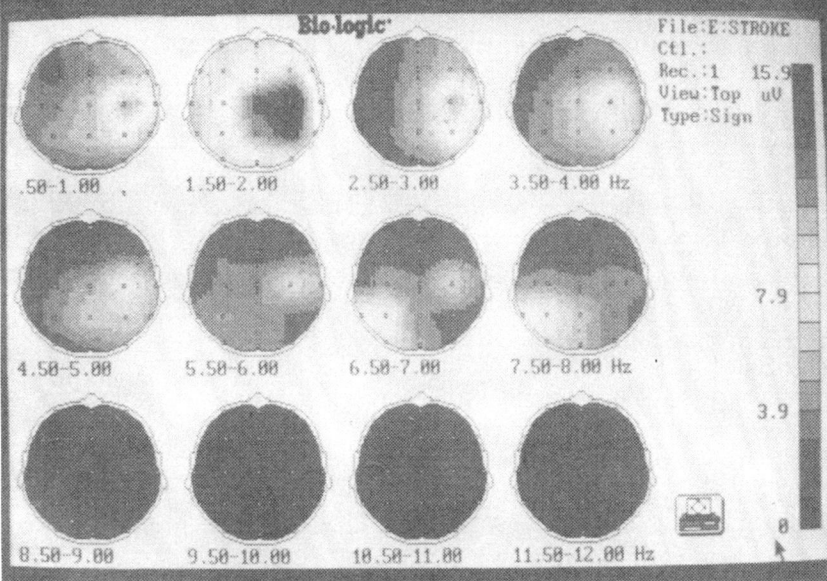

Fig. 3. Presented are examples of topographic displays of electrophysiologic data: a) Integrated voltages of evoked responses for 12 latency windows following stimulus onset are mapped. In this case average evoked response amplitudes to a rare stimulus (oddball P300 paradigm) from a normal subject are shown. Note the posterior maxima in the 288–356 ms latency window. b) Similar data to 2a. but obtained from a schizophrenic patient. When compared with the normal subject, note the overall decreased amplitude as well as the right-sided skew the positive potential has, especially at the 288–356 ms latency window. c) In another example of a voltage map, the map displays the maxima of a spike obtained from an epileptic which is indicated by the red cursor on the continuous EEG display. d) This display is of EEG that has been subjected to frequency analysis and the 12 integrated spectral bands are plotted topographically. In a patient with a right CVA, maximal amplitudes in the delta range (first three maps) are easily appreciated over the right hemisphere.

The application of these techniques to the understanding of human behavior is still in its infancy. We have barely passed the stage of identifying the sensitivity and limitation of some of these methods, and only crude dimensions of behavior have been examined. Here I will describe some of the findings and try to outline where this work could lead us.

When applied to normal subjects, reliable patterns of physiologic activity have been observed. For example, the 133-Xenon technique consistently showed increased rCBF in anterior compared to posterior brain regions, "the hyperfrontal pattern" (e.g., [5]). PET showed higher glucose uptake in frontal regions, as well as in the posterior visual (calcarine) cortex. The question of whether the techniques are sensitive to changes in brain activity produced by sensory stimulation has been also answered affirmatively for the visual, auditory and somatosensory modalities [6].

The next step for determining the applicability of the techniques for behavioral research was to evaluate whether metabolic activity, as measured by the techniques, shows changes during cognition. It was not obvious that they would, since the changes could be smaller than what the techniques could detect. Furthermore, the blood contains excess supply of nutrients, and the increased cell demands during cognitive effort could be accommodated without immediate increase in blood flow. The prospects for finding blood flow increase in specific regions that would presumably become activated by a given cognitive task were even more questionable. This would require a mechanism that controls CBF locally, at the cellular level. However, anecdotal reports of subjects studied with the 133-Xenon technique reported, for example, subjects who showed increased CBF in frontotemporal regions during talk and parietal increase for a musical task. These studies were confined to measures of one hemisphere at a time, and were unable to demonstrate statistical effects.

In our initial attempt to answer this question we measured rCBF with the 133-Xenon inhalation technique, using a 16 detector system, in a sample of right-handed males [7]. We chose right-handed males because this was the group expected to have the greatest extent of hemispheric specialization. The rCBF was measured at rest and during the performance of two standardized cognitive tasks: reasoning (analogies) and spatial closure (gestalt). On the basis of the hemispheric specialization hypothesis, we expected left hemispheric increase for the verbal analogies and right hemispheric increased activity for the spatial closure task. What we found was that both tasks increased rCBF bilaterally. The verbal task, as expected, showed greater increase to the left hemisphere. The spatial task did not show the hypothesized greater right hemispheric increase. Of the 36 subjects, 14 showed greater increase to the right, 2 showed bilaterally symmetric changes, and 14 showed greater increase to the left. This did not necessarily invalidate the hypothesis that cognitive activity produces increased CBF in regions required for its processing. Some earlier studies have shown individual differences in characteristic hemispheric activation, and our subjects have all been highly educated, they may have had a bias to activate the left hemisphere even for spatial tasks. Indeed, the

14 subjects showing greater right hemispheric activation perform better on the spatial task than the subjects showing the reverse pattern.

In a second study we used the same design in right- and left-handed males and females [8]. The verbal task was the same, and the spatial task was replaced by a line orientation task. This time both the verbal and the spatial tasks produced hemispherically asymmetric increase in rCBF, verbal for left and spatial for right. The dimensions of individual differences selected for examination, handedness and sex, also played a role. Females had higher rCBF and left-handers differed from right-handers in the pattern of hemispheric activation. This indicated that rCBF measurement is sensitive not only to the effects of cognitive effort on regional brain activity, but also to individual differences known to affect the direction and degree of hemispheric specialization for cognitive function.

Subsequent studies with rCBF and PET have confirmed and extended these findings. In most cases some of the results related to hypotheses that had been generated from earlier observations, but as would be expected from new technology, some of the results were unexpected and yet others could not have been predicted from earlier theories but the data helped explain behavioral observations. For example, a PET study with the same verbal analogies and spatial line orientation tasks showed asymmetric effects in the expected temporo-parietal regions implicated by the effects of brain damage. However, a hypothesis proposed in 1976 by the British neuropsychologist Colwyn Trevarthen was also supported by the data. Trevarthen suggested that neural activation of lateralized cognitive processes could "spill over" to motor brain regions and produce orientation to the contralateral hemispace. Thus, when people have verbal thoughts they would orient themselves to the right and when they have spatial cognitions they would orient themselves to the left. This hypothesis received some confirmation in studies examining the effects of verbal and spatial tasks on the direction of conjugate lateral eye movements while individuals were reflecting on these tasks. The PET study showed that the effects of the tasks were asymmetric not only in the temporo-parietal regions, but also in the regions controlling the orientation response [9]. Another behavioral observation that received explanation from the new techniques is a "law" first proposed by the results of an animal study of the American neuropsychologists Yerkes and Dodson in 1908, and which was confirmed by numerous subsequent studies in animals and humans. The law postulates a curvilinear, "inverted-U" relationship between anxiety and performance. Performance is not very good when anxiety is extremely low, since the attentional and arousal components required for optimal performance are missing. At extremely high anxiety, however, performance also deteriorates. The brain mechanisms responsible for the operation of this law could not be studied without the availability of the neuroimaging techniques. Initial studies with PET and the 133-Xenon technique showed that this inverted-U relationship between anxiety and performance is paralleled by changes in cortical metabolism and blood flow. This suggests a neural mechanism that reduces cortical activity in high anxiety, perhaps reflecting a shift toward activation of subcortical regions which are more important in fight-or-flight situations. Other PET and 133-Xenon studies have examined regional brain involvement in attention. These studies examined, for example, a network of regions which animal neuroanatomic studies by Marcel Mesulam from Harvard have implicated in attentional processing. It was found that in humans these regions show greater right hemispheric activation. These early and preliminary studies seem to point to the possibility that neuroimaging techniques are sufficiently sensitive to detect the association between regional brain activity and behavior. They encourage more systematic work, using the neuroimaging techniques for testing hypotheses and generating new observations on brain-behavior relationships. This can be done by manipulating behavioral dimensions in normal subjects, and examining the effects of such manipulations on regional brain activity. Thus far, the cognitive dimension has received the greatest attention, particularly in the examination of verbal and spatial tasks in relation to hemispheric activation. But emotion and conative or motivational factors could also be studied with the techniques. Such studies could be done not only in normal populations. Its extension to populations representing a large range of human behavior could be informative in understanding regional brain involvement in the regulation of behavior and of considerable relevance to the diagnosis and treatment of dysfunction. On the one hand, populations with behavioral deficits could be studied. Thus, applying these techniques to patients with destructive brain lesions, such as are produced by stroke, head trauma or brain tumors, could help in determining the extent and topographic distribution of suppressed metabolic activity. There is considerable evidence that metabolism is suppressed even in regions that appear anatomically intact when evaluated by techniques for assessing regional brain anatomy, such as CT scans and magnetic resonance imaging (MRI). This could explain why so frequently patients show behavioral deficits that are more pervasive than what can be explained by regions of anatomic involvement.

Another example is epilepsy, where frequently the CT scan is normal or unrelated to the seizure focus. Yet, there appear to be interictal deficits in behavior that were hitherto seen as reflecting secondary psychological reactions to the presence of a debilitating disease. The metabolic studies could help localize regions with epileptogenic activity and also identify regions of metabolic abnormalities that could explain brain mechanisms responsible for the behavioral deficits observed interictally. Other clinical populations of particular interest include Parkinson's disease and Alzheimer's disease. There is strong evidence that dopamine deficiency is responsible for the symptoms of the former, and some suggestions for the involvement of another neurotransmitter (cholinergic) system in the latter. PET will enable imaging of the distribution of neurotransmitters, and studying the topographic distribution of metabolic abnormalities in these disorders could help understand how these neurotransmitter systems regulate behavior.

A complementary approach would begin with disorders of behavior where the brain pathology is unclear, and the metabolic studies could help identify regional brain involvement. For example, reading disabilities and other learning disabilities could be studied, and this could help test hypotheses on regional brain dysfunction that underly these disorders. Understanding of psychiatric disorders could similarly be enhanced by techniques for measuring regional brain activity. In both psychiatric and neurologic populations it would be particularly informative to measure the physiologic activity not only at rest, but also while patients are engaged in pertinent behavior.

But looking at pathology and deficit is only one side of the coin. Normal individuals vary considerably in behavior and abilities, and studying the relation between this variability and regional brain physiology can shed light on the neural underpinnings of this variability. For example, exceptionally talented individuals in the sciences, art and humanities could be evaluated. Again, this should be done at rest and during behavioral "challenge" procedures. How does regional brain activity of a mathematician differ from that of an architect? Which brain regions does a mathematician activate when he is attempting to develop a calculus for a particular problem? Could we identify mathematical talent early by selecting individuals who show activation patterns similar to talented mathematicians? Could we train individuals to activate appropriate brain regions and thereby enhance their mathematical abilities? The technology permits us to begin answering such questions.

I believe that a key issue for such future work centers on our ability to integrate multifaceted data on regional brain function. In addition to the anatomic information on the integrity of brain regions, such as is now available from X-ray CT and from MRI scans, the PET and 133-Xenon techniques provide information on regional brain physiologic activity and topographic EEG techniques complement our armamentarium of data on regional brain function with information on electric activity. Imaging technology provide means for integrating such multifaceted data in a comprehensible manner, but theory is needed to guide our understanding of how the activity of the brain is related to behavior. Now the challenge is to integrate behavioral theories on regional brain function with the anatomic and physiologic neuroimaging data. One approach toward accomplishing this task is to frame behavioral theories of regional brain function as representing a "behavioral image" of the brain. This can be done by determining, for any particular behavioral measure or set of measures, the probability that each brain region is involved in regulating behavior tapped by this measure. Such regional "behavioral weights" could be used in imaging algorithms that can be validated against the anatomic and physiologic neuroimaging data [10]. For example, we generated a table of regional weights for a standard neuropsychological battery, which included measures of language comprehension and fluency, spatial abilities, verbal and figural memory, attention and sensorimotor functions. When the weight table was applied to the scores of a patient with a right hemispheric stroke (Figure 4), the resulting "behavioral image" showed clear correspondence with the location of lesion.

Within this framework, the availability of the new techniques for imaging the inside of the human brain could lead to improved understanding of how the organ of the mind regulates mental processes by optimizing the regional

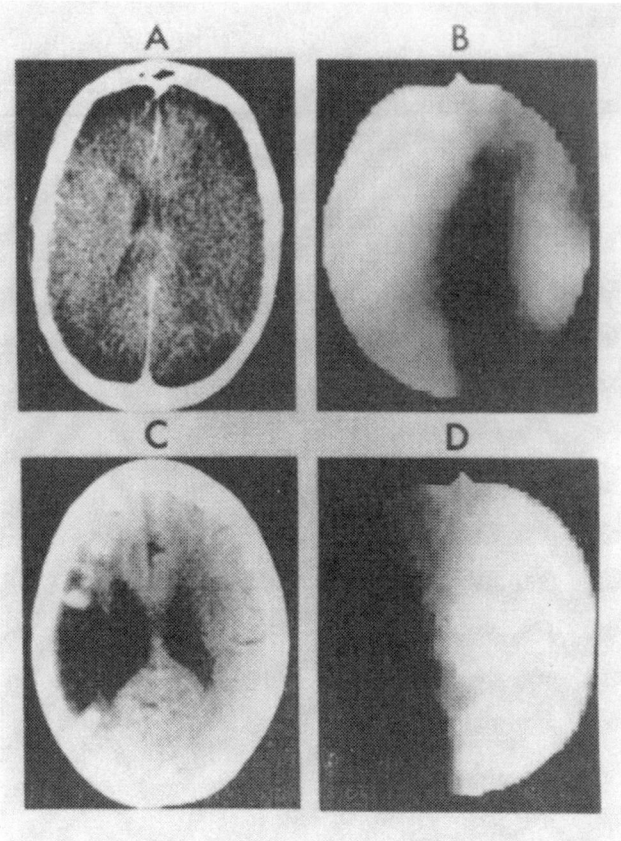

Fig. 4. CT scans and corresponding behavioral images of two patients with cerebral infarcts, one in the right hemisphere (A and B for CT and behavioral image, respectively) and one in the left (C and D). The CT scans were reversed so that the left hemisphere is to the viewer's left. (Figure 4 appears in Gur *et al*, "Behavioral Imaging" – A procedure for analysis and display of neuropsychological test scores: I. Construction of algorithm and initial clinical evaluation, *Neuropsychiatry, Neuropsychology, and Behavioral Neurology* 1988; 1:53).

"behavioral weights" against anatomic and physiologic data. As "behavioral images" are contrasted with the anatomic and physiologic neuroimaging data, theories on brain and behavior can be tested and refined. Understanding of the effects of neural tissue and bone on propagation of photons helped improve the quality of anatomic and physiologic brain images. Analogously, improvement of neuropsychological theories will lead to better clarity and resolution of the "behavioral image".

References

1. Kety SS, Schmidt CF. The nitrous oxide method for the quantitative determination of cerebral blood flow in man: theory, procedure and normal values. J Clin Invest 1948; 27:476.
2. Olesen J, Paulson OB, Lassen NA. Regional cerebral blood flow in man determined by the initial slope of the clearance of intra-arterially injected 133Xe. Stroke 1971; 2:519.
3. Obrist WD, Thompson HK, Wang HS *et al.* Regional cerebral blood flow estimated by 133-Xenon inhalation. Stroke 1975; 6:245.
4. Reivich M, Kuhl D, Wolf AP *et al.* The 18-F-fluorodeoxyglucose method for the measurement of local cerebral glucose utilization in man. Circ Res 1979; 44:127.
5. Risberg J, Ingvar DH. Patterns of activation in the grey matter of the dominant hemisphere during memorizing and reasoning. Brain 1973; 96:737.
6. Reivich M, Gur RC, Alavi A. Positron emission tomographic studies of sensory stimuli, cognitive processes, and anxiety. Human Neurobio 1983; 2:25.
7. Gur RC, Reivich M. Cognitive task effects on hemispheric blood flow in humans. Brain Lang 1980; 9:78.
8. Gur RC, Gur RE, Obrist WE *et al.* Sex and handedness differences in cerebral blood flow during rest and cognitive activity. Science 1982; 217:659.
9. Gur RC, Gur RE, Rosen AD *et al.* A cognitive-motor network demonstrated by positron emission tomography. Neuropsychologia 1983; 21:601.
10. Gur RC, Trivedi SS, Saykin S, Resnick SM, Malamut BL, Gur RE. Behavioral imaging. J of Clinical and Experimental Neuropsychology 1985; 7:633.

9. Computerized EEG in cardiac surgery

E.H.J.F. BOEZEMAN, J.A. LEUSINK and
F.E.E. VERMEULEN

Introduction

EEG analysis is indicated in those cases in which cerebral ischemia may
arise from procedures performed during cardiac surgery. The EEG is extremely
sensitive to brain dysfunction [1] caused, for instance, by cerebral hypoperfusion or changing metabolism caused by different anaesthetics [2, 3]. Due
to its sensitivity, the EEG provides general information concerning the
condition of the patient involved. Observing the EEGs during surgery remains
a hazardous task because of the enormous amount of EEG information
generated from several cases simultaneously. It is obvious that automatic
analysis is essential to interpret this information within the limited period of
the surgical procedure. Automatic analysis of the EEG during cardiac surgery
is focussed on three hallmarks. First is detection of brain dysfunction related
to anaesthesiological and surgical procedures with the shortest possible delay
so that its cause can be discovered and the efficacy of the course of action
can be checked. Second, it is essential to have a built-in warning/alarm system
to indicate when the margins of safety have been reached. Automatic analysis
without such a system is useless and brings one no further than conventional
strip chart recording. Such a warning system is based on the experience of
the clinical neurophysiologist and can be considered an artificial intelligence
system. The third is documentation of brain function in relationship to all other
parameters being monitored; this brings up its capabilities for evaluating the
impact of new anaesthesiological and surgical procedures on brain function
in this fast developing field.

The present analysis pays attention to the following topics: the monitoring
system, crucial moments during surgery, and preliminary results of outcome
at the intensive care unit. The system has been running now for 9 years. This
contribution reflects our overall experience in almost 11,000 cases.

114

The monitoring system

Figure 1 shows a block diagram of the compact monitoring system. It presents the flow of information from the patient to the computer and so to the anaesthesiologist who controls a special function keyboard. The EEG is recorded with an EEG device and transmitted to a computer (DEC PDP 11/03) connected to a minicomputer (DEC PDP 11/34).

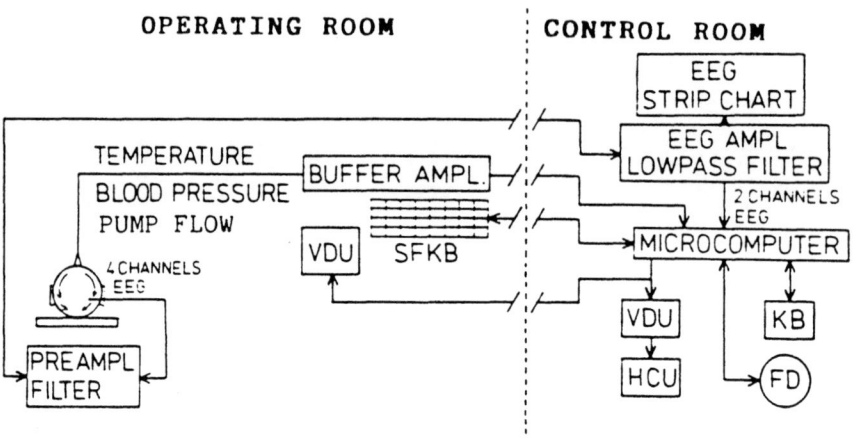

Fig. 1. The configuration of the EEG monitoring system in the operating room and in the control room. The abbreviations indicate: VDU, visual display unit; SFKB, disk drive; HCU: hard copy unit.

Data acquisition

For the recording of the EEG from both hemispheres silver-silver chloride discs are used. These are filled with a conducting paste and are reliable for long term monitoring. To improve electrode stability gauze pads of 2 × 2 cm are fixed with collodion over the electrodes and the surrounding scalp. With this set-up one is able to record a follow-up EEG in the ICU 24 hours later, as needed, without using new electrodes. During anaesthesia and cooling, the electric activity of the brain usually differs little between the scalp regions, so bipolar long distance symmetrical montages are used. Of the 10–20 system, we use for computer analysis F4–P4 (rightside) and F3–P3 (leftside). Needle electrodes are not advisable since the patient is under anaesthesia and there is little time to position them properly. Fixation remains a problem, especially after the operation, if a follow-up EEG is necessary. Further polarisation artifacts may occur quite often. The bio-electric activity from both montages is written on a strip chart to check for artifacts (carried out by an EEG technologist). A special filter was designed for filtering out artifacts caused by electrocautery [4]. A 50 Hz notch filter was used to eliminate the main voltage interference at 50 Hz. If an electrode artifact is observed, data analysis and presentation is briefly interrupted by the EEG technologist. An artifact message is transmitted to the video monitor situated in the operating room. Meanwhile the artifact is repaired.

In addition to the patient's EEG, other important parameters are sampled and presented as well, i.e., the arterial blood pressure, the pump flow and temperature of the perfusion blood, and finally the nasopharyngeal temperature. A special function keyboard, built into the anaesthesiologists front end workspace and connected to the computer, is used by the anaesthesiologist to note the dose related administration of drugs, e.g., Fentanyl, Diazepam, or special events during the operation such as the beginning and end of the cardiopulmonary bypass. These data are displayed on the VDU. For recall, data retrieval is also possible using this keyboard (Figure 2).

SPECIAL FUNCTION KEYBOARD

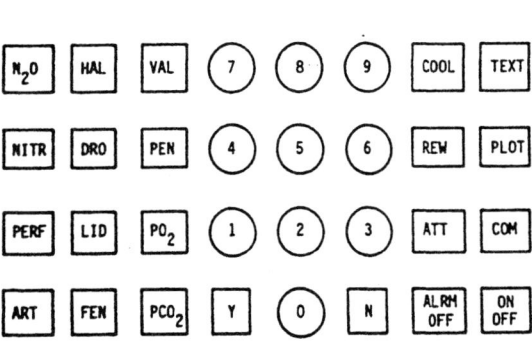

Fig. 2. Special function keyboard with on/off keys for alphanumerical data and numerical data (0–9) for dosage. The abbreviations indicate: N_2O, nitrous oxide/oxygen; NITR, nitroprusside; PERF, arterial perfusion; ART, signal artifacts; HAL, halothane; DRO, droperiodol; LID, lidocaine; FEN, fentanyl; VAL, valium; PEN, pentothal; PO_2, arterial partial pressure of oxygen; pCO_2, arterial partial pressure of carbon dioxide; Y, YES key (dosage); N, NO key (dosage); COOL, cooling of a patient; REW, rewarming of a patient; ATT, attention key for asking attention of the user when an EEG warning and/or alarm is detected; ALRM, key for disabling the EEG warning program; TEXT, key for requesting the retrieval of alphanumerical data; PLOT, key for requesting the retrieval of graphical data; COM, key for storage of special anesthetic and/or surgical events; ON/OFF, on/off key of the monitoring system.

Data processing

After filtering (0.5–30 Hz) and amplifying, the EEG signal is fed into the computer for digitalization (sampling rate 200 Hz). The method of processing is based on the determination of zero-crossing intervals during 15 seconds that are defined by positive direction or negative direction zero-crossings through the baseline of the EEG.

The wave durations are converted into frequency values and stored into a zero-crossing histogram during a 60 second epoch. Asymmetry detection can be performed by sequential analysis of asymmetry indices or values. A simple measure is the difference in EEG zero-crossings of the left and right hemisphere in percentages. We use the relative, i.e., individual differences in EEG zero-crossings, instead of absolute differences because this can be easily compared among different cases. A mean value of the EEG amplitude is determined after rectifying and integrating the EEG signal.

Pronk and Simons [5, 6] investigated which method of analysis was the most appropriate for detecting patterns of abnormal EEG activity. They compared the following pattern recognition methods: special analysis, period-amplitude analysis, autoregressive filtering using Kalman filtering, and Hjorth descriptors. They came to the conclusion that even such a simple method as period-amplitude analysis gives satisfactory results as a data reduction method for long-term perioperative EEG monitoring. Glaria and Murray [7] stress the fact that most workers in this field have found that their techniques produce good results. This is based on the fact that these techniques supply both frequency and amplitude information that are essential for recording reliable EEG trends.

One of the main features of the system concerns the possibility of producing warnings and alarms on which action can be taken. This set-up can be considered an on line automatic EEG interpreter during anaesthesia and surgery (Expert System). Clinical experience obtained from the ongoing EEG forms the basis of the system. The zero-crossing rates and amplitudes of the two recorded EEG signals are checked every 15 seconds for 3 types of abnormal EEG activity:

1) Slow waves (SLOW EEG); i.e., if the average number of zero-crossing falls below 52 (about 1.0 Hz).
2) Slow waves of low amplitude (LOW EEG); i.e., as slow EEG but with an average amplitude that falls below 15 μV.
3) Unilateral slow wave and/or low amplitude activity, i.e., an asymmetry exceeding 8% is called SLIGHT, an asymmetry exceeding 14% is called SEVERE.

The warning and alarm signals are presented in this order of priority. The computer program has a logical decision tree structure. After checking the zero-crossing rates, as well as the amplitude values, the software tests whether the patient is on cardiopulmonary bypass, i.e., cooled or rewarmed or has been given anaesthetics that affect the EEG. If no explanation is found a visual warning, i.e., SLOW EEG, is generated on the VDU followed by an auditory alarm in case the user does not respond by pressing an attention key on the special function keyboard. If simultaneously systolic blood pressure falls below 50 torr an additional LOW PRESS warning signal appears. The warnings are only presented after a steady state of 2 minutes. This software based system makes the immediate supervision of an expert in this field, i.e., a clinical neurophysiologist unnecessary. If artifacts occur that are difficult to distinguish from biological activity, the neurophysiologist can attend to slave monitors situated in the EEG department outside the operating complex showing the histograms and the ongoing EEG.

Data presentation

Figure 3 shows the presentation of the data on the VDU monitor in the operating room. The EEG wavelength histograms of successive 1-minute time intervals are presented from the bottom to the top showing a trend analysis. For signalling relatively fast changes in the patient data, instantaneous numerical values of the parameters are determined and displayed every 15 seconds at the top of the VDU. Figure 4 shows the spatial relationship of the trend analysis (VDU) with the special function keyboard in the operating room.

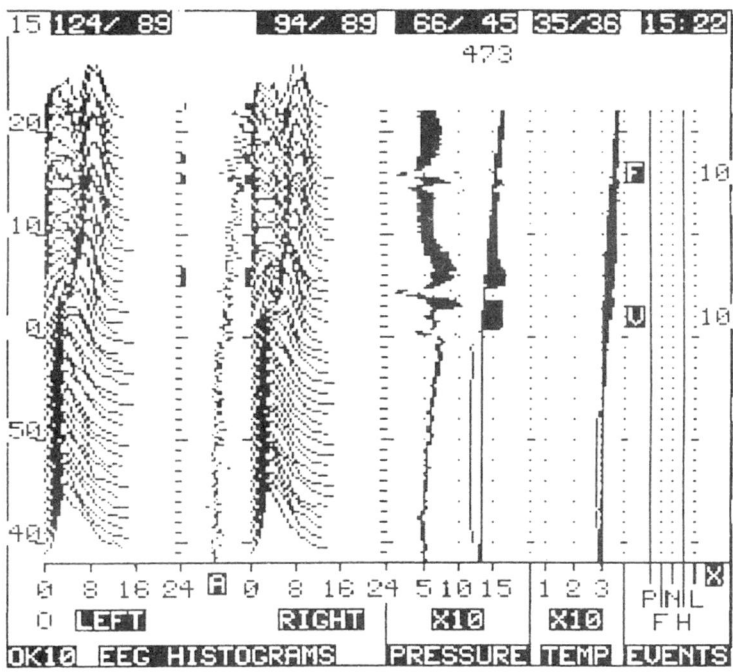

Fig. 3. From left to right are displayed: 1) Time setting from the bottom to the top. 2) EEG wave length histograms of the left hemisphere with a zero crossing rate of 124 (top line) and mean amplitude of 89 uV. 3) Integrated EEG amplitude values (=A) of both hemispheres with an amplitude scale of 0–100 uV. 4) EEG wavelength histograms of the right hemisphere with a zero crossing rate of 94 and mean amplitude of 89 uV. 5) Systolic and diastolic values (66/45 torr) of the arterial blood pressure; horizontal scale 0–200 torr. 6) Pump flow; 4.73 l/min. The curve is presented but the horizontal scaling is not yet modified. A dark area between the theoretical flow – dependent on body surface and temperature of perfusion blood – and the real flow indicates overflow; a white area indicates underflow. 7) Nasopharyngeal temperature (=35° C) and the temperature of the perfusion blood (=36°C); horizontal scale 5–37°C; a dark area between the temperature curves indicates rewarming; a white area indicates cooling. 8) Event marker columns indicating the type and dosage of drugs and their time of administration. F, fentanyl; V, valium; P, arterial perfusion; N, nitrous oxide/oxygen; H, halothane; L, lidocaine.

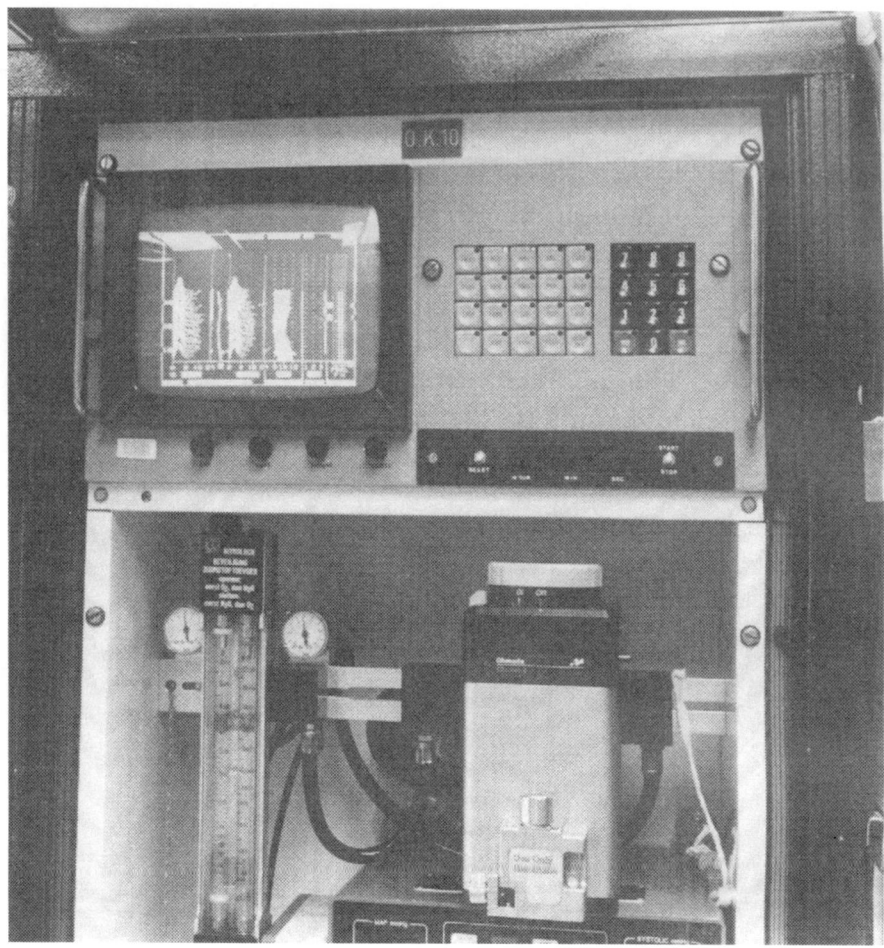

Fig. 4. The spatial relationship of the VDU with the special function keyboard in the operating room on top of the respirator control unit.

Data documentation

Finally, at the end of the procedure, all graphical and alphanumerical data are copied by a hard copy device. A report is provided that focuses on any abnormality and states whether complications are to be expected or not.

Figure 5 shows such documentation.

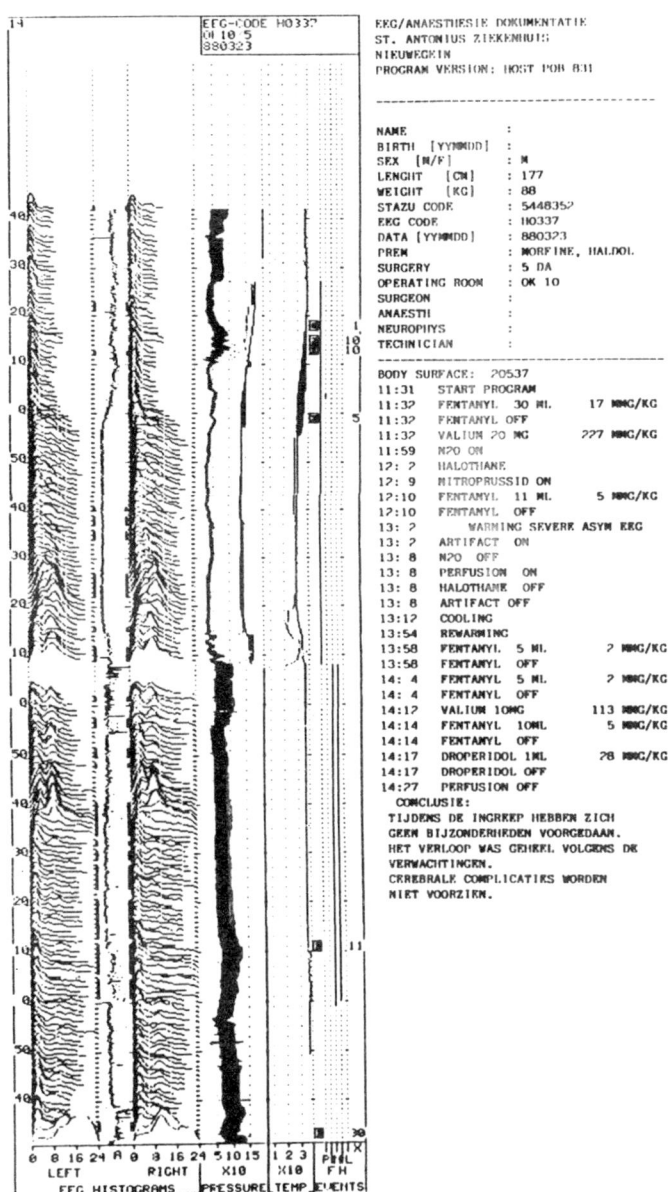

Fig. 5. Documentation of patient data at the end of the operation. On the left hand side, the EEG histograms and the curves of the anesthetic data that are displayed from the bottom to the top. On the right hand side, the alphanumerical data file that is printed from the top to the bottom.

Results

EEG – Normal procedure

Figure 5 shows the typical course of an uneventful procedure. It illustrates the minor alterations that take place under the influence of anaesthetics, cardiopulmonary bypass and hypothermia. It also shows the sensitivity of the system to the patient's state of awareness or anaesthesia-depth. The operation starts at 10.30 (read from bottom to top). The very first histograms show a peak around 9 Hz indicating alpha rhythm. In that period the patient is still awake and on our request had his eyes closed. Alpha, as well as beta activity rapidly disappear following a shot of 1500 μg Fentanyl. The EEG becomes slow. Around eleven o'clock, volatile inhalation agents like N20/02 and halothane are introduced producing a faster and lower voltage EEG. Simultaneously, electrocautery takes place as shown by the interrupted heavy black lines printed alongside the histograms. At 11.40 a change takes place in the patient's state of awareness. As one can see there is an alpha wave coming up around 8 Hz indicating a higher level of awareness. In addition, this alpha bump is preceded by a little bump around 4 Hz. Because of this latter finding it is thought that the patient is still sufficiently anaesthesized and no further action is taken. At 12.00, high voltage changes occur quite suddenly (see A) that are caused by artifacts. The histograms therefore are interrupted for 5 minutes during which time repair takes place. Introduction of the bypass is at 12.08. Cooling is briefly at 20 centigrade and then returns to 29 centigrade blood temperature. The nasopharyngeal temperature lags behind. During that time the EEG histograms show an immediate loss of fast activity (20–24 Hz). The bump around 8 Hz becomes clearer, most likely caused by dilution of the analgesics. Following the bypass, there is a drop in blood pressure (< 50 mm Hg) and a gradual decrease of amplitude develops.

At 12.30 the situation is stable, i.e., a moderately slow EEG around 4 Hz, no clear alpha wave and low amplitude. The nasopharyngeal temperature is 29 centigrade, the blood pressure is around 50 Torr, the pump flow is stable.

At 12.56 rewarming starts followed by a dose of fentanyl. Because of that, the EEG becomes slower. At 13.12 hours this effect becomes more pronounced because of the additional amounts of Droperidol, Fentanyl and Diazepam. At that time the blood pressure is higher. The heart is already beating and a moment later the bypass is disconnected. At the end of the surgery, the EEG is still slow but in an acceptable range because of the drugs given in an earlier phase.

EEG – Abnormal procedure

We have investigated the mortality and morbidity rate in a population of 4500 cases who underwent coronary artery bypass grafting (CABG) and/or replacement of heart valves. We have only looked for gross abnormalities like stroke, encephalopathy, and cardiac failures. Because we monitor nearly all our patients, EEG data are mostly available.

The morbidity rate was 0.44% and the mortality rate was 0.60%. Combined rate was 1.04% (47/4500). If one looks to milder abnormalities the combined rate is of course very much higher [8]. CABG procedures do not produce significantly higher morbidity and mortality rates than the other procedures (0.6% versus 0.4%). Cardiac failures (0.4%) were the main causes for the mortality rate. As to morbidity, neurological injury like stroke and encephalopathy prevailed (0.4%). Of the 47 cases investigated, 16 cases had normal EEG findings peroperatively. These cases however, sustained organ failures following the intervention from hours to days later in the ICU. From a neurophysiological point of view they sustained the procedure very well. In another 8 cases EEG recordings were not available because those were emergency procedures. So finally, 23 cases remained with abnormal EEG findings.

The peroperative EEG findings can be divided in two types, those with diffuse abnormalities (13 cases) and those with focal abnormalities (10 cases). Table 1 shows the relationship with the specific events that caused these abnormalities.

Table 1.

| | Peroperative EEG findings* | | |
	Diffuse	Focal	All
Low perfusion	6	2	8
Emboli	1	7	8
Uncertain	6	0	7
All	13	10	23

*The numerical data represent the number of cases.

Diffuse EEG abnormalities in our material lead generally to a diffuse encephalopathy caused by a haemodynamic instability. Figure 6 shows a diffuse slow and low voltage EEG as a reaction to a sudden drop in blood pressure at 11.35 during rewarming. At 10.03 a similar event occurred with less effect because the brain was still protected by moderate cooling. Increased perfusion (not shown) did not improve brain function. This patient did not recover and subsequently died following a period of a persistent vegetative state. A suddenly decreased perfusion during cardiopulmonary bypass is the main cause of diffuse abnormalities in the EEG. Automatic analysis can detect this on-line and gives insight into the efficacy of the protective measures as shown in Figure 7. Following the introduction of bypass at 9.54, a SLOW EEG appears at 10.00, followed by a LOW EEG at 10.02. The pump flow and blood pressure are both decreased. The perfusion of the brain is seriously diminished at that time. Following the slow increase of perfusion at 10.10, brain function is restored at 10.35 without further complications in the ICU.

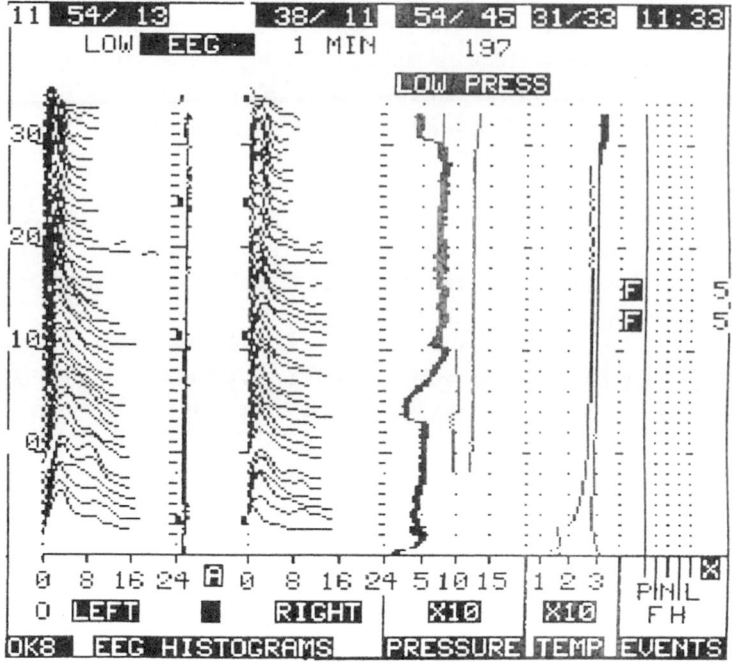

Fig. 6. Low EEG alarm as a consequence of low perfusion during rewarming.

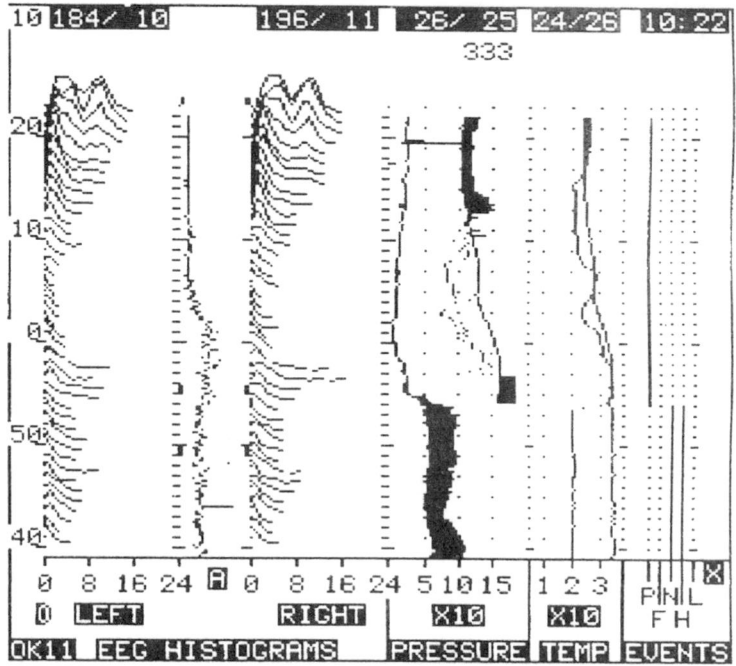

Fig. 7. Improvement of brain function following an increase in perfusion.

There are diffuse abnormalities during bypass (6 cases) of which the causes are uncertain. Figure 8 shows a slow EEG at the end of the rewarming despite the fact that hemodynamic factors like pump flow and blood pressure have apparently sufficient values. This case sustained a prolonged encephalopathy in ICU, for reasons which are unclear. In the literature [9], suggestions have been made that a defective cerebral autoregulation in hypertensive patients with arteriolar disease may be responsible, or an unrecognized stenosis of the carotid artery that may lead to low perfusion. A partial explanation can be found in the preoperative EEG [10, 11] with diffuse abnormalities as we observed in 2 cases that increased throughout the operation without recovery. Both had an encephalopathy.

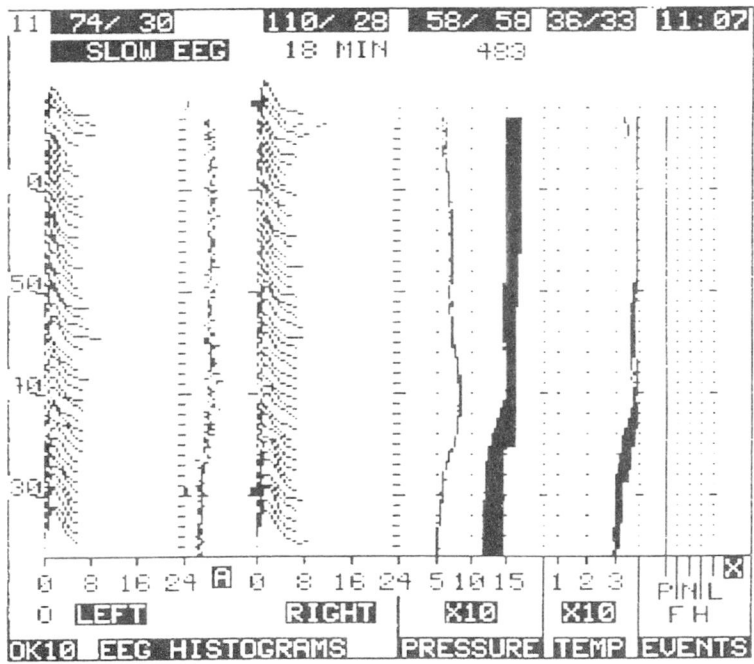

Fig. 8. Slow EEG at the end of rewarming with sufficient values for blood pressure and pump flow.

Focal abnormalities in our material lead mostly to stroke caused by emboliza-tion, i.e., air in the heart or bypass lines; brittle aorta at the side of the clamping or cardiac arrhythmia. Figure 9 shows an example of embolization from air bubbles that were observed too late in the bypass line at the start of the bypass. The left hemisphere lags behind quite suddenly at 15.32. There is a loss of fast waves in the EEG as shown in the histograms around that time. After auto-matic alarming for a severe asymmetric EEG, the pump flow and blood pressure are raised at 15.35. The asymmetry is reduced and the patient awoke

124

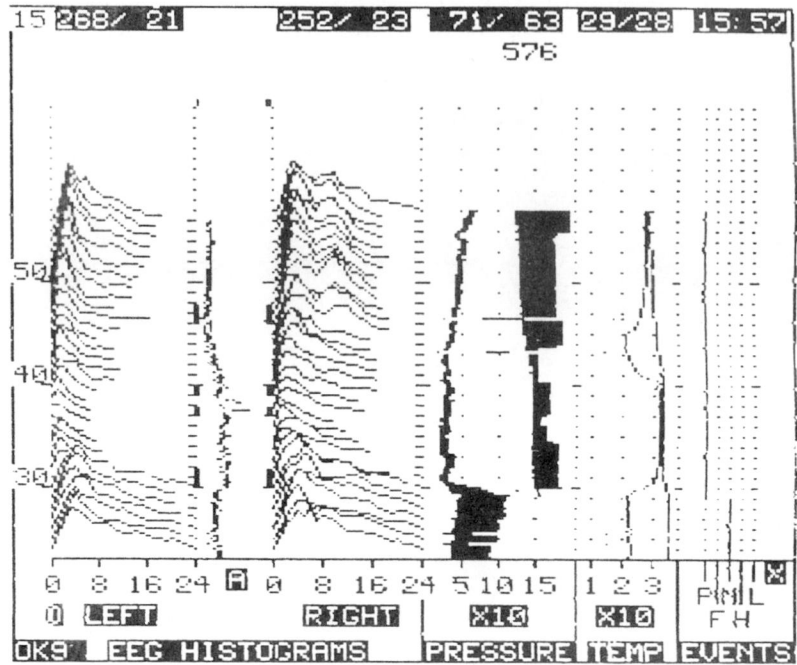

Fig. 9. Asymmetric EEG at the start of the bypass at 15.32 caused by embolization. Improvement follows after increase in blood pressure.

with a slight hemiparesis at the right side that they recovered from. A few focal abnormalities are not explained by the peroperative EEG findings. They are mainly based on preoperative EEG abnormalities like dysfunction of the temporal lobe caused by cerebrovascular disease.

A special remark has to be made about the rewarming procedure. Indeed fact rewarming, i.e., a difference of more than 8 degrees between blood and nasopharyngeal temperature, gives rise to more diffuse EEG abnormalities than slow rewarming [12], as shown respectively in Figures 10 and 11. Fast rewarming starts at 10.47 immediately followed by a slow EEG with high amplitudes while the pump flow and blood pressure have sufficient values. Slow rewarming starts at 15.00. The EEG remains stable throughout this period. Its significance concerning clinical outcome is as yet not quite clear. In our material it has not been taken as a sign of gross clinical abnormalities.

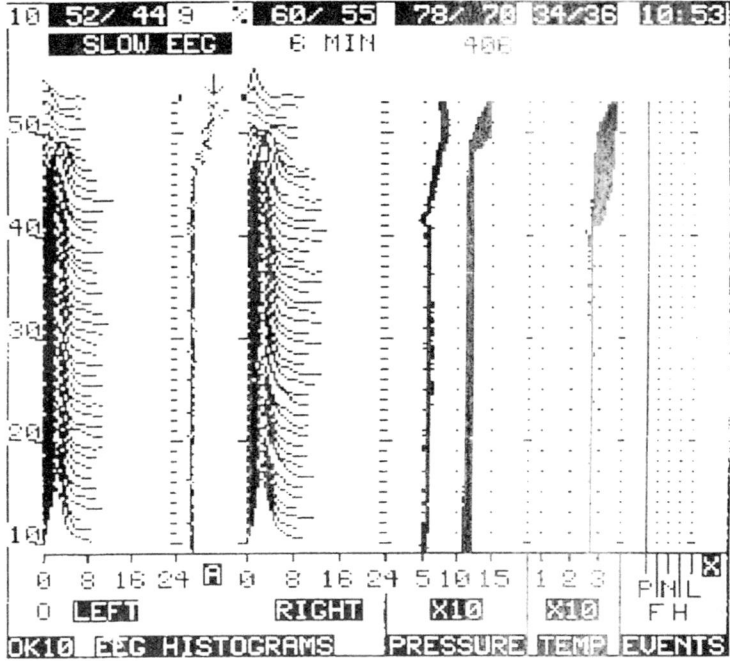

Fig. 10. Fast rewarming at 10.47. Slow EEG warning appears.

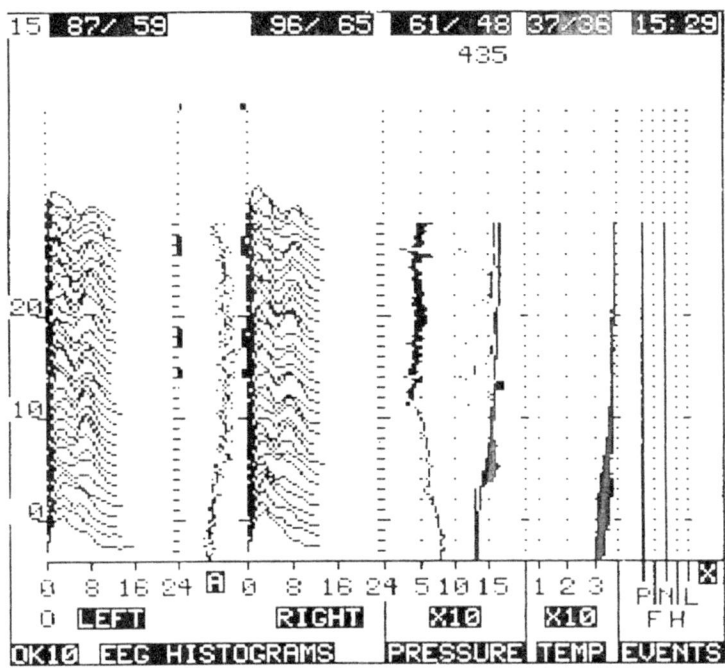

Fig. 11. Slow rewarming at 15.00. The EEG remains stable.

Conclusions

1. Automatic EEG monitoring provides an ongoing measure of brain function in relationship to hemodynamic and anesthetic variables.
2. The Expert system automatically generates warnings based on logical decision procedures concerning the type and the degree of the cerebral change.
3. The Expert system provides guidelines for surgical and anesthetic procedures so that one can work within safe margins. If these are exceeded, however, it shows the impact of the corrective measures on brain function that have to be taken.
4. The anaesthetist does not need to have extensive knowledge of clinical neurophysiology and experience with EEG monitoring.
5. Finally the significance and the value of a monitoring system is dependent on the degree of motivation and attention to its use. All data and events that are important for the automatic decision procedure should be entered into the computer using the special function keyboard.

References

1. Sulg I. Quantitative EEG as a measure of brain dysfunction. In: Pfurtscheller G, Jonkman EJ, Lopes da Silva FH (eds). Brain Ischemia: Quantitative EEG and Imaging Techniques. Progress in Brain Research. Vol. 62. Elsevier Science Publishers B.V., 1984; p. 65.
2. Simons AJR, Pronk RAF. Computing in anaesthesia and intensive care. In: Prakash O (eds). Automatic EEG Monitoring During Anaesthesia. Boston: Martinus Nijhoff Publishers, 1983; p. 227.
3. Simons AJR, Pronk RAF. Les donnees electroencephalographiques pendant la chirurgie a coeur ouvert. Leur analyse automatique en relation avec les parametres anesthesiques et son utilisation pour la surveillance peroperatoire de la fonction cerebrale. Rev EEG Neurophysiol 1982; 12:243.
4. Weide H van der, Pronk RAF. Interference suppression for EEG-recording during open heart surgery. Electroenceph Clin Neurophysiol 1979; 46:609.
5. Pronk RAF, Simons AJR. Automatic recognition of abnormal EEG activity during open heart and carotid surgery. In: Buser PA, Cobb WA, Okuma T (eds.). Kyoto Symposes. Amsterdam: Elsevier Biomedical Press, 1982; p. 590.
6. Pronk RAF, Simons AJR. Processing of the electroencephalogram in cardiac surgery. Computer Programs In Biomedicine. Elsevier Science Publishers B.V., 1984; 18:181.
7. Glaria TP, Murray A. Comparison of EEG monitoring techniques: an evaluation during cardiac surgery. Electroenceph Clin Neurophysiol 1985; 61:323.
8. Shaw PJ, MRCP, Bates D, FRPC, Cartlidge NEF, FRCP, French JM, BSc, Heaviside D, FFARCS, Julian DG, MD, FRCP, Shaw DA FRCP. Neurologic and neuro-psychological morbidity following major surgery: comparison of coronary artery bypass and peripheral vascular surgery. Stroke 1987; 18:700.
9. Furlan AJ, Breuer AC. Central nervous system complications of open heart surgery. Stroke 1984; 15:912.
10. Sotaniemi K. Five-year neurological and EEG outcome after open-heart surgery. J Neurol Neurosurg Psychiatry 1985; 48:569.
11. Sotaniemi K. Clinical and prognostic correlates of EEG in open-heart surgery patients. J Neurol Neurosurg Psychiatry 1980; 43:941.
12. Levy WJ, MD. Quantitative analysis of EEG changes during hypothermia. Anesthesiology 1984; 60:291.

10. Clinical electroencephalographic assessment of cerebral impairment

FREDERICK A. STRUVE

The relationship between cardiovascular integrity and optimal cerebral functioning is both intimate and complex. The brain constantly consumes the body's available oxygen and glucose in prodigious amounts which are clearly disproportionate to its own weight, and its most recently evolved structure – the cortical mantle – is uniquely sensitive to metabolic compromise [1–3]. Clearly a variety of disturbances of cardiac function might be expected to produce measurable alterations in brain function ranging from the dramatic and catastrophic to effects which are subclinical and quite subtle. Not infrequently cardiovascular induced compromise of cerebral metabolic needs will result in alterations of one kind or another in the ongoing electrical activity of the brain.

The history of electroencephalography (EEG) extends back 114 years to 1875 when Caton recorded fluctuating electrical activity from the brains of living rabbits and monkeys [4]. His conviction that the rhythmic cyclical potentials he observed were directly related to *functional* activity of the brain presaged the emergence over fifty years later of EEG as a useful tool for the study of human brain function. Other early studies [5, 6] using animal models and equipment primitive by today's standards confirmed Caton's findings and in 1892 Beck and Cybulski [7] demonstrated that the brain electrical activity of the dog could be altered by localized cortical injury – thus providing perhaps the first experimental result predictive of subsequent uses of EEG in detecting localized structural, vascular, or traumatically induced damage to the brain in humans. Although many other animal studies successfully demonstrating alterations of brain electrical activity under various conditions continued to appear, such empirical findings were, as the Gibbs' have noted [8], not readily accepted and were often ignored by the "leaders of neurology and neurophysiology" of the time. It was not until the persevering German psychiatrist Hans Berger began publishing his classic series of investigations [9] on the "Elektrenekphalogramm des Menschen" from 1929 through 1938 that EEG much as we now recognize it began to be accepted and used. Berger was completely dedicated to the quest for understanding the physiological basis for psychic and cognitive function and his empirical studies in this respect were far ranging and varied. Long before his outstanding studies of the human EEG he was probing into the effects of intracranial blood circulation [10] and one suspects that, were he alive today, his approval of a volume focusing on cerebral damage before and after cardiac surgery would be assured.

The basic parameters of EEG recording methodology and the electroencephalographic findings expected with normal individuals have been well documented over many years and are well summarized in standard reference works [8, 11–19]. Furthermore over the years there has emerged a general acceptance of the relevance of EEG recording methods in the study of a truly wide variety of cerebral dysfunctions extending well beyond their original applications in epilepsy [20–21] and cerebral tumor detection [22]. In addition to seizure disorders and neoplastic structure lesions, the visually analyzed EEG can undergo change and alteration with: head trauma, vascular disorders of the brain, coma, degenerative disorders, infective and noninfective encephalopathies and cerebral inflammatory processes, dementias, metabolic and endocrinological dysfunctions impacting on cerebral function, heavy metal exposures, electrolytic imbalances, toxic reactions to abused or prescribed substances or industrial solvents, cerebral effects of nutritional deficits and many other variables which either directly or indirectly affect the brain's neurophysiological substrate. Certainly such a large scope of application cannot be detailed here and interested readers must consult available specialty texts in the field [12–14, 16–18, 22–27]. The previously referenced [18] large volume edited by Niedermeyer and Lopes da Silva is a particularly comprehensive desk volume which many will find useful in this respect. Understandably many clinical areas where strong EEG-clinical correlations exist are not germane to issues of cardiac disease and cerebral impairment and they cannot be covered in this space.

Methodological and conceptual issues

There seems to be an inherent human tendency to think in dichotomous terms and in the case of EEG evaluations one frequently is asked simply if the recording is normal or abnormal. Such a dichotomy is an artificial one and if unchecked will lead to conceptual confusion in a number of ways. By itself the term "abnormal EEG" has little meaning and without further clarification it cannot even be presumed to have clinical relevance. Instead we must recognize that the EEG can be "abnormal" in a great variety of ways all of which may have considerably different implications. Some EEG findings are associated with such low symptom expressivity that it is difficult to establish what, if any, diagnostic relevance they possess while other patterns instill truly grave clinical concern. Most are somewhere in-between.

A serious conceptual problem arises when a normal-abnormal dichotomy is applied to normal population studies. One frequently hears it stated that 10, 15 or 20% of the normal population have "abnormal" EEGs. Such statistical offerings are common in discussions related to the use of EEG in psychiatry [28–34]. However, those EEG findings in normals are largely accounted for by minor and clinically inconsequential patterns existing at the borderland of clinical relevance. In a previous paper [35] we reviewed sixteen available EEG studies of adult normal control subjects and collectively these studies involved 6,752 "normal" individuals. A weighted average of all EEG "abnormalities" reported by the various authors was 18% for the combined subject population. However, when only clinically moderate to serious EEG abnormality was allowed to remain (we removed all minor findings) the control percentage of EEG abnormality shrunk to about 3%. In the same paper we also generated similar findings in an analysis of sixteen studies of EEG abnormality in normal control children which collectively involved 1,898 normal youngsters. Clearly opinions suggesting that a high percentage of the normal population have abnormal EEGs rests on EEG inclusion criteria of unrealistic leniency.

Ideally control populations for EEG studies should be screened rigorously to eliminate all subjects with current or past histories of relevant medical, neurological, and neuropsychiatric conditions as well as instances of head trauma. Unfortunately only a few investigators have attempted to do this [36–37]. In fact so called normal control groups often have not been comprised of normal individuals at all but have consisted of psychiatric outpatients [38], patients referred for EEG study who were not epileptic [39] or patients hospitalized for a variety of conditions felt to be unrelated to brain damage [40–42]. Some investigators have re-examined normal control groups more carefully and when they did so, significant proportions of subjects, ranging from 3.4% to 22.8%, were found to have antecedent conditions that could have affected the EEG [43–46]. Those wishing to include EEG measures in research studies of cardiac patients would be wise to ensure that comparison or control subjects are screened specifically by history and examination to eliminate cardiovascular as well as other conditions (including neuropsychiatric) that could alter EEG activity.

Electroencephalographic interpretation involves a complex process of pattern recognition which becomes fully developed only after long periods of consistent practice. It cannot be achieved simply by "reading a few records" now and again and it represents a skill which may atrophy through disuse. Differences in interpretive accuracy and acumen do exist between electro-encephalographers and, at least in some instances, poorly recorded and/or poorly read tracings have occurred. For example, ten years ago Hooshmand reviewed 96 clinical EEG tracings and their accompanying reports which he had obtained from 41 different electroencephalographers and found [47] that 17.7% of the EEG reports contained major interpretive errors and 7.2% of the tracings were so poorly taken that accurate interpretation was not possible. Interpretive error was not at all subtle but instead involved interpreting signals such as pulse, loose electrode, and eye movement artifact as abnormal potentials of brain origin. In other fields, problems of observer measurement error are addressed by demonstrating satisfactory levels of either inter-rater or intra-rater reliability figures. Both are appropriate for EEG interpretation assessment but unfortunately neither are often attempted. When reliability studies of EEG interpretation have been done sometimes the results have been regrettably poor [48–51]. However, among experienced interpreters high levels of interpretive reliability sufficient for both clinical and research purposes can be achieved [52–58]. While reliability of EEG interpretation can never be taken for granted, it is certainly obtainable given the motivation to develop it. It should be expected by investigators using clinical laboratory services and it should be pursued by laboratories engaged in investigative research.

One final methodological consideration involves the completeness of the electroencephalographic study. Since many EEG findings associated with cardiac disease will primarily involve alterations of frequency, amplitude or composition of background activity, it is tempting to view long wake EEG studies as adequate. Perhaps in many cases they will be all that is needed. However, focal spike and spike-wave activity with or without overt seizure development can occur as sequelae of localized or regional cerebral ischemia following cardiovascular cerebral embarrassment. Because of such possibilities, sleep recording should always be considered because it potentiates the appearance of paroxysmal dysrhythmic activity [33, 59, 60]. A variety of other activating techniques including sensory, cognitive and pharmacological activators are given comprehensive discussion by Takahashi [61]. With a fragile cardiac patient certain activation procedures (i.e. strenuous hyperventilation, 24 hour sleep deprivation) are best avoided. Certain activating methods specific for cardiac and cerebrovascular induced EEG change will be discussed later.

Limitations of noninvasive scalp EEG

Clinical EEG assessment can not be used properly unless the very real limitations of the method are seriously taken into account. Not all abnormal electrical discharges within the brain are detectable with current technology and normal tracings must be construed as at least having the potential to be false negatives.

The primary constraint in noninvasive clinical EEG is that the recording electrodes are insulated from the brain's activity by the impedance of the protective bony skull and dura. Even the brain tissue itself imposes impedance to the propagation of those electrical signals we seek to see. Restricted as we are to the surface of the head we are allowed a reasonable degree of recording coverage from only about one third of the outer convexity of the cortex – the so called "electroencephalographically accessible cortex" spoken of by Gibbs [22] or the "outer cortical mantle" described by Glaser [62]. If, for example, electrical dysregulation occurs in mesial, inferior and deep buried cortical tissue – as well as subcortical areas – the surface scalp EEG may be normal. Even within the accessible cortex events may occur which because of signal strength, location and other factors are not faithfully detected – or even detected at all – by scalp recordings. Based on comparative recordings made from scalp, cortex surface, and within brain locations it has been known for many years that both depth electrodes and cortical surface electrodes will reveal events not evident at the scalp [63–69].

A second limiting constraint involves the way in which paroxysmal dysrhythmias appear during the EEG recording. The term "paroxysmal" is used here to refer to frank generalized or focal spike and spike-wave discharges, many of which have strong correlations with seizures, as well as minor episodically occurring dysrhythmic patterns. Frequently these kinds of abnormal EEG features are not present during most of the recording period. Instead they may appear only infrequently and briefly [13, 14, 16, 20, 22] or they may occur only during certain levels of consciousness such as at the transition from wake to drowsy or during spindle sleep. Consequently the only safe recording strategy is to record for long periods of time to provide a fair chance for paroxysmal events to occur.

Because of these limitations, as well as others discussed elsewhere [35], a normal wake, sleep and activated EEG can only provide "presumptive evidence" that a scalp recordable EEG abnormality does not exist. A normal EEG can never be construed as positive evidence of lack of damage to the brain.

Just about all standard reference volumes stress that the majority of discrete EEG abnormalities are nonspecific as to cause. While there are exceptions in which certain characteristic EEG wave forms are pathognomonic of specific disease [70] (i.e., Jakob-Creutzfelt Disease, Herpes Simplex Encephalitis, Subacute Sclerosing Pan encephalitis), most EEG findings unfortunately will not point to a specific etiology. There are some who are sufficiently dismayed at EEG's failure to denote etiology that they would avoid its use on that limitation alone. A more useful view would be that positive test results suggest that something is wrong – even if the then required search for the cause may not turn out to be the easiest of tasks.

EEG and preoperative cardiac and cerebrovascular disease

Sufficient blood must circulate through the brain to sustain neuronal function and that blood at all times must contain sufficient oxygen and glucose to satisfy the metabolic needs of brain tissue. If for any reason blood volume is decreased or its contents become compromised, the neurons in the affected brain regions will begin to function improperly and symptoms of physical and/or cognitive dysfunction will emerge. Should the deficiency be severe or persist the neurons will eventually die and permanent brain damage (or death) may result. Compromised cardiac and/or cerebrovascular integrity represents a potent class of causes of such insults to the brain. With some of these insults, the resulting cerebral impairment will be associated with EEG change.

Cogenital and acquired heart disease

Clear broad generalizations about EEG correlates of cogenital heart disease are difficult to make because cerebral effects may depend heavily upon individual variation in pathology, severity of dysfunction and the specifics of hemodynamic change. Reports of high incidence of EEG abnormality among cogenital heart disease patients have been made [71–73] although in commenting on these studies and others, Niedermeyer has cautioned [74] that selection factors may inflate incidence figures in that patients with neurological complications are most often studied. Diffuse slowing may be seen with hypoxia [13] and may involve generalized delta activity in severe cases in which lethargy and coma occur [74]. Should localized brain abscesses or thrombotic lesions develop, the EEG will usually show focal slowing and epileptogenic paroxysmal activity may subsequently develop from areas of regional or focal hypoxic lesion [13, 73, 74].

EEG findings in acquired heart disease are also variable depending upon the nature of the pathophysiological processes involved and the degree to which clinical symptoms of cerebral involvement are present. When a high degree of cognitive integrity is maintained with little in the way of symptomatic cognitive difficulty, slowing of the EEG or other abnormal EEG features are not likely. In one study [75] we found that patients scheduled for mitral valve replacement had normal waking EEGs but displayed a marked interhemispheric asynchrony and/or shifting asymmetry of sleep spindles which suggested that subcortical effects might have been present. However their exact nature and the implications of such disordered sleep pattern findings remain unclear. Cardiac decompensation, when it occurs, is often associated with cerebral hypoxia and generally this would cause some degree of diffuse slowing to emerge in the EEG. However, those EEG changes stemming from oxygen compromise caused by cardiac impairment are not easily distinguishable from similar EEG effects associated with respiratory disease [76]. Initial EEG slowing, which may only involve a decrease in alpha frequency, would not be expected to correlate with clear cognitive difficulty even though it may denote early hypoxic change [77]. With later diffuse hypoxic encephalopathy increased severity of EEG slowing is seen, cognitive and attentional capabilities may suffer and eventually change in level of consciousness will occur. Some cardiac disease, such as bacterial endocarditis may at times be associated with secondary cerebral involvement (meningitis, brain abscess) and when this happens many focal or diffuse EEG abnormalities may appear – each dependent on the nature of the underlying cerebral event [74]. When rheumatic endocarditis results in embolic cerebral lesions with ensuing symptoms, the EEG may contain focal or generalized paroxysmal activity with or without focal slowing.

Cardiovascular and cerebrovascular syncope

Naquet and Vigouroux [78] have defined syncope as a sudden and brief loss of consciousness during transient generalized cerebral ischaemia associated with acute cerebral circulatory insufficiency. There are a variety of mechanisms which produce this response including several reflex syncopes, syncopal episodes related to cardiac disease including heart block and arrhythmias as well as impaired compensation for acute decrease in peripheral vascular resistance found in myocardial and cogenital heart disease, syncope from orthostatic hypotension and others [78, 79]. During a spontaneous or provoked syncopal episode, bilateral slow waves will appear in the EEG tracing and may consist of high voltage delta activity prior to loss of consciousness [14, 22, 78–80]. Following the syncopal attack normal EEG frequencies are restored. Between syncopal episodes the EEG is often normal [22] and cognitive signs of cerebral dysfunction would not be expected. However, since syncope is not uncommon in cardiovascular or cerebrovascular disorder EEG abnormalities related to those chronic ongoing conditions may be encountered [79]. EEG assessment of the syncopal complaint should be polygraphic with simultaneous recording of electrocardiographic data [79, 81–83].

Episodic syncopal attacks as well as brief episodes of dizziness, vertigo, light-headedness, visual changes (blurring, dimness), ataxia and the like without loss of consciousness are common in people past age 40 or 50 with basilar or carotid artery insufficiently. Such pathophysiological processes can also produce brief transient focal neurological signs or temporary confusion and cognitive distress. Often the EEG is within normal limits if recorded from patients who are clinically asymptomatic during intervals between discrete attacks. However, if ongoing neurological findings are present then the incidence of generalized or focal slowing or spiking may exceed eighty percent [84]. Some studies have reported low voltage tracings in basilar artery compromise [85]. It should be mentioned that should EEG abnormality be seen it may also relate to other ongoing chronic cardio-cerebral vascular disease as well.

Because normal EEGs are not uncommon during symptom free intervals there have been efforts to develop procedures which would precipitate EEG change in persons with symptoms suspected to rest on such insufficiency states. A long time ago Meyer and associates [86] used a tilt-table to induce varying speed postural tilts to 70 degrees in patients with cerebrovascular disease as well as a variety of comparison control subjects. It was reasoned that temporary postural reduction in cardiac output and collateral circulation would produce transient localized cerebral insufficiency with visible EEG alteration effects. Overt clinical symptoms during the tilt process were infrequent (about 6%) however postural tilt produced EEG changes (slowing bitemporally or over temporal region ipsilateral to occluded artery) in 91.3% of patients with carotid artery insufficiency and posterior slowing in 69.2% of patients with basilar artery compromise. Nearly half (45%) of patients referred for syncope without prior clinical evidence of cerebrovascular abnormality had positive tilt induced EEG change-usually compatible with carotid artery problems. Others have not reported the same experience [87]. Digital carotid artery compression has also been suggested as an activating procedure to assess functionally collateral circulation in patients with known or suspected insufficiency [88]. However, while the procedure is relatively safe with asymptomatic young people [88] it may be associated with considerable risk in clinical populations [89–92]. Only those with solid experience in this area should attempt this procedure and Kooi [13] has cautioned that the possibility of neurologic complications must be considered.

Neurogenic versus cardiogenic transient disturbances of autonomic/ cerebral function

Syncope, brief cognitive dysfunction or autonomic symptomatology (flushing, sweating, pallor, dizziness, viceral and sensory events) can be complex issues for some patients because symptom constellations in this domain can have either primary cardiological or cerebral origins.

In what Blumhart [93] refers to as "cardiogenic neurology", confusion arises when intermittent cardiac irregularities produce clinical events which resemble true primary brain lesion seizure phenomena. Not only can some of the symptoms seen with complex partial seizures emerge from arrhythmic cardiac dysfunctions but tonic-clonic seizures can have such causes as well [94, 95]. The distinction is not without clinical relevance because cardiogenic seizures may be refractory to traditional anticonvulsant treatment [94, 96] and require cardiac management instead. An electrocardiogram (which is usually of brief duration) and even prolonged Holter monitor studies will not capture all arrhythmic events. In this respect, Espinosa and associates [97] have taken advantage of long EEG recordings to include a single channel for simultaneous ECG monitoring as well. They have noted that in some patients referred for syncopal attacks who had prior normal cardiac evaluations, ECG arrhythmias correlating with clinical symptoms occurred during prolonged EEG study. As illustrations they describe two patients with normal cardiac studies who displayed spontaneous asystolic pauses of up to 3.9 and 6.0 seconds (which led to subsequent treatment with implanted pacemaker). Their recommendation that concomitant ECG registration be included in EEG studies seems sensible indeed and has been recognized by others [98, 99].

A clinical reality which is probably more often neglected by cardiology is the fact that primary paroxysmal epileptic discharges within the brain can sometimes trigger cardiac arrhythmias with their attendant overt physical symptoms. Using animal models [100, 101] it has been shown that stimulation of the diencephalon or orbitral cortex will induce cardiac arrhythmias and with humans a wide variety of cardiac arrhythmias have been seen to occur as secondary effects of primary brain originating seizure discharges [102–110]. In an important experiment Blumhardt and associates [111] secured 24 hour combined EEG and ECG ambulatory monitoring of 50 temporal lobe epilepsy patients who had no present or past evidence of cardiac disease. They found that 91% of the captured EEG seizures produced abrupt accelerations of heart rate and that with 30% of the EEG paroxysms tachycardia exceeding 140 BPM (up to 200 BPM) occurred. In cases of EEG seizure produced symptomatic cardiac arrhythmias, patients may be refractory to cardiac antiarryhythmic drugs [109] but helped instead by anticonvulsant medications [102, 109]. It would seem that more frequent use of combined EEG-ECG monitoring could have an increasingly positive impact on clinical care.

Sequelae of cardiac arrest

With continuing medical advances in cardiology and the technology for dealing with medical catastrophe, successful resuscitation from cardiac arrest is increasingly common. Fortunate patients will be clinically asymptomatic upon recovery or they will experience only minor neurological and/or cognitive problems. Many, however, will develop either transient or persistent neurological/cognitive dysfunctions covering a wide range of severity and impairment of functional capacity. Failure to survive is also a consequence for some. These wide gradations in clinical outcome result largely from differences in the duration of complete cerebral ischemia when cardiac output ceases and they speak to the profound effects or cerebral anoxia on brain function. Brain neurons seem to withstand the first few seconds of anoxia without obvious EEG change. However, after seven or so seconds brain waves become increasingly slow in frequency with some increase in amplitude and eventually they become flat (no activity) if anoxia is prolonged [112]. Animal studies [113, 114] have shown that EEGs will become isoelectric within 25 seconds of anoxic challenge caused by cardiac failure. EEG recording before and throughout a period of cardiac arrest in the human patient is an uncommon occurrence however reports have appeared [115–117] and in one case EEG activity became isoelectric after fifteen seconds of ventricular asystole but returned after successful resuscitation twelve seconds later. Whenever the animal or human EEG is lost, if the period of EEG flattening is not too long in duration a return of circulation will result in a re-emergence of brain waves which may or may not – depending on the length of the ischemic interval-return to normal frequencies.

Clinical EEG study can be accomplished soon after resuscitation from cardiopulmonary arrest (CPA) in most patients. Furthermore, it can be secured in serial fashion at multiple time points following the re-establishment of stable circulation thus allowing change, if any, in cerebral electrical activity over time to be detected. Several investigators [118–126] have examined the relationship between post CPA EEG findings and subsequent clinical course. In general, the severity of EEG abnormality encountered will depend both upon the duration of anoxic insult to the brain and how soon after resuscitation the EEG was secured. An EEG taken a short time after resuscitation is not likely to be normal although should this be the case it would be an excellent prognostic sign for recovery without neurological/cognitive deficit. Most EEGs secured within only hours of resuscitation are very abnormal and considered as single findings have limited or no real prognostic relevance. However, the degree of improvement (or lack of it) in the EEG over the initial 20 to 30 post-resuscitation hours or the status of a single EEG secured a day or two after the CPA event may have considerable prognostic importance. If an EEG secured 24 or more hours following CPA is found to contain dominant alpha activity, the probability that an asymptomatic recovery or one with only minor neurological/cognitive consequence will take place is very high. In one study [124] 94% of patients with post CPA normal EEGs made a recovery free of significant neurological or cognitive impairment (present author's calculations). If, following resuscitation, EEGs persist in showing very abnormal patterns such as continual delta activity, continuous spike or spike-wave activity, or continual or intermittent isoletric periods the prospect for survival is limited and of those surviving, postanoxic encephalopathy and other severe impairments are likely to be present.

The potential for significant improvement of the EEG following CPA is influenced by the duration of the anoxic period. Should the anoxic episode last beyond four or five minutes EEG improvement will probably not occur. When there is no detectable EEG activity at all immediately after resuscitation, the duration of the time elapsed until some EEG trace reappears is of critical importance. Recently Prior has combined and summarized [126] data collected by Jørgensen and Malchow-Møller [127, 128] which shows that if a continuous EEG signal has not reappeared within the first 10.5 hours following resuscitation, recovery of consciousness may not occur and at least intermittent EEG activity must reoccur within three hours if full recovery is to be even possible. The prognostic importance of EEG study following cardiopulmonary arrest has been questioned [129] and Bauer [112] has noted that EEGs which are only mildly abnormal and those which remain severely abnormal have the most prognostic clarity. In the individual case, in-between grades of EEG abnormality are not as reliably predictive of outcome.

Ischemia from embolic obstruction

Emboli of cardiac origin may at times cause obstruction of cerebral blood vessels [130] thus producing localized cerebral ischemic trauma. The type and magnitude of transient or persistent brain damage from embolic obstruction varies considerably with the location of the arterial blockage, its degree and its duration. Furthermore, while EEG abnormality is a common consequence of localized brain ischemia, the EEG findings themselves do not permit differentiation between embolism versus other types of causality.

Occlusive processes involving the middle cerebral artery and the internal carotid artery may be electroencephalographically silent if they are small and nonproductive of clinical symptoms. In symptomatic ischemia involving either of these arterial routes decreased amplitude of intrinsic EEG rhythms over the ipsilateral affected side may appear as an initial sign or as the only change following mild involvement. However, with more moderate or pronounced ischemic insult mixed delta and theta activity – or rhythmic high voltage delta alone – will appear over either the centrolateral, frontotemporal or temporal region of the involved ipsilateral hemisphere [13, 14, 92, 131]. Posterior cerebral artery involvement will produce regional slowing in the delta or theta-delta range over the parietal-posterior temporal-occipital area on the involved side although mild occulsive insult may only lead to an ipsilateral reduction of alpha amplitude or even to no EEG change at all [13, 131]. Slowing of the EEG over the frontal area of one hemisphere may accompany cases of ischemia from anterior cerebral artery obstruction [92, 131]. Seizure type paroxysmal discharges may be seen with embolic ischemia and in some patients overt clinical seizures can occur [132]. Persistent spike foci can develop and with persistent lateralized or regional slow wave abnormalities correlations with cognitive deficits may be sought.

Transient ischemic attacks

It is not uncommon for an EEG laboratory to be asked to evaluate patients who have had known or suspected transient ischemic attacks (TIA). However, whether or not an abnormal EEG will be found depends upon how severe or for how long a period of time the symptoms of the attack persisted as well as on how soon after symptom resolution the EEG was recorded. If because of fortunate circumstance the EEG is secured during the TIA there is a high probability that some degree of EEG abnormality will be seen over the hemisphere ipsilateral to the ischemia. In mild TIA it may be that only minor asymmetries of the background activity will be seen while the introduction of theta activity or even regional delta frequencies signify increasingly serious ischemic insult. EEG findings seen *during* the TIA itself do not permit determination of whether the attack is a transient one or one which will progress to become a clinically threatening event. Assuming the attack is a transient episode, the degree of EEG abnormality encountered may correlate with the rate of recovery with longer periods of symptom presence being associated with the more severe EEG findings. Since most of the time patients with TIA are seen in the EEG laboratory a day or several days after the attack, the EEG is not surprisingly normal in the majority of cases [92, 131, 133, 134].

Hemorrhagic cerebrovascular accident

In hemorrhagic CVA involving the cortical mantle the EEG very rapidly becomes profoundly abnormal with a focus of high voltage delta activity developing over the damaged side [12–14, 16, 18, 22] and these EEG changes may actually precede the more delayed CT scan evidence of stroke by a considerable period of time [135]. However, if the vascular rupture is small and confined to deeper brain areas visible EEG abnormality may not appear in scalp leads at all [22, 131]. A salient feature of EEG findings in hemorrhagic stroke is that they are dynamic and changing over time. The general trend is toward a normalization of the EEG and this process can continue for as long as six months or more. In a great many cases a complete or near complete resolution may occur [14, 22] however, neurological or cognitive impairment may persist despite normalization of the EEG [22]. Spike foci may develop in some patients as the focal slow wave dysfunction resolves and this is one reason why sleep EEG recording – which activates spike dysrhythmias [20, 22, 35] – is important in evaluating the post CVA case. If paroxysmal dysrhythmias fail to develop during the first six months post CVA, the probability is high that the patient will be spared an epileptic process.

Cerebral vascular insufficiency

Generalized insufficiency from cardiogenic or arteriosclerotic pathophysiology can alter the clinical EEG but the magnitude of change will depend upon the severity of the underlying process. Mild insufficiency may produce no EEG signs or perhaps only a slight slowing of the intrinsic alpha frequency while more moderate depression of cerebral metabolism may be associated with EEGs containing varying degrees of generalized slowing, bitemporal slowing or anterior bradyrhythmia [14, 22, 77, 131]. Cognitive changes and impairments of attention, concentration and memory may be seen in patients who show such EEG change.

EEG and cardiac surgery

While open heart surgery provides substantial promise of benefit it also involves a degree of cerebral risk. The period of artificial extracorporeal circulation required by open heart surgical repair offers opportunities for a number of events (hypoxia, inadequate perfusion, creation and release of microemboli, etc.) to occur which can adversely effect cerebral homeostasis. Furthermore, some surgical patients (for example those with congenital cardiac defect) may already have sufficient cerebral change stemming from cardiac problems to render them less able to tolerate any additional adverse effects of the perfusion period. There have been numerous papers [136–144] describing the kinds of neurological or cerebral impairments, not always lasting or permanent, which can follow open heart operative procedures and they will not be detailed here.

In this problem area, EEG might be useful in three ways. First, preoperative EEG findings correlating with risk of postoperative complications would be important to know about because they might allow identification of patients who should be watched especially closely. A normal preoperative EEG argues for preoperative cerebral integrity but this only suggests a favorable outcome provided that unusual perfusion difficulties do not produce cerebral compromise during the intraoperative period. An abnormal preoperative EEG suggests that some degree of cerebral impairment already exists and therefore tolerance for perfusion stress may be lessened. Over 70% of patients with preoperative EEGs containing either slowing of the intrinsic alpha rhythm and/or very slow intermittent delta activity may show clinical disorders and neurological signs at a ten month postoperative follow-up [145]. The above report also suggests that lateralized sharp wave discharges in the preoperative EEG may correlate with same side hemispheric dysfunction at follow-up. Generally most cases of preoperative EEG abnormality are seen in patients with serious congenital cardiac dysfunction [146] while non-congenital cases tend to have normal baseline EEG studies [143].

A second role played by EEG involves the use of this technique in ongoing monitoring of brain wave activity throughout the intraoperative period and especially while the patient is on bypass circulation. Significant EEG deterioration during surgery may denote impaired postoperative recovery. Since intra-operative EEG procedures, especially those which are computer assisted, are presented in depth elsewhere in this volume they will not be discussed here.

Finally, the postoperative EEG may provide valuable information on just how well the brain has fared throughout the surgical, anesthetic, and perfusion procedures. In this respect, the most valuable protocol by far would involve both pre and postoperative studies so that one could determine whether postoperative findings were new or simply pre-existing abnormalities. Pre and post comparison tracings are also the only way to detect that slight slowing or amplitude changes of normal intrinsic rhythms have occurred. Since EEG abnormalities caused by cardiac surgery may, of course, resolve or improve over time, securing more than one postoperative tracing is always advisable. Postoperative EEGs which are normal are good prognostic indicators [143, 145]. A decrease in frequency of intrinsic background EEG rhythms correlates positively with postoperative cerebral complications [145] which often will resolve while serious EEG abnormality not present before surgery may denote risk of residual impairment and even disability and death if the EEG abnormality continues to worsen on postoperative serial EEG studies [143, 145].

Postscript

Because the EEG is altered by changes in brain homeostasis produced by a wide variety of variables, it is useful as a measure of brain dysfunction. The sensitivity of EEG to problems of hypoxia and ischemia make it especially relevant to the study of the cardiac impaired who seek surgical intervention. Those who wish to use EEG methods in the study of open-heart surgery patients should, however, recognize the serious limitations of the technique and the conceptual confusions which have plagued the field. It is important to address

140

issues of interpretive reliability in exactly the same manner as one would with any measurement instrument. Furthermore, decisions about when and how often to record deserve careful consideration and in postoperative studies the value of multiple serial EEG studies is stressed. In the final analysis, the development of a close working relationship – a partnership if you will – between open heart surgery clinicians and researchers on the one hand and the electroneurophysiology laboratory team on the other offer the best hope of optimal use of EEG methods in this important medical area.

References

1. Himwich HE. Brain Metabolism and Cerebral Disorders. Baltimore, Williams and Wilkins, 1951.
2. Meyer JS, Sakamoto K, Akiyama M, Yoshida K, Yushitake S. Monitoring cerebral blood flow, metabolism and EEG. Electroenceph Clin Neurophysiol 1967; 23:497.
3. Siesjö BK. Brain Energy Metabolism. New York, John Wiley, 1980.
4. Caton R. The electric currents of the brain. Br Med J 1875; 2:278.
5. Beck A. Die Bestimmung der Localisation der Gehirn-und Ruckenmarksfunctionen vermittelst der elektrischen Erscheinungen. Zentralbl f Psysiol 1890; 4:473.
6. Fleischl von Marxow E. Mittheilung betrefferd die Physiologie der Hirnrinde. Zentralbl f Psysiol 1890; 4:437.
7. Beck A, Cybulski N. Weitere Untersuchungen uber die elektrischen Erscheinungen in der Hirnrinde der Affen and Hunde. Zentralbl f Physiol 1892; 6:1.
8. Gibbs FA, Gibbs EL. Atlas of Electro-encephalography Volume 1: Methodology and Controls. Cambridge, MA: Addison-Wesley, 1950.
9. Berger H. Ueber das Elektrenkephalogramm des Menschen. Arch f Psychiat 1929–1938; 1-14.
10. Berger H. Zur Lehre der Blutzirkulation in der Schadelhöhle des Menschen. Jena, G. Fischer, 1901.
11. Fois A, Lo NL. The Electroenrephalogram of the Normal Ghild. Springfield, IL Charles Thomas, 1961.
12. Hill D, Parr G (eds). Electroencephalography New York, Macmillian, 1963.
13. Kooi KA, Tucker RA, marshall RE. Fundamentals of Electroencephalography. 2nd ed. New York, Harper and Row, 1978.
14. Kiloh LG, McComas AJ, Osselton JW. Clinical Electroencephalography. 3rd ed. London, Butterworths, 1972.
15. Rémond A, Lairy TC, Chatrian GE (eds). Handbook of Electroencephalography and Clinical Neurophysiology, Vol. 6. The Normal EEG Throughout Life. Amsterdam, Elsevier, 1975.
16. Klass KW, Daly DD. Current Practice of Clinical Electroencephalography. New York, Raven Press, 1979.
17. Kellaway P and Petersen I (eds). Clinical Electroencephalography of Children. Stockholm, Almquist and Wiksell, 1980.
18. Niedermeyer E, Lopes da Silva F (eds). Electroencephalography – Basic Principles, Clinical Applications and Related Fields. Baltimore – Munich, Urban and Schwarzenberg, 1987.
19. Gibbs FA, Davis H, Lennox WG. The electroencephalogram in epilepsy and conditons of impaired consciousness. Arch Neurol Psychiat 1935; 34:1133.
20. Gibbs FA, Gibbs EL. Atlas of Electroencephalography, Vol. 2. Epilepsy. Reading, MA, Addison-Wesley, 1952.
21. Walter WG. The location of cerebral tumors by electroencephalography. Lancet 1936; 2:305.
22. Gibbs FA, Gibbs EL. Atlas of Electro-encephalography, Vol. 3. Neurological and Psychiatric Disorders. Reading, MA, Addison-Wesley, 1964.

23. Rémond A, Harner R, Naquet R (eds). Handbook of Electroencephalography and Clinical Neurophysiology, Vol. 12. Altered States of Consciousness, Coma, Cerebral Death. Amsterdam, Elsevier, 1975.
24. Wilson WP. The electroencephalogram in endocrine disorders. In: Wilson WP (ed). Applications of Electroencephalography in Psychiatry. Durham, NC, Duke University Press, 1965; p. 102.
25. Green RL. The electroencephalogram in alcoholism, toxic psychoses, and infection. In Wilson WP (ed.) Applications of Electroencephalography in Psychiatry, Durham, NC, Duke University Press, 1965; p. 123.
26. Rémond A, Radermecker FJ (eds). Handbook of Electroencephalography and Clinical Neurophysiology, Vol. 15A, Infections and Inflammatory Reactions, Allergy and Allergic Reactions. Degenerative Diseases. Amsterdam, Elsevier, 1977.
27. Rémond A, Glaser GH (ed). Handbook of Electroencephalography and Clinical Neurophysiology, Vol. 15C, Metabolic, Endocrine and Toxic Diseases. Amsterdam, Elsevier, 1977.
28. Ellingson RJ. The incidence of EEG abnormality among patients with mental disorders of apparently nonorganic origin: A critical review. Am J Psychiat 1954; 111:263.
29. Bergman PS, Green MA. The use of electroencephalography in differentiating psychogenic disorders and organic brain diseases. Am J Psychiat 1956; 113:27.
30. Hanretta AG. Psychiatric utilization of electroencephalography. Dis Nerv Syst 1965; 26:409.
31. Wender PH. Minimal Brain Dysfunction in Children. New York, John Wiley and Sons, 1971.
32. Satterfield JH. EEG issues in children with minimal brain dysfunction. Semin Psych 1973; 5:35.
33. Solomon S. Neurological evaluation. In: Kaplan HI, Freedman AM, Sadock BM (eds). Comprehensive Textbook of Psychiatry, Vol. 1, 3rd ed. Baltimore, Williams and Wilkins, 1980.
34. Kolb LC, Brodie HKL. Modern Clinical Psychiatry. Philadelphia, W. B. Saunders, 1982.
35. Struve FA. Clinical electroencephalography as an assessment method in psychiatric practice. In: Hall RCW, Beresford TP (eds). Handbook of Psychiatric Diagnostic Procedures, Vol. 2. New York, Spectrum, 1985; p. 1.
36. Eeg-Olofsson O, Petersén I, Sellden V. The development of the electroencephalogram in normal children from the age of 1 through 15 years: Paroxysmal activity. Neuropaediatrie 1971; 2:375.
37. Eeg-Olofsson O. The development of the EEG in normal young persons from the age of 16 to 21 years. Neuropaediatrie 1971; 3:11.
38. Taterka JH, Katz J. Study of correlations between electroencephalographic and psychological patterns in emotionally disturbed children. Psychosom Med 1955; 17:62.
39. Cure C, Rasmussen T, Jasper H. Activation of seizures and electroencephalographic disturbances in epileptic and in control subjects with "metrazol". Arch Neurol Psychiat 1948; 59:691.
40. White PT, DeMyer W, DeMyer M. EEG abnormalities in early childhood schizophrenia: A double-blind study of psychiatrically disturbed and normal children during promazine sedation. Am J Psych 1964; 120:950.
41. Whitehouse D, Pappas JA, Escala PH, Livingston S. Electroencephalographic changes in children with migraine. N Eng J Med 1967; 276:23.
42. Herrlin KN. EEG with photic stimulation: A study of children with manifest or suspected epilepsy. Electroenceph Clin Neurophysiol 1954; 6:573.140140
43. Stevens JR, Sachdev K, Milstein V. Behavior disorders of childhood and the electroencephalogram. Arch Neurol 1968; 18:160.
44. Kooi KA, Güvener AM, Tupper CJ, Bagchi BK. Electroencephalographic patterns of the temporal region in normal adults. Neurol 1964; 14:1029.
45. Pacheco e Silva A. Value of the electroencephalogram in the selection of 1,000 aviators. Clin Electroenceph 1977; 5:545.

46. Williams D. The significance of an abnormal electroencephalogram. J Neurol Psych 1941; 4:257.
47. Hooshmand H. A look at the EEG report. Clin Electroenceph 1978; 9:118.
48. Blum RH. A note on the reliability of electroencephalographic judgments. Neurol 1954; 4:143.
49. Woody RH. Intra-judge reliability in clinical electroencephalography. J Clin Psychol 1966; 22:150.
50. Woody RH. Inter-judge reliability in clinical electroencephalography. J Clin Psychol 1968; 24:251.
51. Volavka J, Matousek M, Roubicek J, Feldstein S, Brezinova V, Prior P, Scott D, Synek V. The reliability of visual EEG assessment. Electroenceph Clin Neurophysiol 1970; 31:294.
52. Houfek EE, Ellingson RJ. On the reliability of clinical EEG interpretation. J Nerv Ment Dis 1959; 128:425.
53. Walker AE, Jablon S. A follow-up study of head wounds in World War II. VA Medical Monograph. Washington, DC, US Government Printing Office, 1961.
54. Little SC, Raffel SC. Intra-rater reliability of EEG interpretations. J Nerv Ment Dis 1962; 135:77.
55. Majkowski J. The reliability of visual EEG assessment. Polish Med J 1971; 10:1223.
56. Rose SW, Penry JK, White BG, Sato S. Reliability and validity of visual EEG assessment on third grade children. Clin Electroenceph 1973; 4:197.
57. Struve FA, Becka DR, Green MA, Howard A. Reliability of clinical interpretation of the electroencephalogram. Clin Electroenceph 1975; 6:54.
58. Small JG, Milstein V, DeMyel MK, Moore JE. Electroencephalographic (EEG) and clinical studies of early infantile autism. Clin Electroenceph 1977; 8:27.
59. Struve FA, Pike LE. (1974). Routine admission electroencephalograms of adolescent and adult psychiatric patients awake and asleep. Clin Electroenceph 1974; 5:67.
60. Gibbs FA, Gibbs EL. How much do sleep recordings contribute to the detection of seizure activity. Clin Electroenceph 1971; 2:169–172.
61. Takahashi T. Activation methods. In: Niedermeyer E, Lopes da Silva F (eds). Electroencephalography – Basic Principles, Clinical Applications and Related Fields, Second Edition, Baltimore-Munich, Urban and Schwarzenberg, 1987; p. 209.
62. Glaser GH. The normal electroencephalogram and its reactivity. In: Glaser GH (ed). EEG and Behavior. New York, Basic Books, 1063; p. 3.
63. Abraham A, Ajmone-Marsan C. Patterns of cortical discharges and their relation to scalp electroencephalography. Electroenceph Clin Neurophysiol 1958; 10:447.
64. Heath RG, Mickle WA. Evaluation of 7 years experience with depth electrodes studies in human patients. In: Hamey E, O'Doherty D (eds). Electrical Studies on the Unanesthestized Brain. New York, Paul B. Hoeber, 1960.
65. Walter WG, Crow HJ. Depth recording from the human brain. Electroenceph Clin Neurophysiol 1964; 16:68.
66. Cooper R, Winter AL, Crow JH, Walter WG. Comparison of subcortical, and scalp activity using chronically indwelling electrodes in man. Electroenceph Clin Neurophysiol 1965; 18:217.
67. Niedermeyer E, Rocca U. The diagnostic significance of sleep electroencephalogram in temporal lobe epilepsy. Europ Neurol (Basal) 1972; 7:119.
68. Heath RG. Brain function and behavior. J Nerv Ment Dis 1975; 160:159.
69. Spencer SS, Spencer DD, Williamson PD, Mattson RH. The localizing value of depth electroencephalography in 32 patients with refractory epilepsy. Ann Neurol 1982; 12:248.
70. Westmoreland BF. The EEG in cerebral inflammatory processes. In: Niedermeyer E, Lopes da Silva F (eds). Electroencephalography – Basic Principles, Clinical Applications and Related Fields. Second Edition. Baltimore-Munich, Urban and Schwarzenberg, 1982; p. 259.
71. Shev EE, Robinson SJ. Electroencephalographic findings associated with cogenital heart disease. Electroenceph Clin Neurophysiol 1958; 10:253.
72. Lesny' I, Bor I, Vlach V. EEG changes in children suffering from cogenital heart disease: Influence of O_2 inhalation. Electroenceph Clin Neurophysiol 1961; 13:173.

73. Kalyanaraman K, Niedermeyer E, Rowe R, Wolfe K. The electroencephalogram in cogenital heart disease. Arch Neurol 1968; 18:98.
74. Niedermeyer E. The EEG in cardiac diseases. In: Remond A (ed). Handbook of Electroencephalography and Clinical Neurophysiology, Vol. 14A Cardiac and Vascular Diseases. Amsterdam, Elsevier, 1972; p. 65.
75. Struve FA. Marked increase in interhemispheric asynchrony of parietal sleep spindles in patients receiving aortic or mitral value replacement: Preliminary empirical findings. World Psychiatric Association Regional Symposium, Helsinki, Finland, June 18–21, 1984.
76. Davidson LAG, Jefferson JM. Electro-encephalographic studies in respiratory failure. Brit Med J 1959; 2:396.
77. Engel GL, Romano J. Delirium, a syndrome of cerebral insufficiency. J Chron Dis 1959; 9:260.
78. Naquet R, Vigouroux RA. Acute cerebral anoxia and syncopal attacks. In: Remond A (ed). Handbook of Electroencephalography and Clinical Neurophysiology, Vol. 14A, Cardiac and Vascular Diseases. Amsterdam, Elsevier, 1972; p. 68.
79. Niedermeyer E. Nonepileptic attacks. In: Niedermeyer E, Lopes da Silva F (eds). Electroencephalography – Basic Principles, Clinical Applications and Related Fields, Second Edition. Baltimore-Munich, Urban and Schwarzenberg, 1982; p. 511.
80. Gastaut H, and Fisher-Williams M. Electro-encephalographic study of syncope, its differentiation from epilepsy. Lancet 1957; 2:1018.
81. Gastaut H, Vigouroux RA, Deli MG. Polygraphyic study of carotid sinus hypersensitivity produced by extra-sinus stimulation. In: Gastaut H, Meyer JE (eds). Cerebral Anoxia and the Electroencephalogram. Springfield, IL, Thomas, 1961; p. 185.
82. Andriola M. Pseudo-seizures secondary to cardiac asystole and apnea. Electroenceph Clin Neurophysiol 1983; 56:7 (Abstract).
83. Dinner DS, Lesser RB, Morris HH, Lueders H. Electro-clinical study of convulsive syncope: A case report. Electroenceph Clin Neurophysiol 1984; 57:44 (Abstract).
84. Schlagenhauff RE, Megahed SM. Electroclinical correlation in the syndrome of vertebrobasilar artery insufficiency. Clin Electroenceph 1970; 1:63.
85. Niedermeyer E. The electroencephalogram and vertebro-basilar artery insufficiency. Neurology 1963; 13:412.
86. Meyer JS, Leiderman H, Denny-Brown D. Electroencephalographic study of insufficiency of the basilar and carotid arteries in man. Neurology 1956; 6:455.
87. Weiss S, Froelich W. Tilt table electro-encephalography in insufficiency syndromes. Neurology 1958; 8:686.
88. Roger J, Naquet R, Gastaut H, Lechner H, Fernandez-Guardiola A, Bostem F. Electroencephalographic and electrocardiographic manifestations provoked by carotid compression in cerebral circulatory insufficiency. In: Gastaut H, Meyer JE (eds). Cerebral Anoxia and the Electroencephalogram, Springfield, IL, Thomas, 1961; p. 439.
89. Marmor J, Sapirstein MR. Bilateral thrombosis of the anterior cerebral artery following stimulation of a hypersensitive carotid sinus. JAMA 1941; 117:1089.
90. Askey JM. Hemiplegia following carotid sinus stimulation. Am Heart J 1946; 31:131.
91. Zeman FD, Siegal S. Monoplegia following carotid sinus pressure in the aged. Am J M Sc 1947; 213:603.
92. Van der Drift JHA, Kok NKD. The EEG in cerebrovascular disorders in relation to pathology. In: Rémond A (ed). Handbook of Electroencephalography and Clinical Neurophysiology Vol. 14 A. Amsterdam, Elsevier, 1972; p. 12, p. 47.
93. Blumhardt LD. Ambulatory ECG and EEG monitoring in the differential diagnosis of cardiac and cerebral dysrhythmias. In: Gumnit RJ (ed). Advances in Neurology Vol. 46: Intensive Neurodiagnostic Monitoring. New York, Raven, 1986; p. 183.
94. Driver MV, Solby PJ. Apparent epilepsy due to intermittent tachyarrhythmia (Romano-Ward syndrome). Electroenceph Clin Neurophysiol 1977; 43:289.
95. Ballardie FW, Murphy RD, Davis J. Epilepsy: a presentation of the Romano-Ward syndrome. Brit Med J 1983; 287:896.
96. Sulg ZA. Dependency between cerebral and cardiac activity in physiological as well as

144

in abnormal conditions. In: Busse E (ed). Cerebral Manifestations of Episodic Cardiac Arrhythmias, Amsterdam, Excerpta Medica, 1979; p. 30.

97. Espinosa R E, Klass D W, Maloney J D. Contributions of the electroencephalogram in monitoring cardiac dysrhythmias. Mayo Clin Proc 1978; 53:119.

98. Gilchrist J M. Arrhythmic seizures: diagnosis by simultaneous EEG/ECG recording. Neurology 1985; 35:1503.

99. Lai C W, Ziegler D K. Syncope problem solved by continuous ambulatory simultaneous EEG/ECG recording. Neurology 1981; 31:1152.

100. Fuster J M, Veinberg S J. Bioelectrical changes of the heart cycle induced by stimulation of diencephalic regions. Exper Neurol 1960; 2:26.

101. Lown B, Verrier R L. Neural activity and ventricular fibrillation. N Eng J Med 1976; 294:1165.

102. Phizackerley P, Poole E, Whitly C. Sinoauricular heart block as an epileptic manifestation. Epilepsia 1954; 3:89.

103. Van Buren J M. Some autonomic concomitants of ictal automatism. Brain 1958; 81:505.

104. Delgado J M R, Mihailovic L, Sevillano M. Cardiovascular phenomena during seizure activity. J Nerv Ment Dis 1960; 130:477.

105. White P T, Grant P, Mosier J, Craig A. Changes in cerebral dynamics associated with seizures. Neurology 1961; 11:354.

106. Mathew N T, Taori G M, Mathai V V, Chandy J. Atrial fibrillation associated with seizure in a case of frontal meningioma. Neurology 1970; 20:725.

107. Walsh G O, Masland W, Goldensohn E S. Relationship between paroxysmal atrial tachycardia and paroxysmal cerebral discharges. Bull Los Angeles Neurol Soc 1972; 31:28.

108. Rush J L, Everett B A, Adams A H, Viusske J A. Paroxysmal atrial tachycardia and frontal lobe tumor. Arch Neurol 1977; 34:578.

109. Pritchett E L C, McNamara J O, Gallagher J J. Arrhythmogenic epilepsy: An hypothesis. Am Heart J 1980; 100:683.

110. Marshall D W, Westmoreland B F, Sharbrough F W. Ictal tachycardia during temporal lobes seizures. Mayo Clin Proc 1983; 58:443.

111. Blumhardt L D, Smith P E M, Owen L. Electrocardiographic accompaniments of temporal lobe epileptic seizures. Lancet 1986; 1:1051.

112. Bauer G. Cerebral anoxia. In: Niedermeyer E, Lopes da Silva F (eds). Electroencephalography – Basic Principles, Clinical Applications and Related Fields, Second Edition. Baltimore-Munich, Urban and Schwarzenberg, 1982; p. 511.

113. Safar P, Stezoski W, Nemoto E M. Amelioration of brain damage after 12 minutes of cardiac arrest in dogs. Arch Neurol 1976; 33:91.

114. Myers R B, Yamaguchi S. Nervous system effects of cardiac arrest in monkeys. Arch Neurol 1977; 33:65.

115. Moss J, Rockoff M. EEG monitoring during cardiac arrest and resuscitation. JAMA 1980; 244:2750.

116. Morrison D, Goldman S, Labadie E, Hager W D. Primary VF during EEG in a psychiatric patient. Amer Heart J 1982; 103:1081.

117. Young W L, Ornstein E. Compressed spectral array EEG monitoring during cardiac arrest and resuscitation. Anesthesiology 1985; 62:535.

118. Prior P F, Volavka J. An attempt to assess the prognostic value of the EEG after cardiac arrest. Electroenceph Clin Neurophysiol 1958; 10:367.

119. Pampiglione G. Electroencephalographic studies after cardiorespiratory resuscitation. Proc R Soc Med 1962; 55:653.

120. Hockaday J, Potts F, Epstein E, Bonazzi A, Schwab R S. Electroencephalographic changes in acute cerebral anoxia from cardiac or respiratory arrest. Electroenceph Clin Neurophysiol 1965; 18:575.

121. Pampiglione G, Harden A. Resuscitation after cardiocirculatory arrest. Prognostic evaluation of early electroencephalographic findings. Lancet 1968; 1:1261.

122. Binnie C D, Prior P F, Lloyd D S L, Scott D F, Margerison J H. Electroencephalographic pre-

diction of fatal anoxic brain damage after resuscitation from cardiac arrest. Brit Med J 1970; 4:265.

123. Prior PF. The EEG ín Acute Anoxia. Amsterdam, Excerpta Medica, 1973.

124. Møller M, Holm B, Sindrup E, Nielson L. Electroencephalographic prediction of anoxic brain damage after resuscitation from cardiac arrest in patients with acute myocardial infarction. Acta Med Scan 1978; 203:31.

125. Ducasse J, Marc-Vergnes J, Cathala B, Genestal M, Lareng L. Early cerebral prognosis of anoxic encephalopathy using brain energy metabolism. Critical Care Med 1984; 12:897.

126. Prior PF. EEG monitoring and evoked potentials in brain ischaemia. Brit J Anaesth 1985; 57:63.

127. Jørgensen EO, Malchow-Møller A. Cerebral signs during cardiopulmonary resuscitation. Resuscitation 1978; 6:217.

128. Jørgensen EO, Malchow-Møller A. Natural history of global and critical brain ischaemia. Part I and II, Resuscitation 1981; 9:133.

129. Allen N. Life or death of the brain after cardiac arrest. Neurology 1977; 27:805.

130. Lhermitte F, Gautier JC. Sites of cerebral arterial occlusions. In: Williams D (ed). Modern Trends in Neurology. London, Butterworths, 1975; p. 123.

131. Niedermeyer E. Cerebrovascular disorders and EEG. In: Niedermeyer E, Lopes da Silva F (eds). Electroencephalography-Basic Principles, Clinical Applications and Related Fields, Second Edition. Baltimore-Munich, Urban and Schwarzenberg, 1982; p. 511.

132. Rasheva M. Epileptic seizures in the acute stage of embolic stroke. Electroenceph Clin Neurophysiol 1981; 52:78 (Abstract).

133. Birchfield RI, Wilson WP, Heyman A. An evaluation of electroencephalography in cerebral infarction and ischemia due to arteriosclerosis. Neurology 1959; 9:859.

134. Silva A, Gross PT. Use of EEG in the evaluation of TIAs. Electroenceph Clin Neurophysiol 1983; 56:13 (Abstract).

135. Keilson MJ, Miller AE, and Drexler ED. Early EEG and CT scanning in stroke – a comparative study. Electroenceph Clin Neurophysiol 1985; 61:21 (Abstract).

136. Gilman S. Cerebral disorders after open-heart operations. N Eng J Med 1965; 272:489.

137. Sachdev NS, Carter CC, Swank RL, Blachly PH. Relationship between post-cardiotomy delirium, clinical neurological changes and EEG abnormalities. J Thorac Cardiovasc Surg 1968; 54:557.

138. Javid H, Tofo H. Najafi H, Dye WS, Hunter TA, Julian OC. Neurological abnormalities following open heart surgery. J Thorac Cardiovasc Surg 1969; 58:502.

139. Tufo HM, Ostfeld AM, Shekelle R. Central nervous system dysfunction following open-heart surgery. JAMA 1970; 212:1333.

140. Aguilar JJ, Gerbode F, Hil D. Neuropathologic complications of cardiac surgery. J Thorac Cardiovasc Surg 1971; 61:676.

141. Branthwaite MD. Neurological damage related to open-heart surgery. Thorax 1972; 27:748.

142. Witoszka MM, Tamura H, Indeglia R, Hopkins RW, Simeone FA. Electroencephalographic changes and cerebral complications in open-heart surgery. J Thorac Cardiovasc Surg 1973; 66:855.

143. Hansotia PL, Myers WO, Ray JF, Greehling C, Sautter RD. Prognostic value of ßelectroencephalography in cardiac surgery. Ann Thorac Surg 1975; 19:127.

144. Sotaniemi KA. Brain damage and neurological outcome after open-heart surgery. J Neurol Neurosurg Psychiat 1980; 43:127.

145. Sotaniemi KA. Clinical and prognostic correlates of EEG in open-heart surgery patients. J Neurol Neurosurg Psychiat 1980; 43:941.

146. Torres F, Frank GS, Cohen M, Lillehi CW, Kasper N. Neurologic and electroencephalographic studies in open heart surgery. Neurol 1959; 9:174.

11. The promise and the peril of topographic mapping of quantified brain electrical activity: Technical and interpretive considerations affecting validity

FREDERICK A. STRUVE

Attempts to develop topographic visual displays of EEG data go back over thirty years [1]. In fact, the entire history of quantitative methods in electroencephalography has been sprinkled with efforts to devise useful graphic displays of EEG variables over schematic head representations. Interested readers will find salient historical research developments leading to today's impressive topographic EEG mapping technology succinctly summarized by Etevenon [2]. More recently in 1979 Duffy and associates presented [3] a sophisticated system (Brain Electrical Activity Mapping or "BEAM") which allowed a variety of quantitated EEG measures to be displayed topographically over a head representation with high quality color graphics. Furthermore, they selected choice examples (i.e., tumor localization when the traditional EEG was normal or nondiagnostic) which suggested high potential utility for their graphic EEG mapping displays.

In the single decade since Duffy introduced his system, interest in topographic mapping of EEG activity has grown at an increasingly rapid rate [4–12]. A recent volume [13] released only two years ago contains research and critical commentary from over 40 current investigators in this newly emerging field. Computed EEG topographic mapping techniques are being applied to an expanding range of topics including dyslexia [14, 15], epilepsy [4, 16, 17], atrophic and mass lesions [18], cerebral ischemia, stroke and transient ischemic attacks [19–25], dementia [26], CNS effects of lead exposure [27], neonate studies [28], sleep research [29], pharmacology [30, 31], cerebellar syndrome [32], porencephaly and arachnoid cysts [33] and substance abuse [34] among others. Psychiatry attracts considerable attention from those using these EEG techniques [35–41]. In many of these studies the topographic displays of various quantified EEG variables are shown to convey temporal-spatial EEG information not readily assimilated from the complex multichannel "squiggly line" traditional ink writing tracing. It is this ability to synthesize and visually portray complex regional and focalized EEG phenomena more effectively that gives EEG mapping techniques their rich promise as investigative tools for the study of brain function. It is

147

certain that these approaches will be more frequently used in the assessment of functional and dysfunctional brain states in cardiac surgery patients as well.

Topographic display of quantitative EEG variables

There are many ways to generate topographic representations of EEG variables from original raw EEG signals but it would not be productive to detail numerous variations in approach at this time. In most commercially available mapping units certain common features are found and for present purposes we may consider them typical. However, it must be understood and underscored that the "hard numerical" output generated, along with its topographical display, is simply *not* more "objective" than the original EEG tracing. It cannot be more "objective" than the primary raw EEG because it is only a transformation of that EEG itself. As we hope to see later, errors in the original traditional EEG can (if one is not careful) be impressively magnified in the final mapping of quantified data. Furthermore, decisions made in initial selection of EEG epochs for quantitative analyses can have profound influences on the topographic maps produced.

Initially a series of brief multichannel artifact free raw EEG epochs are selected for quantitative analyses. Depending on the program used, single EEG epochs may range from one or two to over ten seconds in length with 2.5 seconds being a common choice. An analog to digital conversion program then digitizes each second of raw wave form EEG in the sample epoch into multiple individual points on the voltage gradient and assigns a value to each point. Typically a number of "digitized" EEG epochs are then combined or averaged at a later point in subsequent data processing. The number of combined digitized epochs underlying the final numerical output may range from only a few to over 50 or 60 epochs, again depending on the program, purpose, and degree of "user-selection" control of the operation. Spectral subdivision into basic EEG bandwidths is accomplished with a Fast Fourier Transform applied to each epoch with results averaged across epochs and the frequency bands used in subsequent quantitative analyses usually conform to the four "traditional" EEG bands of Delta, Theta, Alpha, and Beta frequencies. The option to "user-define" and hence alter frequency bandwidths selected for analyses is always desirable but not available on all units.

Now that the raw analog EEG trace at each electrode site has been broken into presumably artifact free segments or "epochs" and these have been "digitized", combined together, and characterized by spectrum and signal strength, a number of quantitative measures are computed which presumably describe the EEG activity which has been recorded at each electrode site on the head. One of these, Absolute Power, is analogous to amplitude or signal strength and is the average amount of power in picowatts within each frequency band computed separately for each electrode site. With the typical situation involving the four traditional EEG bands and 21 scalp electrodes, 84 numerical values are generated for Absolute Power alone. Percent Relative Power is also commonly computed. It involves a calculation of the percentage of total overall power distributed into each of the EEG frequency bands selected and hence is analogous to the "abundance" or relative amount of each frequency band activity at each electrode site. Many commercial units also estimate the degree of difference in measures of electrical activity between homologous brain areas. This variable, termed Asymmetry, is generally the percent difference in Absolute Power between homologous scalp electrodes for each of the traditional EEG frequency bands. Some units compute a measure (methods may vary) of interhemispheric coherence as well. Essentially Coherence is a measure, expressed in percentage terms, of the degree of timing and phase agreement of EEG activity between homologous electrode pairs for each of the EEG frequency bands examined.

For a given quantitative variable – say Absolute Power of delta – actual values are known only for each recording electrode site on the head. Therefore, prior to displaying absolute power of delta activity over a schematic representation of the scalp, *estimates* of its value must be obtained for all areas *between* recording electrode sites. Such estimates are generated by mathematical interpolation of values for each "pixel" on the head diagram using the known numerical values of the 2, 3, or 4 electrodes closest to that spot (complexities of such interpolation are many and are discussed elsewhere [2, 42–44]). With the head schematic divided into numerous pixels, each pixel in turn is assigned an interpolation derived estimate of delta absolute power – or a known value if the pixel corresponds to a recording electrode site. The range of numerical values are then assigned positions on a color bar scale with the resulting gradations in color over head regions thus corresponding to areas of maxima and minima of the quantitative EEG measure selected. In this fashion, multicolored topographic displays of all common quantitative EEG variables can be produced for a variety of EEG frequency bands, and fine gradations in magnitude of each quantitative variable over brain areas can be visually appreciated. Other frequently available features may involve expressing a subject's quantitative EEG variables in terms of z-score departures from reference group mean values. The resulting topographic map of z-scores allows visual recognition of head areas where meaningful differences between subject and reference group may be found. Furthermore one can topographically map mean quantitative EEG variable values obtained from a group of patients or even display some statistical measure of between group difference of the EEG variable selected.

The steps which transform the traditional raw "squiggly line" EEC tracings into such compelling and impressive multicolored brain maps are complex and arduous. The promise they truly offer must be balanced by the peril of real distortions which can easily be produced.

Distortions from technical considerations

The technical parameters of many commercially available EEC mapping devices may be set and not user-definable. While they may well be adequate for most recording purposes the user typically is not made aware of the relationship between such features as epoch length, number of collected epochs, choice of reference, analog to digital conversion sampling rate, bandwidth selection and the like and the accuracy or validity of the topographic maps produced. That variation in such parameters can produce results which can be misleading has been detailed in an excellent recent paper of concern by Kahn and associates [45].

Although not often appreciated, the choice of reference electrode can affect topographic EEG map generation in much the same way it affects the traditional ink EEG tracing. Topographic mapping commonly involves monopolar or common reference recordings although bipolar topographic maps are easily generated and often useful. Frequently (but not always) linked ears are used for common reference purposes. High voltage activity near any selected common reference location may be picked up by this reference electrode and made to appear in all recording channels – and hence throughout large areas of the topographic map. Furthermore use of more distant common reference locations such as the nose or chin may introduce biological electrical potentials of non-brain origin into all topographically mapped regions. In such instances the map appearance may not always be easily identified as distorted or influenced by artifact. Montage and reference selection is not an automatic and "trouble free" operation. Because of this no one should generate and interpret quantitative variable EEG topographic maps without first acquiring complete familiarity with issues of montage and reference selection in traditional EEG methods. One must frequently examine the raw EEG tracing when distortions in topographic maps are suspected.

The length of single EEG epochs used in quantitative analysis as well as the total number of epochs combined together can affect mapping results in subtle ways. Not uncommonly, the length of EEG sample epochs will be fixed in commercially sold units. The longer the length of the individual epoch, the higher will be the degree of resolution of the Fast Fourier Transform. To resolve EEG activity to 0.5 Hz the sample epoch must be at least two seconds long. Epoch lengths less than this will offer poor resolution. For optimal stability of results a large number of epochs should be collected and care should be taken that the patient maintains the same level of alertness throughout the collection period. In our laboratory, we attempt to collect at least 60 artifact free epochs for each analysis and will not accept less than 40. Estimates of coherence will suffer if less than 30 epochs are used while maps generated from only a small number of epochs may lack representativeness or be unduly altered by inclusion of one or two atypical epochs.

The sampling rate used to "digitize" the original raw analog EEG signal must be within defined limits. One must know the upper EEG frequency needed to be seen and the sampling rate must be at least twice that frequency if information is not to be lost [46]. More troublesome is the problem called "aliasing" in which raw EEG frequencies (or non EEG activity such as muscle potentials or 60 Hz. artifact) which exceed one-half the sampling rate may be falsely identified as much lower frequencies. Furthermore the EEG bandwidths used in quantitative EEG analyses may or may not be user definable. Significant changes can occur within a given bandwidth and not be detected in the final topographic maps and this may sometimes result in loss of relevant clinical information. For example, a person may have a baseline alpha frequency of 11 to 12 Hz. but this frequency may slow to 8 or 9 to 10 Hz. as a result of cardiological or cardiac surgery induced brain ischemia or hypoxic challenge. Topographic mapping using a single alpha band of 8 to 12 Hz. would not detect this change at all.

Distortions from medications and substances

Many medications and substances alter the EEG spectrum and will, of course, alter topographic maps of EEG activity as well. Soporifics will introduce lower beta frequencies into the spectrum while benzodiazepine type compounds will produce large amounts of 20–25 Hz. activity over bilateral frontal-central areas. High blood levels of some medications (i.e. Dilantin) may decrease alpha frequency and introduce generalized theta activity. In a study using traditional EEG recordings we have shown [47] that about one third of patients receiving lithium may develop generalized and/or paroxysmal EEG slowing even though blood levels are within therapeutic range limits. There are even preliminary suggestions [34] that marihuana use, which is not socially uncommon, may lead to persistent alterations of the topological distribution of alpha activity. It must be stressed that topographic EEG mapping only clearly represents an individual's underlying EEG characteristics if that individual is totally medication and substance free. In our pharmacological oriented clinical world this requirement may not be obtainable in all cases.

A related concern involves quantitative EEG and topographic map comparisons between an individual subject and a normative reference group. Maps and statistical indices reflecting a subject's degree of departure from normative group means are only valid when the subject is recorded under exactly the same conditions as the controls. This almost always means testing the subject in a drug and substance free state.

Distortions from EEG epoch selection decisions

1. Paroxysmal discharges

Topographic mapping of quantitative EEG variables is designed to show in fine detail a subject's characteristic background EEG activity over all head regions during an alert and relaxed awake state. Subjects will be found, however, in which this background ongoing EEG is interrupted episodically by brief duration (a few seconds) paroxysmal dysrhythmic events. Such clinical discharges may involve frank focal or diffuse spike or spike-wave activity or they may involve a variety of minor paroxysmal dysrhythmic discharges. Frank spike activity will not necessarily be confined to seizure populations and minor paroxysmal patterns can sometimes be seen in normal clinically asymptomatic individuals. These dysrhythmic events are not characteristic of an individual's ongoing EEG activity but instead are sharp departures from it. Should any of the EEG epochs used for quantitative analyses and EEG map production contain paroxysmal dysrhythmic activity the resulting topographic map may be seriously distorted. More unfortunately, the nature of the distortion may not at all be apparent from visual inspection of the maps alone.

In Figures 1 and 2, we present two cases to illustrate this point. In the first case, the ongoing EEG of a 52 year old woman with a diagnosis of Atypical Depression contained infrequent episodic diffuse bursts of paroxysmal slowing [48] with frequencies in the theta-high delta range. The duration of each discharge was brief, lasting only a few seconds.

We collected 58 artifact free EEG epochs from this patient; however, by accident, 8 of these epochs (13.8% of the total) contained the paroxysmal activity just described. The first two topographic maps display, for Absolute Power of Theta, this patient's raw absolute power values (Map A) and z-score departures from a normative data base (Map B). As can be seen, power within the theta band is essentially increased over all head regions. Clearly these maps are misleading (although this cannot be gathered from the maps alone) and they do not indicate that the theta activity was episodic, brief and infrequent as opposed to ongoing as might be the case in an organic, metabolic, or toxic condition. When this patient's map was reconstructed (Map C) by removing the eight epochs containing paroxysmal activity the widespread marked elevation in Absolute Power of Theta disappears. Figure 2 shows a man whose EEG contained paroxysmal runs of slow [48] in the bi-occipital area. The initial epoch collection contained several epochs containing this activity and the resulting map suggests elevated theta focal to the occipital region. Again the maps alone (Map A and B) do not allow us to know that this represents only infrequent episodic activity and for this reason it is misleading. Reconstructing the map (Map C) by eliminating epochs which contain paroxysmal activity results in a picture more truly representative of the patient's ongoing EEG activity.

It is recognized that for certain specific reasons one may want to include paroxysmal activity into a quantitative analysis or topographic map. However, this would be an act of deliberate choice done for specific purpose. The casual and unrecognized inclusion of such EEG events in epochs collected for topographic EEG mapping may produce distortions which are serious indeed. Ongoing *clinical interpretation* by an electroencephalographer of the EEG used for quantitative analyses and map generation is necessary if such error is to be avoided.

153

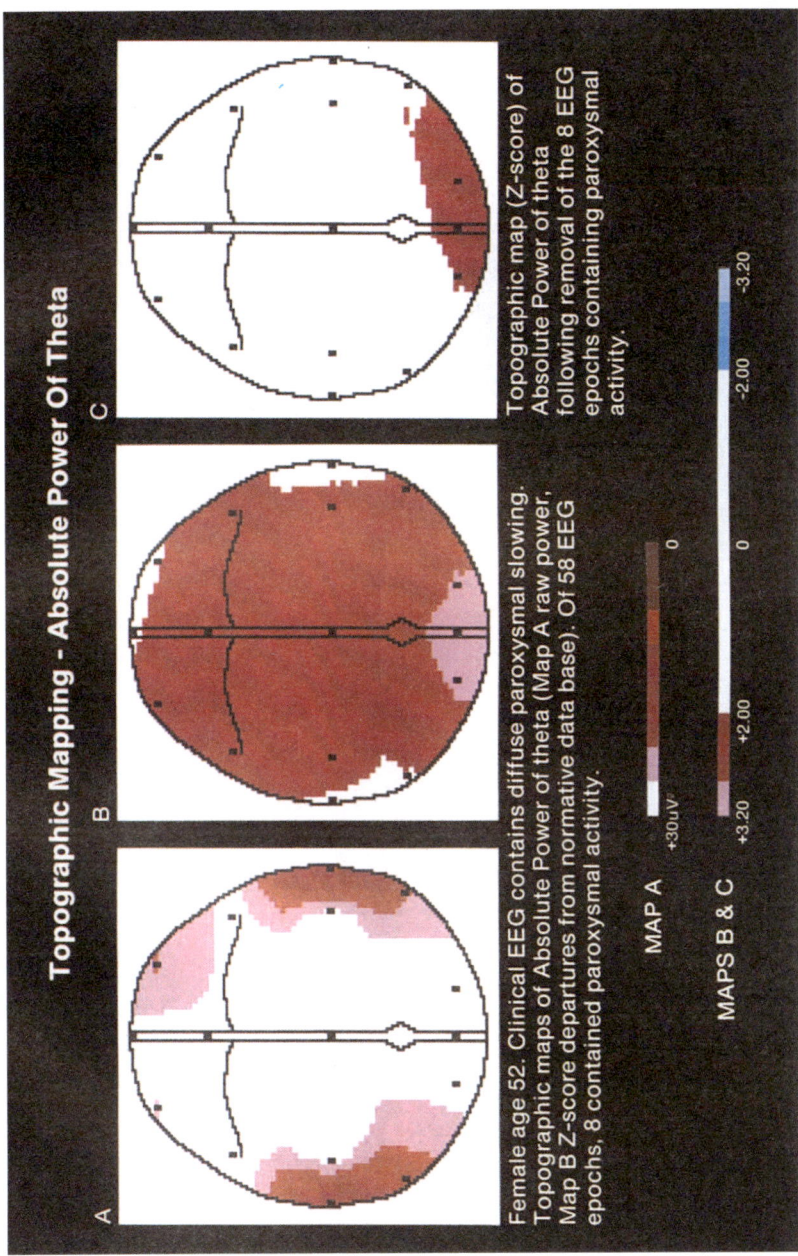

Fig. 1. Distortion of topographic EEG map produced by inclusion of epochs containing Diffuse Paroxysmal Slowing.

154

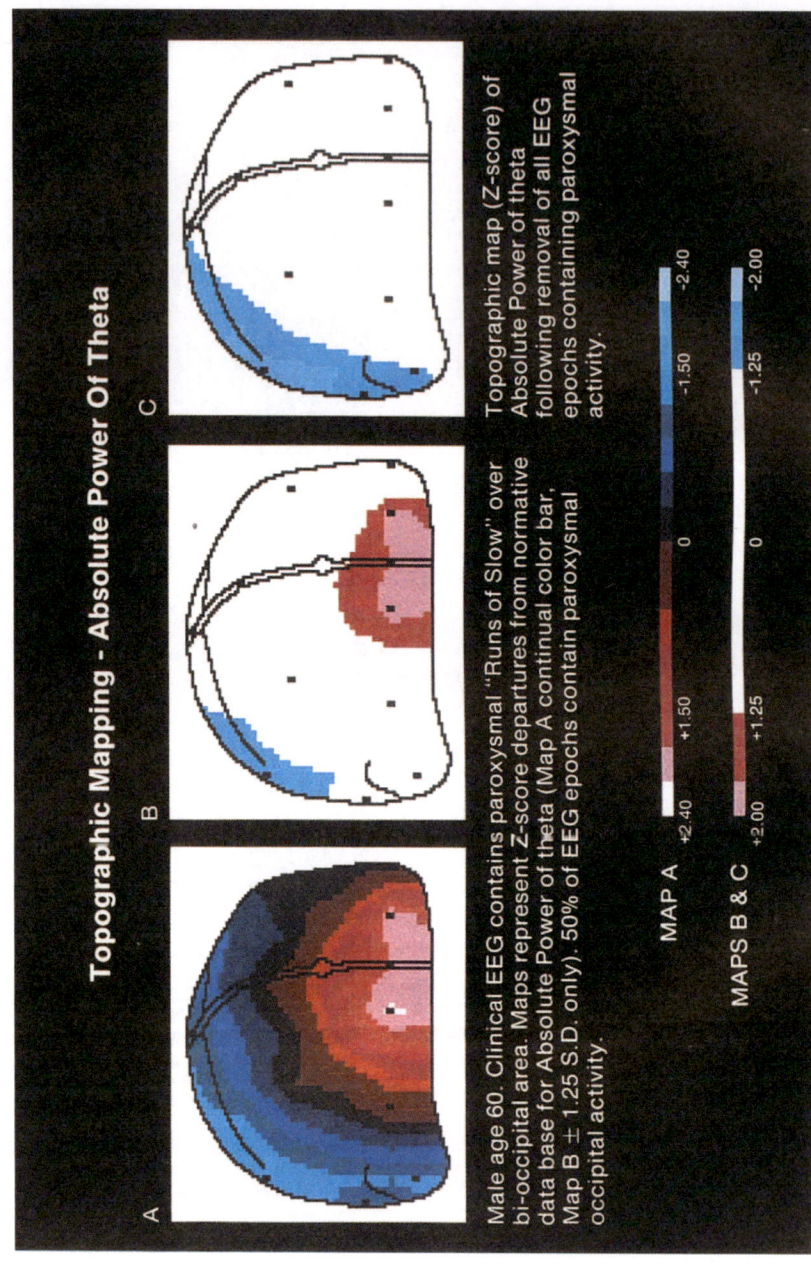

Topographic Mapping - Absolute Power Of Theta

A B C

Male age 60. Clinical EEG contains paroxysmal "Runs of Slow" over bi-occipital area. Maps represent Z-score departures from normative data base for Absolute Power of theta (Map A continual color bar, Map B ± 1.25 S.D. only). 50% of EEG epochs contain paroxysmal occipital activity.

Topographic map (Z-score) of Absolute Power of theta following removal of all EEG epochs containing paroxysmal activity.

MAP A   +2.40   +1.50   0   -1.50   -2.40

MAPS B & C   +2.00   +1.25   0   -1.25   -2.00

Fig. 2. Distortion of topographic EEG map produced by inclusion of epochs containing Bi-occipital Paroxysmal Runs of Slow.

Distortions from epoch selection decisions

2. Artifact rejection

Artifacts of various kinds produce fluctuating potentials which can be registered by EEG leads on the scalp and which totally or partially fall within the frequency range of brain wave activity. Common biological artifacts include eye blinks, vertical and lateral eye movement under closed lids, eye flutter, EKG, muscle potential, and electrodermal artifact as well as others. Electrode and amplifier artifacts are nonbiological but can often mimic brain wave activity. An exhaustive discussion of artifacts and the different strategies used to eliminate them from quantitative EEG analyses is given by Barlow [49].

In the traditional EEG tracing the most common and frequently occurring artifacts are easily identified by the experienced electroencephalographer due to their often characteristic wave forms and/or locations. Subtle atypical or low voltage artifact may at times elude detection. However, in the finished topographic EEG map this is no longer the case because wave form is no longer accessible and features identifying focal, regional or lateral topographic spectral variations as artifact generated do not exist. Some have recognized that topographic mapping techniques can emphasize the effect of artifact [43] while others have been more forceful in stating that ". . . topographic mapping techniques are so powerful that artifact recognition is extremely difficult" (Ref. 50, p. 395). A topographical map of absolute power of delta activity (z-score departures from a normative sample) for a 27 year old woman tested in our laboratory is shown in Figure 3. The apparent right occipital delta focus with considerable spread to surrounding area (Maps A, B, C) appears to be genuine although it resulted from episodic delta potentials caused by a faulty right occipital electrode. This was suspected but not proven by interpretation of the raw analog EEG tracing. When the patient was re-tested with the electrode problem corrected, the delta focus vanished (Maps D, E, F).

At the present time, there is a strong consensus [40, 43, 46, 50–53] among major investigators that experienced electroencephalographic interpretation of the raw multichannel analog EEG tracing is an essential process in either on line or off line artifact elimination. Often interpretation of the topographic EEG map can only be clarified by concurrent interpretation of the traditional analog EEG as well. A common further recommendation is that recordings used for topographic map generation should be supplemented by several non-cephalic special electrode placements used to record directly those non-brain biopotentials from eyes, face, muscles, tongue and the like [40, 42, 50, 54]. This is a suggestion to be viewed seriously. For example, when Small and her team [40] used visual inspection of analog EEG tracings plus analog output from non-scalp artifact detecting electrodes to insure collection of artifact free epochs, their maps did not show the increased bilateral frontal delta activity in unmedicated schizophrenics which previously had been reported [35, 36, 38, 39] in brain mapping studies conducted by others.

156

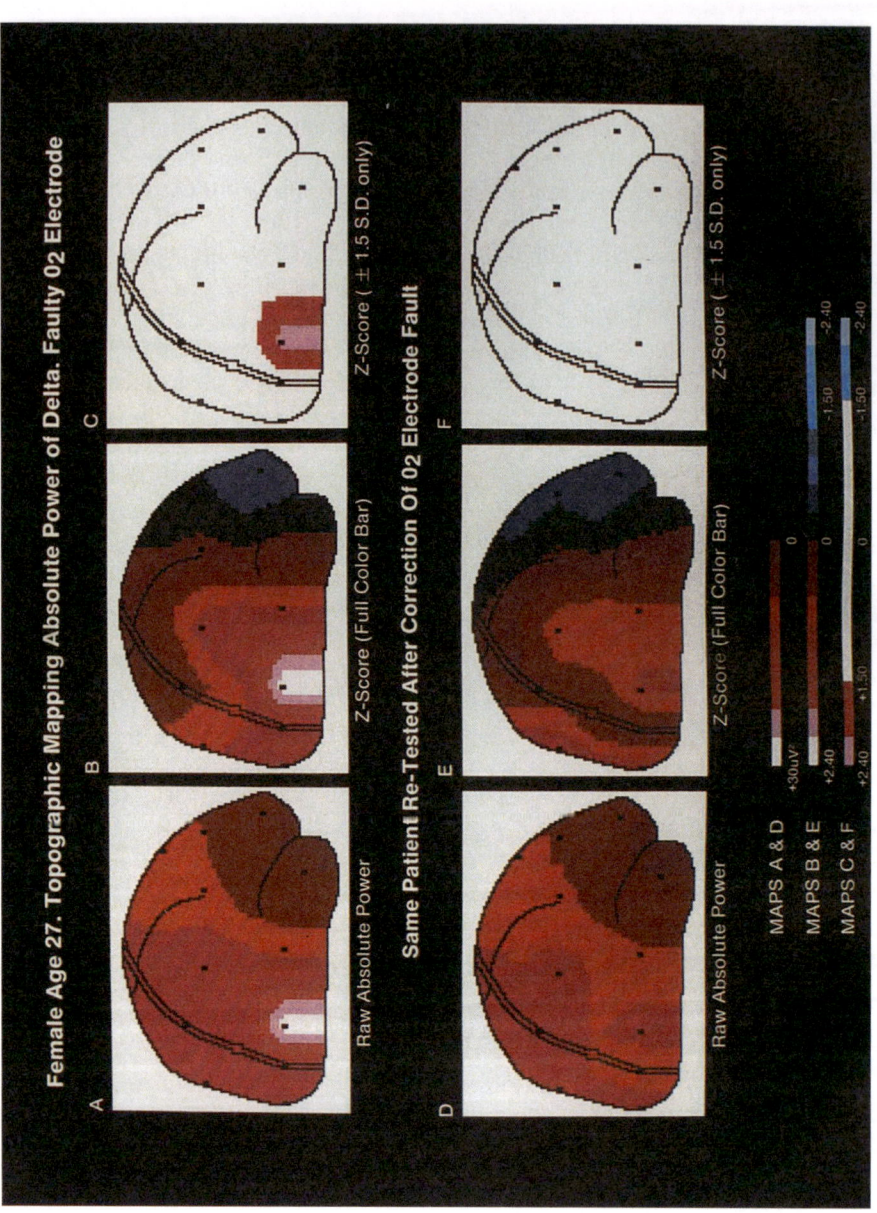

Fig. 3. Distortion of topographic EEG map produced by inclusion of epochs containing artifact from faulty O_2 electrode.

Almost all commercial EEG mapping units now incorporate a program for automatic machine rejection of artifact contaminated EEG epochs. Methods of automatic artifact detection can be quite complex [49], however most commercial units rely on some variation of creating an amplitude "window" around a user selected presumably artifact free reference epoch. Activity within this window is accepted as "artifact free" whereas that exceeding window limits is rejected. Such developments carry an unfortunate implication, even if not stated explicitly that artifact free topographic EEG maps can, in fact, be generated by automated programs not requiring electroencephalographic interpretive skill. While automated programs do eliminate some artifact, especially that which is of high voltage, they do so very imperfectly and the rate of automated machine acceptance of artifact contaminated epochs may be high.

Currently we are carefully looking at the issue of automated artifact

Table 1. Clinical versus automated EEG epoch selection – various measures of agreement

	Standard deviation settings for "window" around artifact free reference EEG epoch				
	4.0 SD	4.5 SD	5.0 SD	5.5 SD	All combined
Total number of EEG epochs reviewed	1,379	2,376	2,347	1,856	7,958
% of total epochs accepted by automated program	11.8%	20.2%	23.1%	51.0%	26.8%
Percent agreement: automated vs clinical acceptance or rejection of EEG epoch	73.6%	73.7%	71.2%	63.5%	70.6%
H1C coefficients: automated vs clinical acceptance or rejection	0.34	0.36	0.28	0.32	0.28
Proportion of automated accepted epochs which are clinically rejected: automated selection false positives	23.9%	32.8%	45.8%	60.0%	47.5%
Proportion of automated accepted epochs also clinically accepted: automated selection true positives	76.1%	67.2%	54.2%	40.0%	52.5%
Proportion of clinically rejected epochs receiving automated acceptance	4.2%	9.9%	15.3%	41.5%	18.4%
% of clinically judged drowsy epochs accepted by automated selection	24%	41.9%	53.8%	77.4%	51.9%

Note: This is preliminary data from an empirical study still in progress and hence incomplete.

rejection. For example, in Table 1 we show a comparison of clinical versus automated machine accept/reject decisions for a total of 7,958 EEG epochs secured live from a variety of patients. The sample is broken down by the width, in standard deviation units, of the "window" surrounding each patient's selected artifact free reference epoch. Neither percent agreement or phi coefficients are very high. However, most important is the observation that the proportion of automatic machine accepted EEG epochs which in fact do contain artifact is high and ranges from 23.9 to 60% as the selection window widens. Our empirical observations follow the views expressed by Shipton [52] that truly effective automated discrimination between brain and extra cerebral potentials is not yet possible.

Distortions from epoch selection decisions

3. Spontaneous drowsiness

With a subject relaxed with his or her eyes closed it would be remarkable if drowsiness did not often intrude. Even the traditional EEG drowsy activity is dramatically different from EEG activity recorded during the awake state. During drowsiness alpha is attenuated or disappears and theta activity over central regions becomes prominent. In many subjects central or vertex sharp waves appear as well. In the majority (but not all) of cases, drowsy activity is readily identified in the traditional EEG. However, its representation in the topographically mapped EEG is not identifiable as to cause at all. Even a few EEG epochs containing unrecognized drowsiness will seriously distort quantitative EEG analyses and produce topographic maps with a theta dominent organic appearing quality. In our experience 78% of the patients tested in our laboratory at one time or another display drowsiness during quantitative EEG epoch collection procedures. Of the 7,958 EEG epochs reviewed in Table 1, 8.3% consisted of frank drowsy activity. It is also clear that automated machine epoch selection programs do not do well in separating out and rejecting drowsy epochs from analysis. In our program (see Table 1) automated artifact rejection systems *accepted* from 24 to 77.4% of drowsy contaminated EEG epochs. Again it becomes imperative that skilled clinical electroencephalographic interpretation of the raw analog EEG tracing be employed in the process of ensuring that collected epochs contain representative alert waking artifact free EEG activity.

Distortions produced by scaling decisions

The maximum and minimum values on a color bar used in topographic EEG mapping are almost always user definable. How one selects these maximum and minimum values will often produce rather dramatic changes in map appearance. Adjustments that either expand scaling limits to permit color identification and hence visualization of extreme values or constrict scale range to enhance small numerical values at the expense of larger ones can also produce maps which at first glance seem to contain the most impressive foci or regional changes of activity when in fact the underlying electroencephalographic phenomena are unimpressive and without statistical or clinical relevance. This occurs most often when a narrow constricted range of numerical values is selected and then represented topographically with a full spectrum color bar scale creating a dazzling enhancement of differences which in reality are quite small. If collected by the uninformed and then conveyed to the even less informed of other disciplines this type of misleading information can spread more easily than one can imagine.

Postscript

Topographic mapping of brain electrical activity involves a complex combination of techniques which in truth hold substantial promise for the future of neuroscience and the study of brain function. Use of EEG brain mapping technology is expanding with extreme rapidly but not all of this expansion is within the field of experienced neurophysiologic and electroencephalographic investigation. The maps are compelling, often striking in their impact, and to the uninitiated who review attractive product brochures or see demonstrations, they may appear to be based on "objective" and automatic data collection procedures. In truth, however, topographic mapping is a complex process highly subject to profound distortions which can only be avoided or minimized by a deep understanding of electroencephalography and a solid electroencephalographic interpretive scrutiny of the raw EEG phenomena out of which the maps are made. Concern that this may not always be appreciated and that abuse may occur has been voiced recently by the American Electroencephalographic Society [55].

Topographic EEG brain mapping should offer considerable promise to the study of brain function in cardiac disease and in the assessment of patients prior to and following open heart surgery. This is because such techniques would be expected to be highly sensitive to those frequency and amplitude alterations – even subtle changes – following transient or reoccurring ischemic or hypoxic brain compromise. One hopes that as application of mapping techniques extends into this important clinical area the perils of unrecognized error and map distortion will be avoided and the positive value of topographic mapping will be realized.

References

1. Walter WG, Shipton HW. A new toposcopic display system. Electroenceph Clin Neurophysiol 1951; 3:281.
2. Etevenon P. Applications and perspectives of EEG cartography. In: Duffy FH (ed).

Topographic Mapping of Brain Electrical Activity. Boston, London, Butterworths, 1986; p. 113.

3. Duffy FH, Burchfiel JL, Lombroso CT. Brain electrical activity mapping (BEAM): A new method for extending the clinical utility of EEG and evoked potential data. Ann Neurol 1979; 5:309.

4. Lombroso CT, Duffy FH. Brain electrical activity mapping as an adjunct to CT scanning. In: Canger R, Angeleri F, Perry JK (eds). Advances in Epileptology: Proceedings of XIII Epilepsy International Symposium. New York, Raven Press, 1980; p. 83.

5. Duffy FH. Brain electrical activity mapping (BEAM): Computerized access to complex brain function. Int J Neurosci 1981; 13:55.

6. Duffy FH, Bartels PH, Burchfiel JL. Significance probability mapping: An aid in the topographic analysis of brain electrical activity. Electroenceph Clin Neurophysiol 1981; 51:455.

7. Buchsbaum MS, Rigal F, Coppola R, Cappelleti J, King C, Johnson J. A new system for gray-level surface distribution maps of electrical activity. Electroenceph Clin Neurophysiol 1982; 53:237.

8. Friedman LR. Unwrapping the riddle of the brain-injured patient by utilizing the BEAM EEG. Am J Forensic Psychiat 1982; 3:467.

9. Persson A, Hjorth B. EEG topogram: An aid in describing EEG to the clinician. Electroenceph Clin Neurophsyiol 1983; 56:399.

10. Duffy FH, Albert MS, McAnulty G, Garvey AJ. Age related differences in brain electrical activity in healthy subjects. Ann Neurol 1984; 16:430.

11. Etevenon P, Gaches J, Debouzy C, Gueguen B, Peron-Magon P. Electroencephalographic cartography. Neuropsychobiol 1985; 13:141.

12. Jarrett SA, Corsak J. Clinical utility of topographic EEG brain mapping. Clin Electroenceph 1988; 19:134.

13. Duff FH (ed). Topographic Mapping of Brain Electrical Activity. Boston, London, Butterworths, 1986.

14. Duffy FH, Denckla MB, Bartels PH, Sandini G, Keissling LS. Dyslexia: Automated diagnosis by computerized classification of brain electrical activity. Ann Neurol 1980; 7:421.

15. Duffy FH, Denckla MB, Bartels PH, Sandini G. Dyslexia: Regional differences in brain electrical activity by topographic mapping. Ann Neurol 1980; 7:412.

16. Lombroso CT, Duffy FH. Brain electrical activity mapping in the epilepsies. In: Akimoto H, Kazamatsuir H, Seino M, Ward A (eds). Advances in Epileptology, Proceedings of the XIII Epilepsy International Symposium. New York, Raven Press, 1982; p. 173.

17. Popoviciu L, Tudosie M, Pepelea P, Baciulescu I, Bagothy I, Roman V, Foisareanu V. Comparative aspects of the electroencephalographic map in various forms of epilepsy. Neurol Psychiat 1984; 22:9.

18. Duffy FH, Jensen F, Erba G, Burchfiel JL, Lombroso CT. Extraction of clinical information from electroencephalographic background activity – the combined use of brain electrical activity mapping and intravenous sodium thiopental. Ann Neurol 1984; 15:22.

19. Nagata L, Mizukami M, Araki G, Kawase T, Hirano M. Topographic electroencephalographic study of cerebral infarction using computed mapping of the EEG. J Cerebral Blood Flow Metabol 1982; 2:79.

20. Popoviciu L, Tudosie M, Schiopu M, Pepelea R, Baciulesco I, Bagothay I, Pascu I, Roman V. The contributionof the electroencephalographic computerized map in setting down the topography of the cerebral infarctions. Neurol Psychiat 1984; 22:117.

21. Nagata K, Yunoki K, Araki G, Mizukami M. Topographic electroencephalographic study of transient ischemic attacks. Electroenceph Clin Neurophysiol 1984; 58:291.

22. Buchsbaum MS, Kessler R, King A, Johnson J, Cappelletti J. Simultaneous cerebral glucography with positron emission tomagraphy and topographic electroencephalography. In: Pfurtscheller G, Jonkman EJ, Lopes da Silva FH (eds). Brain Ischemia: Quantitative EEG and Imaging Techniques. Amsterdam, Elsevier, 1984; p. 263.

23. Nagata K, Yunoki K, Araki G, Mizukami M, Hyodo A. Topographic electroencephalographic study of ischemic cerebrovascular disease. In: Pfurtscheller G, Jonkman EJ, Lopes

da Silva FH (eds). Brain Ischemia: Quantitative EEG and Imagining Techniques Amsterdam, Elsevier, 1984; p. 271.

24. Pfurtscheller G, Ladurner G, Maresch H, Vollmer R. Brain electrical activity mapping in normal and ischemic brain. In: Pfurtscheller G, Jonkman EJ, Lopes da Silva FH (eds). Brain Ischemia: Quantitative EEG and Imaging Techniques. Amsterdam, Elsevier, 1984; p. 287.

25. Nuwer MR, Jordan SE, Ahn SS. Evaluation of stroke using EEG frequency analysis and topographic mapping. Neurology 1987; 37:1153.

26. Duffy FH, Albert MS, McAnulty G. Brain electrical activity in patients with presenile and senile dementia of the Alzheimer's type. Ann Neurol 1984; 16:439.

27. Burchfiel JL, Duffy FH, Bartels PH, Needleman HL. The combined discriminating power of quantitative electroencephalography and neuropsychiatric measures in evaluating central nervous system effects of lead at low levels. In: Needleman HL (ed). Low Level Lead Exposure: The Clinical Implications of Current Research. New York, Raven Press, 1980.

28. Duffy FH, Als H. Neurophysiological assessment of the neonate: An approach combining brain electrical activity mapping (BEAM) with behavioral assessment. In: Brazelton JB, Lester BM (eds). New Approaches to Developmental Screening of Infants. New York, Elsevier, 1983; p.175.

29. Buchsbaum MS, Mendelson WB, Duncan WC, Coppola R, Kelsoe J, Gillin JC. Topographic cortical mapping of EEG sleep stages during daytime naps in normal subjects. Sleep 1982; 5:248.

30. Buchsbaum MS, Coppola R, Cappelletti J. Positron emission tomography, EEG and evoked potential topography: New approaches to local function in pharmaco-electroencephalography. In: Herrman E (ed). EEG in Drug Research. Stuttgart, New York, Gustav Fisher, 1982; p. 192.

31. Buchsbaum MS, Cappelletti J, Coppola R, Regal F, King AC, Vankammen DP. New methods to determine the CNS effects of antigeriatric compounds: EEG topography and glucose use. Drug Develop Res 1982; 2:489.

32. Rodin E, Nigro M. The cerebral electrical fields in cerebellar syndrome. Clin Electroenceph 1987; 18:142.

33. Takaesu E, Watanabe K, Inokuma K, Matsumoto A, Sugiura M, Negoro T. EEG topography in porencephaly and arachnoid cyst. Clin Electroenceph 1985; 16:21.

34. Struve FA, Straumanis JJ, Patrick G, Price L. Topographic mapping of quantitative EEG variables in chronic heavy marihuana users: Empirical findings with psychiatric patients. Clin Electroenceph 1989; 20 (in press).

35. Morihisa JM, Duffy FH, Wyatt RJ. Brain electrical activity mapping (BEAM) in schizophrenic patients. Arch Gen Psychiat 1983; 40:719.

36. Morstyn R, Duffy FH, McCarley RW. Altered topography of EEG spectral content in schizophrenia. Electroenceph Clin Neurophysiol 1983; 56:263.

37. Pockeberger H, Petsche H, Rappelsberger P et al. On-going EEG in depression: A topographic spectral analytical pilot study. Electroenceph Clin Neurophysiol 1985; 61:349.

38. Guenther W, Breitling D. Predominant sensorimotor area left hemisphere dysfunction in schizophrenia measured by brain electrical activity mapping. Biol Psychiat 1985; 20:515.

39. Morihisa JM, McAnulty GB. Structure and function: Brain electrical activity mapping and computed tomography in schizophrenia. Biol Psychiat 1985; 20:3.

40. Small JG, Milstein V, Small IF, Miller MJ, Kellams JJ, Corsaro C. Computerized EEG profiles of haloperidol, chlorpromazine, clozapine and placebo in treatment resistant schizophrenia. Clin Electroenceph 1987; 18:124.

41. John ER, Prichep LS, Fridman J, Easton P. Neurometrics: Computer-assisted differential diagnosis of brain dysfunctions. Science 1988; 239:162.

42. Coppola R. Issues in topographic analysis of EEG activity. In: Duffy FH (ed). Topographic Mapping of Brain Electrical Activity. Boston, London, Butterworths, 1986; p. 339.

43. Duffy FH. Brain electrical activity mapping: Issues and answers. In: Duffy FH (ed). Topographic Mapping of Brain Electrical Activity. Boston, London, Butterworths, 1986; p. 401.

44. Walter DO, Etevenon P, Pidoux B, Tortrat D, Guillou S. Computerized topo-EEG spectral maps: Difficulties and perspectives. Neuropsychobiol 1984; 11:264.
45. Kahn EM, Weiner RD, Brenner RP, Coppola R. Topographic maps of brain electrical activity – Pitfalls and precautions. Biol Psychiat 1988; 23:628.
46. Cooper R, Osselton JW, Shaw JC. EEG Technology, 3rd edition. London, Butterworths, 1980.
47. Struve FA. Lithium – specific pathological electroencephalographic changes: A successful repliction of earlier investigative results. Clin Electroenceph 1987; 18:46.
48. Gibbs FA, Gibbs EL. Atlas of Electroencephalography, Vol. 3, Neurological and Psychiatric Disorders. Reading MA, Addison-Wesley, 1964.
49. Barlow JS. Artifact processing (Rejection and minimization) in EEG data processing. In: Lopes da Silva FA, van Leewen WS, and Rémond A (eds). Handbook of Electroencephalography. Revised Series Volume 2, Clinical Applications of Computer Analysis of EEG and Other Neurophysiological Signals. Amsterdam, New York, Elsevier, 1986; p. 15.
50. Chiappa KA. Progress in topographic mapping of neurophysiological data: Comments. In: Duffy FH (ed). Topographic Mapping of Brain Electrical Activity. Boston,London, Butterworths, 1986; p. 393.
51. Bickford RG, Allen B. A simple add-on personal computer procedure for color displays of electrophysiological data: Advantages and pitfalls. In: Duffy FH (ed). Topographic Mapping of Brain Electrical Activity. Boston, London, Butterworths, 1986; p. 203.
52. Shipton HW. From entertainment to education, from education to enlightenment. In: Duffy FH (ed). Topographic Mapping of Brain Electrical Activity. Boston, London, Butterworths, 1986; p. 217.
53. Harner RN. 1986. Clinical application of computed EEG topography. In: Duffy FH (ed). Topographic Mapping of Brain Electrical Activity. Boston, London, Butterworths, 1986; p. 347.
54. Torello MW, McCarley RW. The use of topographic mapping techniques in clinical studies in psychiatry. In: Duffy FH (ed). Topographic Mapping of Brain Electrical Activity. Boston, London, Butterworth, 1986; p. 383.
55. American Electroencephalographic Society. Statement on clinical use of quantitative EEG. J Clin Neurophysiol 1987; 4:75.

12. Real time multichannel quantitative EEG monitoring

ROBERT J. CHABOT, E. ROY JOHN,
LESLIE S. PRICHEP, PIERRE M. LANDAU,
WAYNE O. ISOM and LAVERNE D. GUGINO

Estimates of the incidence of central nervous system (CNS) damage during cardiopulmonary bypass (CPB) surgery vary greatly and are dependent upon a number of factors including: (1) the measure of CNS function utilized, (2) whether the study was retrospective or prospective, (3) the time span over which CNS function was monitored postoperatively, (4) the nature of the population studied, and (5) the type of cardiac procedure performed. The incidence of focal neurological damage due to confirmed stroke in the immediate postoperative period ranges from 2 to 5% [1–3]. This finding has remained relatively constant over the past 10 years. Although the overall benefits of coronary artery bypass graft (CABG) and valve replacement procedures have been confirmed [4], the actual number of patients suffering focal CNS damage due to confirmed stroke is substantial, even using the lowest figure suggested in the literature (137,000 CABG procedures per year in the U.S. at 2% = 2740 strokes) [3].

A review of the current literature indicates that subtle CNS damage as estimated by neurological and neuropsychological deficits are even greater, affecting from 11 to 61% of patients within the first 10 days after surgery [1, 5, 6]. Long-term follow-up studies using the same measures indicate that signs of CNS dysfunction persist in approximately 5 to 9% of patients up to one year after surgery [1, 5, 7]. The higher incidence of subtle generalized rather than focal neuronal damage has also been documented in CPB patients by measures showing decreased regional cerebral blood flow [8], increased adenylate kinase in cerebral spinal fluid [9], and significant EEG slowing (i.e., increase of activity in the delta and theta frequency bands) which persisted well into the postoperative period [4, 10]. It is of particular interest that Sotaniemi and his associates [4] showed that early signs of CNS dysfunction predicted CNS decline 5 years postoperatively, despite improved CNS function 1 year after surgery. Similarly, Hammeke and Hastings [7] suggest that subtle neuropsychological dysfunction may appear 2 to 8 years after CPB surgery. Since higher cortical functions play a major role in determining the quality of life [4], these findings have resulted in a widespread call for the development of reliable, objective, and sensitive quantitative techniques to detect impending neuronal damage during CPB surgery so that attempts can be made to reverse these changes prior to the development of permanent damage [4, 11, 12].

Prior to a critical review of currently utilized CNS monitoring techniques and the presentation of a newly developed real-time quantitative EEG technique, a brief discussion of the putative causes of CNS damage and its correlates is in order.

Causes and correlates of CNS damage during CPB

CNS damage during CPB procedures results from one or a combination of the following factors; (A) macroemboli released from athromatous vessels, air in the perfusion circuit or thrombus, (B) microemboli of air, fat, particulate matter, and/or platelet/fibrin clumps formed during CPB, and (C) altered cerebral blood flow during CPB causing inadequate cerebral and capillary bed perfusion resulting in ischemic damage to underperfused cerebral regions [2, 6, 11, 13–15]. Current controversy concerns the relative importance of microemboli and hypoperfusion as the major cause of CNS dysfunction [10, 16]. Real-time quantitative EEG monitoring might correlate with specific surgical or anesthesiologist maneuvers and could play an important role in determining causal relationships. Treatment would vary depending upon the particular factor implicated (i.e., increasing perfusion flow or blood pressure for hypoxic conditions or injecting thiopental or future compounds with the anti-platelet effect of prostacydin without its hypotensive effects for microembolic conditions [17].

Prospective studies of CNS dysfunction after CPB have indicated significant correlations between the presence of CNS damage and the following factors; (1) increasing patient age [13, 18], (2) increasing duration of CPB [13, 18], (3) pre-existing cerebrovascular disease (CVD) associated with concomitant carotid artery disease [6, 10, 19], EEG abnormalities [20, 21], and/or a prior history of stroke or TIA's with or without neurological symptoms [5, 6, 11, 18, 19], and (4) pre-existing hypertension which may cause a shift in cerebral hemodynamic autoregulation making the patient more vulnerable to ischemic events during periods of decreased cerebral perfusion pressure. Surprisingly, several studies have failed to find a significant correlation between CPB perfusion pressure and postoperative CNS dysfunction. This may be due to the fact that most of these studies selectively excluded elderly patients as well as those with pre-existing cerebrovascular disease.

Current monitoring techniques

Several groups of investigators have suggested that at present the electroencephalogram (EEG) is the only objective, non-invasive measure of CNS function during CPB procedures [1, 10, 22–24]. This belief arose from experience in EEG monitoring during carotid endarterectomies [21, 25, 26], and research findings that computer extracted EEG features were sensitive indicators of rCBF and cerebral metabolism [1, 21, 23, 25–27]. Studies during carotid endarterectomy (CE) have indicated the sensitivity, reliability, and utility of computer EEG feature monitoring in preventing permanent cerebral ischemic damage and have shown the following:

a) In 386 CE procedures no permanent neurological dysfunction occurred without significant EEG changes. These changes included decreased amplitude, and/or ipsilateral or bilateral increases in power in the theta and delta frequency range [25].

b) When rCBF fell below 12 ml/100/gm/min EEG changes always occurred within 20 seconds [25], and

c) patients with angiographically confirmed decreased CBF and multiple small vessel occlusions showed impaired cerebral autoregulation and often became passively dependent upon perfusion pressure [21]. In fact, Sundt and associates [21] state that under conditions of pre-existing CVD, ischemic events may lead to an increased susceptibility to CNS damage as a result of microemboli. The preceding findings suggest that there may be no a priori universally safe level of cerebral perfusion during CPB procedures unless intimate knowledge is available about the degree of pre-existing cerebrovascular disease, the extent of autoregulation impairment, as well as an understanding of the relationships between rCBF, cerebral metabolic needs, body temperature, anesthetic type and level as well as $PaCO_2$. pressure [28]. Evidence also exists that computer extracted QEEG features may be extremely sensitive indicators of pre-existing ischemic conditions even in asymptomatic individuals [27]. Thus, there appears to be a role for QEEG testing to determine pre-operative risk of CNS dysfunction, to monitor CNS function intraoperatively, and to monitor CNS function during the postoperative period.

Despite statements to the contrary [29, 30], QEEG monitoring is not accepted routine practice during cardiac surgery. However, research and experience using EEG monitoring during CPB has been accumulating since 1957 [31]. With the advent of computerized EEG monitoring systems there has been a resurgence of interest. This has occurred in part due to a belief (probably erroneous) that these computerized systems will not require extensive EEG knowledge and experience. There are some who believe that minimal numbers of EEG channels (4 or less) are adequate and that only EEG features which reflect amplitude and frequency within these channels are necessary [15, 22, 23, 29, 32–34]. These beliefs are based upon an assumption that minimal EEG channels will suffice to show global ischemic changes, and/or changes within the posterior watershed region. Perhaps because of the hope to decrease the complexity of EEG set-up and monitoring procedures, this belief persists despite the known incidence of false positive and false negative QEEG findings when monitoring with few channels during CPB [30, 31]. In contrast, Sundt and associates [21] failed to find any false positive findings while monitoring CE procedures using 16 channels of conventional EEG. Bashen et al. [31] point out that studies have not yet determined the appropriate number, optimal placement of electrodes and optimal EEG features to be monitored. However, since there are three major cerebral arteries plus the watershed region on each hemisphere, it seems highly unlikely that less than eight channels could suffice.

Disadvantages of current EEG monitoring systems

Despite much data reduction and the loss of valuable information, success in monitoring CPB surgery has been reported using such equipment as the cerebral function monitor (CFM) and the cerebral function analyzing monitor (CFAM) [15, 29, 30, 32, 34]. The CFM system was quickly determined to be inadequate since it monitored only a single channel and only the single EEG feature of amplitude change. It readily became apparent that EEG amplitude and frequency changes could occur independently of one another and this led to the development of CFAM [15, 29, 30]. This system monitors two channels, yielding information about a variety of EEG features including minimum, maximum, mean, 10th and 90th centile amplitude as well as relative percent power in the beta, alpha, theta and delta frequency bands. Although reports of the utility of CFAM monitoring during CPB can be found [30, 34], this system has serious limitations and its clinical utility has recently been questioned [22, 30]. In our viewpoint the most serious limitation of this system as well as other currently available monitoring systems [22, 23, 33] is the reliance on minimal numbers of EEG channels and an inability to quantify changes in EEG features either in a clinically relevant or statistical way. The reliance on monitoring only 2 channels is based upon the erroneous assumption that primarily global EEG changes will occur during CPB and that the posterior watershed areas will reliably be affected [35]. Recent reports suggest not only that the watershed regions between all major cerebral arteries may be at risk [22], but that no specific cortical region shows selective susceptibility to ischemic disturbance [20]. The reliance on 2 channel systems and minimal extracted features of EEG amplitude and frequency (whether compressed spectral array [23, 33], density spectral array and/or spectral edge frequency) [22] has made it difficult if not impossible to define the critical EEG features and the extent and duration of the changes which will be reliably associated with CNS dysfunction [20, 30, 31, 36]. The remainder of this paper will consist of the following: (a) a brief presentation of our relevant findings using a quantitative 20-channel EEG system called a Brain State analyzer, (b) a description of a real-time quantitative EEG monitoring system, called CIMON, whose development was based upon this initial experience, and (c) examples of the sensitivity of the new system to ischemic changes.

Multi-channel QEEG and CPB

During the development of the Brain State Analyzer (BSA),[1] we did preoperative, intraoperative and/or postoperative QEEG testing on 80 CPB patients [10].[2] Several observations from this experience and other related BSA studies have particular relevance to the arguments being presented.

Nineteen monopolar channels (International 10/20 system) of 20 seconds to 2 minutes of artifact-free EEG were collected under control of the microprocessor in the BSA using an on-line automatic artifact detection algorithm [37]. From these 19 channels, an additional 8 bipolar derivations were computed (F_7T_3/F_8T_4, T_3T_5/T_4T_6, C_3C_z/C_4C_z, P_3O_1/P_4O_2). Univariate and multivariate features were calculated for all monopolar and bipolar derivations [38] after spectral analysis using the Fast Fourier Transform [39]. Univariate features extracted included the absolute (μV^2) and relative (%) power in the delta, theta, alpha and beta frequency bands for each derivation and power asymmetry and coherence for each frequency band across homologous unipolar and bipolar derivations. Multivariate features statistically removed the correlations among univariate features and compressed across univariate features within a region, as well as across various regions for a given univariate feature. The raw values of each extracted QEEG feature were either compared against normative values obtained from a larger data base which spanned the ages 6–90 years or compared to the feature values obtained from the same ·patient in a prior QEEG session. In both instances this comparison was made using a Z-transformation. All features were mathematically transformed to obtain gaussian distributions and then age – regressed prior to Z-transformation. Please see John *et al.* [40] for a more detailed discussion of these techniques.

Comparisons between an individual patients' preoperative and/or postoperative QEEG findings and the normative data base could be made to detect pre-existing CVD or postoperative damage due to CPB [41]. Comparisons between preoperative and postoperative findings within a patient could also be used to determine the effects of CPB surgery on the brain. Comparisons between initial intraoperative baseline QEEG sessions and additional sessions during the surgical procedure could be utilized to monitor brain function during CPB.

Relevant findings using the brain state analyzer (BSA)

The possibility that preoperative QEEG evaluation could be used for determining the pre-existence of ischemic cerebral damage was evident from a collaborative study using our QEEG techniques [27]. Four groups of patients were studied 14 days after an ischemic event, having had either completed strokes, persisting neurological symptoms, reversible ischemic neurological deficits or transient ischemic attacks. The relative utility of 133-Xenon measures of rCBF, conventional EEG and QEEG features for detecting cerebrovascular abnormality was evaluated. QEEG features were consistently the most sensitive measures, particularly in the asymptomatic RIND and TIA patients. The multivariate QEEG features proved to be particularly sensitive indicators of these ischemic abnormalities since they indicate disturbances of normal EEG relationships between cortical regions rather than focal changes. This finding suggests that multivariate features may play a critical role in monitoring cortical function during CPB procedures as well as in assessing possible risk to the brain from intraoperative ischemia.

In another study, risk for developing CNS dysfunction was evaluated in 11 coronary artery bypass patients for whom QEEG data had been obtained before preoperative medication. Our prior research as well as numerous other studies had indicated that cerebral ischemia was associated with increased relative power in the delta frequency range seen most clearly when comparisons were made to age-regressed population norms [10]. Significant preoperative elevations of relative delta power were found in 5 of the 11 patients tested. In three, the abnormal delta excess was focal and in two, the delta excess was generalized. These five patients would be considered at risk for intraoperative cerebral damage since abnormal QEEG findings [20, 21] and associated pre-existing CVD [6, 19] have been shown to predict post-operative neurological deficits.

The clinical utility of QEEG monitoring during CPB procedures depends upon the ability to distinguish between QEEG changes which are the signals of impending cortical damage and those which are the predictable biophysical consequence of changes in the CPB parameters. Our experience with the BSA has indicated that it is possible to mathematically predict changes in QEEG measures that occur as a normal consequence of changes in blood flow and body temperature. Thus, changes of potential clinical significance can be defined as those which are greater than predictable from the ongoing changes in CPB parameters [10].

An adequate test of the clinical utility of intraoperative QEEG monitoring for preventing postoperative cortical dysfunction requires a prospective study of neurological and neuropsychological function in matched groups of monitored and non-monitored CPB patients. Appropriate control groups to rule out the detrimental effects of surgical variables other than CPB would also be necessary. Although we did not perform functional testing and lacked desirable control groups, we were able to obtain a preliminary estimate of the clinical utility of QEEG monitoring by examining postoperative QEEG indices of cortical ischemic changes (increases in relative (%) delta power) in a group of 10 patients who were monitored with appropriate interventions and a group of 10 matched patients who were not monitored. In all patients, QEEG testing was accomplished pre-CPB surgery and 7–10 days post surgery in the absence of medication. The results of this preliminary study were encouraging. Comparisons of preoperative with postoperative QEEG revealed no significant change in Z-relative delta power for the monitored group but a significant (0.01) increase in postoperative Z-relative delta power for the non-monitored group. Since increased relative delta power indicates cortical dysfunction and ischemic damage [20, 21, 27], this study indicates that the monitored group did not suffer ischemic damage, whereas ischemic damage did occur within the non-monitored group.

The BSA utilized to collect the data described in the preceding sections was not designed primarily as an intraoperative QEEG monitoring device. All BSA data were collected and analyzed in separate sessions which included between 20 seconds (intraoperative) and 2 minutes (pre and post-operative) of artifact-free EEG. Intraoperative monitoring was not optimal because data collection had to be stopped during analyses and only intermittent (every 7–10 minutes) feedback to the surgeon and/or anesthesiologist was possible. For this reason a new Cardiovascular Intraoperative Monitor (CIMON) was developed by Dr. E. Roy John[3] which makes virtual real-time QEEG monitoring possible. This device is currently being evaluated during CE and CPB procedures[4] and only preliminary findings are available. The remainder of this paper will be used to describe this system and present illustrative examples of its sensitivity to developing ischemic cortical events.

CIMON system description

Hardware

The EEG data were collected on a Cadwell Spectrum-32 system. The 19 leads of the 10/20 system and a differential eye channel were attached to the scalp and recorded referentially relative to linked earlobes. Later in the study, an EKG channel was added. The amplifiers had a bandpass from 0.5 to 70 Hz (3 dB points), with a notch filter at 60 Hz. The data were digitized at 200 Hz with twelve bit resolution. The central processor was a 16-bit microprocessor with 2 MB of RAM, an optical disk and a 70 MB hard disk, on which all recorded data were stored. A color display controller with a resolution of 1024×800 with five color planes was used for the real-time display.

Software

CIMON was designed with the idea of monitoring a complete set of EEG features in real-time during cardiovascular surgery. Thus, unlike traditional systems in which a data collection phase of several minutes is followed by an analysis phase, we wanted a display which could be used for direct real-time feedback to the surgeon. An additional requirement was that though we would only be able to view a small number of features on the display screen at any one time, the system would continuously monitor all other features and warn if significant changes occurred in any features off-screen. Data were collected in 2.56 second "segments". We used a scrolling historical display in which successive measures are calculated over an average of the last N segments including the current data segment. As each new segment is collected, the oldest segment is dropped from the average and a new average is computed and displayed below the previous average, yielding a "sliding average". The size of this average will determine its variability. This parameter N is chosen by the operator to optimizer stability ("large enough") while preserving sensitivity ("but not too large"). In practice, N is usually in the range 6 to 9.

Calculated features

The feature set which was calculated was:

Absolute power. This was calculated for low delta (0.5–1.5 Hz), delta (1.5–3.5 Hz), theta (3.5–7.5 Hz), alpha (7.5–12.5 Hz), beta (12.5–25 Hz), high beta (25–50 Hz), and total (1.5–25 Hz).

Relative power. This was calculated for delta, theta, alpha, beta and represented the percentage of total power within each frequency band.

Asymmetry. The power ratio was calculated between homologous derivations separately for each band and for total.

Coherence. The variance of the normalized cross spectral power between homologous derivations was calculated separately for each band and for total.

Dominant frequency. The centroid of the power spectrum in the Total band (1.5–25 Hz) was calculated. We had earlier calculated this measure for individual bands, but did not find it helpful in monitoring.

Each of these features was calculated for each of the original 19 monopolar, 8 computer bipolar and several multivariate derivations, as described below. Each feature could be represented in any one of 3 ways:

- a raw value which could be displayed directly, or compared via Z-transformation either to
- age-regressed population norms or to
- a "self-norm" previously obtained from the patient preoperatively or intraoperatively during an earlier stage of the surgery.

No matter which of these representations is selected, the resulting value is encoded as a color (see "QEEG Feature Display").

Artifacting algorithms
It was deemed dangerous to rely on a voltage threshold artifact detection algorithm as this might exclude segments containing high-amplitude slow waves, sharp waves, or spikes. Two artifact detection algorithms were included, though the first was primarily used in the study. We looked first for sharp waves, as explained in the next section, and segments which contained sharp waves were automatically accepted. We computed a "tracking artifact level", based on the previous 15 seconds of data, and rejected segments which had no sharp waves but exceeded this threshold. This might be conceptualized as a "floating threshold" method.

The second algorithm considered a segment artifact contaminated if the high beta exceeded its self-norm by two standard deviations, indicating muscle artifact, or the low delta exceeded its self-norm by two standard deviations, indicating eye or head movement. This presupposed that an appropriate self-norm had been constructed with a quiescent patient.

Sharp wave detection

In view of an observed correlation between increase in sharp wave activity and ischemia, we included a sharp wave detector, triggered by any event which significantly exceeded the mean sharpness (N standard deviations above the mean second derivative). Candidate sharp waves were then tested using criteria for slope, gross morphology, duration, anatomical field, surrounding alpha, and surrounding beta activity prior to confirmation as 'true' sharp waves.

QEEG feature display

Two principal types of display were defined. The first was a traditional scrolling EEG display, which could be used to display the EEG segments one at a time, showing either actual monopolar or constructed bipolar derivations. The second was a new type of display, termed the CIMON display, which implemented a historical map.

To visualize the CIMON display (Figures. 1–3), imagine a map, in which each lead is represented by a rectangle of the display screen, in a topographically mapped fashion. This give us a "mosaic" containing the same amount of information as a conventional topographic map, albeit without the interpolation. Now suppose each rectangle is divided vertically into a set of columns, one for each frequency band: Delta, theta, alpha, and beta. Each column has a color which encodes the value of the feature for that frequency

172

Z Relative Power (self-norm)   Z Absolute Power (self-norm)

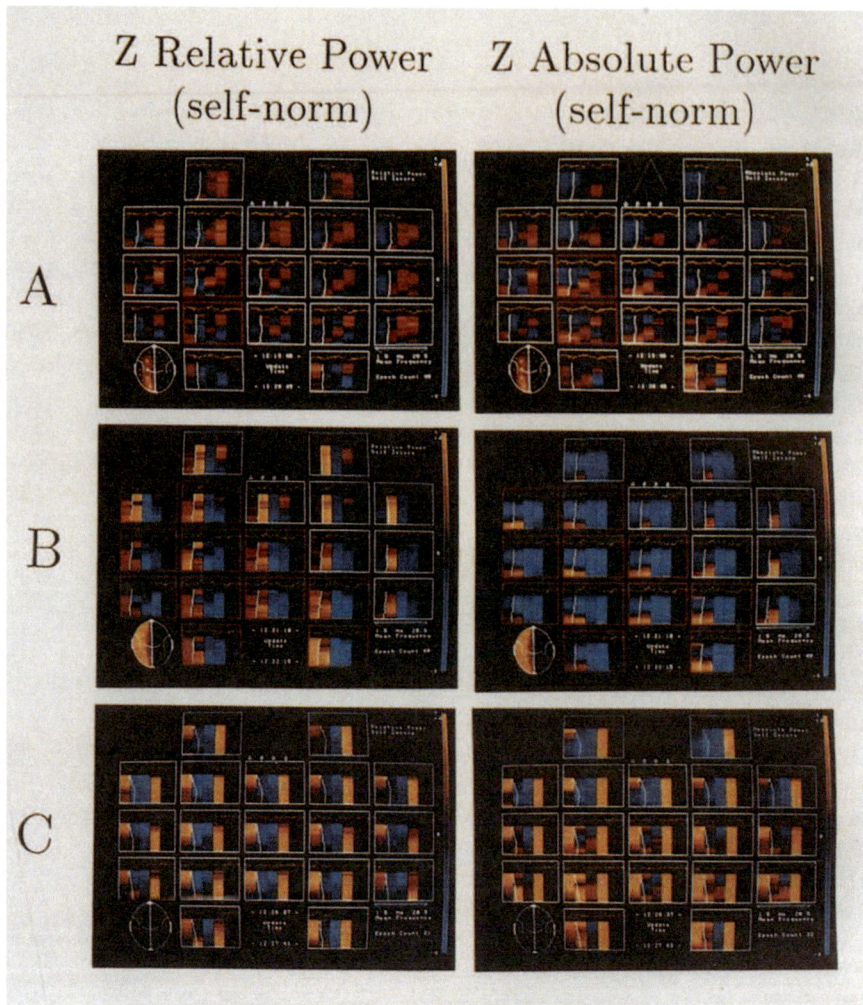

A

B

C

Fig. 1A–C. CIMON displays of Z-transformed relative (left side) and absolute power (right side). Each rectangle represents an electrode position based upon the International 10/20 system. Within each rectangle are four separate scrolling bands representing the self-normed Z-transform (0 to 4 standard deviations from an initial baseline) of relative or absolute power in the delta, theta, alpha and beta frequency range. Each strip within a band represents the appropriate EEG measure calculated over the last 22.5 seconds of EEG with an overlap of 5/6. Rectangles outlined in white represent regions at baseline levels. Those outlined in red represent monopolar warnings due to statistically significant changes from baseline condition. The white line within each rectangle shows mean frequency over the display interval. The small headmap in the left corner remains blank unless significant multivariate changes occur, and persist for two minutes. When multivariate changes occur a topographic display of their extent and significance is presented. Figure 1 shows changes in Z-transformed relative and absolute power immediately after test clamping of the left ICA (1a), two to three minutes after clamping (1b) and two to three minutes after removal of the test clamp (1c).

Z Relative Power
(self-norm)

Z Absolute Power
(self-norm)

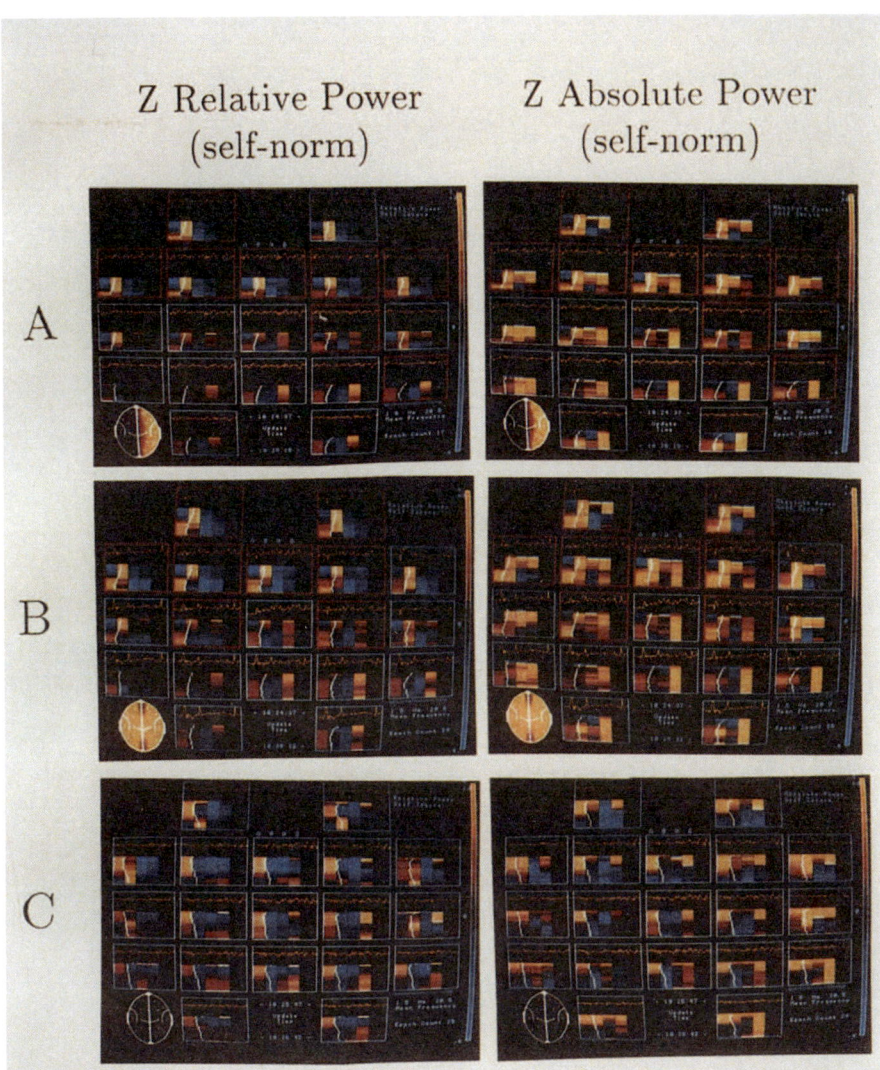

A

B

C

Fig. 2A–C. CIMON displays of actual relative and absolute power changes without Z-transform and monopolar or multivariate warnings. The time periods shown are identical with those seen in figures 1a–1c.

band and location. We are thus viewing a topographic representation of the values of all the features selected for display. Now we add the element of time. We decompose each vertical column into a set of 40 small horizontal segments, corresponding to the feature value at 40 successive times and allow the display to scroll upward. The rectangle now simultaneously displays the values for each frequency band, for each lead, as they occurred during the past 40 time intervals. The overlap in the sliding averages which create the displayed values make most transitions appear smooth. An additional column is included which flags whether sharp waves were detected in a lead at that time.

A CIMON display can be selected to represent any of the 24 available

Relative Power
(%)

Absolute Power
(μV^2)

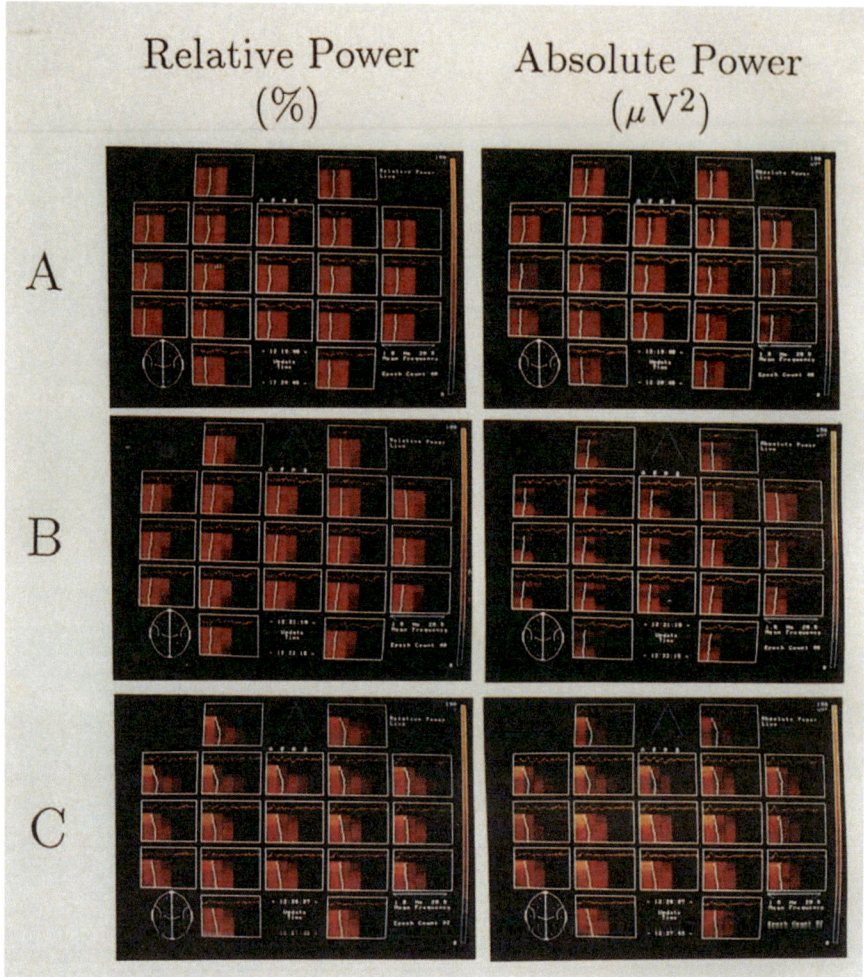

A

B

C

Fig. 3A–C. CIMON displays of Z-transformed relative and absolute power shown; (a) immediately after back-bleeding from the right ICA, (b) the first minute and half after back-bleeding, and (c) the first minute and half after back-bleeding was controlled.

feature sets: monopolar or bipolar absolute power, relative power, asymmetry, or coherence, displayed as raw, population normed, or self-normed values.

In addition, the user can display the EEG traces for the current sample within the top portion of the rectangle corresponding to each electrode, and outline the rectangle with a margin which can be made to blink red when the machine feels that the lead warrants attention (see Warnings, below). The display also warns of significant changes in any feature set other than the one displayed, and of potential problems within the perfusion fields of the major cerebral arteries (see Multivariate Feature Set, below).

Multivariate feature set

In addition to calculating univariate features for 19 monopolar and 8 bipolar derivations, the feature set was expanded to include multivariate features across selected cortical regions. Multivariate features were calculated separately for the left and right cerebral hemispheres and across the sets of leads corresponding to the perfusion fields of the left and right anterior, middle, and posterior cerebral arteries. These features are not displayed continuously but are used in the computation of warnings and then displayed in a topographic manner on a small head in the left corner of the display screen.

Additionally, a multivariate collapse of the bands is computed, taking into account their covariance, called the "combined" band. It is hoped that this condensed information may be more sensitive then any of the individual band measures.

Warnings

Warnings exist for features calculated from individual monopolar and bipolar derivations as well as for the multivariate features associated with the major arterial perfusion fields. Generally, a warning is flagged when the affected area shows signs of ischemia persisting long enough to cause concern. The warning process parameters are user-controllable, but are by default set to trigger a warning if there is an increase of greater than two standard deviations above the value of self-norm delta, and/or a similar decrease in dominant frequency, and these persist for over two minutes of clock time. This is calculated using a t-test of the current set of samples versus the self-norm. To compensate for the unpredictable delays due to artifacting, the size of the current set is determined exclusively by the wall clock. The warning is reset when, similarly, the values have reverted to normal range for the preceding two minutes. Obviously, the current warning settings represent our best guess and definitive settings must await empirical research findings.

Illustrative CIMON cases[5]

Case history 1
The patient was a 64 year old female with a history of hypertension, angina and coronary artery disease. Fifteen days prior to surgery she experienced transient right arm and leg weakness. Angiography revealed total occlusion of the right internal carotid artery (ICA) at its origin, and a 60% stenosis of the left ICA which also had an ulcerated plaque believed to have been the source of the previous TIA. There was reconstitution of the supraclinoid portion of the right ICA by retrograde flow from the ophthalmic artery via internal maxillary collaterals. In addition, there was excellent cross feeding of the right

anterior circulation via the left side. A preoperative neurological exam was within normal limits.

Surgical intervention included a left carotid endarterectomy with excision of the ulcerated plaque. EEG monitoring using CIMON was initiated at the beginning of the surgical procedure. An EEG baseline was computed after the initiation of anesthesia with N_2O/O_2, 0.5% forane, and fentanyl. The stability of this baseline was confirmed during 15 minutes of monitoring using Z-transformed relative power, prior to test clamping of the left ICA. One minute and 14 seconds after application of the test clamp on the ICA, significant EEG slowing occurred. This resulted in the initiation of univariate warnings at C_3 and P_3 and a multivariate warning within the perfusion fields of the left middle and posterior cerebral arteries. These changes are readily apparent in Figure 1A which presents CIMON displays of Z-transformed relative and absolute power during this time period. The C_3 and P_3 regions are outlined in red to represent the monopolar warning and the multivariate warning is displayed on the small headmap in the left bottom portion of each figure. Figure 2A displays, for the same time period, the conventionally used measures of relative and absolute power for each frequency band without Z-transform and the monopolar and multivariate automatic warning systems. Note that significant changes are not apparent in these displays nor are they apparent as changes in the overall mean frequency of the EEG displayed as the white line at each cortical region. Over the next minute and 30 seconds this significant slowing evolved to include all but one left hemisphere region, the central and parietal midline regions, and the parietal and occipital regions over the right hemisphere. Again, these changes are clearly seen in the displays of Z-transformed relative and absolute power (1B) but are not apparent in the displays of actual relative and absolute power (2B). The temporary clamp was removed at 12:24:47 and over the following 3 minutes the EEG returned to baseline values. Corresponding maps are illustrated for Z-transformed relative and absolute power (1C) as well as for relative and absolute power without Z-transform (2C). An identical sequence of changes occurred with subsequent clamping of the left ICA during the shunt placement which preceded the endarterectomy. The EEG returned to baseline values after shunt flow was initiated and remained at baseline levels throughout the procedure. The postoperative neurological exam was within normal limits.

This case illustrates the utility of using a Z-transformed display relative to an appropriate baseline EEG in order to identify significant intraoperative changes. Conceivably, we might have chosen display scales for relative and absolute power without Z-transform that would have shown these changes as clearly. However, we had no *a priori* basis for selecting a display scale which would have allowed us to see the changes which occurred. The use of Z-transformed measures solves the problem of having to decide on appropriate display scales on an *a priori* basis as well as providing a statistical criterion for quantifying change.

Case history 2
The patient was a 38 year old male with a pulsatile mass located in the right neck. CT scan and MRI revealed a 5 cm diameter extracranial aneurysm at the junction of the right common and internal carotid arteries. Preoperative arteriography showed excellent filling of the right middle cerebral artery distribution from the left ICA through widely patent anterior communicating vessels. Surgical excision of the aneurysm was planned with either primary reconstruction or ligation of the right ICA dependent upon surgical circumstances and EEG monitoring changes encountered. A baseline EEG was collected after anesthesia was stabilized, using N_2O/O_2 at induction and a continuous fentanyl drip. The stability of this baseline was verified by monitoring Z-transformed relative power prior to occlusion of the right common and external carotid arteries. For the first 12 minutes after occlusion the EEG remained stable and showed no signs of developing cerebral ischemia. However, when the aneurysm sac was opened significant back-bleeding occurred, accompanied by an immediate increase in Z-transformed relative and absolute delta power, resulting in bilateral frontal, right central and posterior temporal monopolar warnings. Multivariate warnings over the entire right hemisphere also occurred. These changes are apparent in Figure 3A which displays both Z-transformed relative (left side) and absolute (right side) power. Over the following minute sharp waves appeared and the increases in delta relative and absolute power affected both the left and right hemispheres (Figure 3B). These signs of cerebral ischemia persisted until back-bleeding was controlled by placement of a Fogarty embolectomy catheter into the distal right ICA. This resulted in a return of the EEG to initial baseline values (Figure 3C). In the absence of further EEG changes, the right ICA was ligated after the aneurysm was removed. The patient's neurological status remained within normal limits postoperatively. As in the preceding case, these intra-operative changes were not readily apparent if actual values of relative and absolute power without Z-transform were monitored.

The above examples illustrate the sensitivity of Z-transformed relative and absolute power measures across frequency bands for identifying significant ischemic events. Clearly the judicious selection of a baseline signal after anesthesia had been stabilized was critical. Both cases show that monitoring either absolute or relative power across the frequency bands with Z-transform to a self-norm makes it easier to identify significant deviations. The Z-transformation of EEG measures to a self-normed appropriate baseline condition provides the user a statistically defined criterion for identifying significant changes which may warrant intervention. Obviously, research during C.E. and CPB surgery will be necessary to define the critical limits and duration of EEG changes which can be tolerated without serious neurological consequence. At the least, CIMON offers the user QEEG procedures which should make it easier for this research question to be answered.

At this time, our experience with the current CIMON monitoring system during CPB surgery is limited. However, we used the prototype of this system during 20 CPB procedures. We found that Z-transformed relative delta power (self normed to an earlier baseline) was particularly sensitive to changes in both perfusion rate and blood pressure [10]. Prospective monitoring studies with this instrument are being developed and an evaluation of the clinical utility of CIMON should emerge from these endeavors.

Advantages of CIMON:

CIMON offers several distinct advantages for intraoperative monitoring:

1. Z-transformation of the results of preoperative QEEG evaluation relative to age regressed population norms provides an objective criterion to estimate whether the patient is at risk as well as to identify which specific cortical regions might be at risk. Postoperative testing can be easily accomplished and compared to preoperative self-norm baselines to determine the effects of the surgical procedure.
2. CIMON utilizes 19 monopolar and 8 bipolar derivations, thus allowing for the monitoring of focal as well as global changes.
3. The ability to calculate a self-normed baseline and to statistically compare all subsequent EEG samples to this baseline via Z-transform provides a quantitative tool for estimating the statistical significance of changes. The ability to re-calculate the norming baseline easily and quickly if surgical or anesthetic maneuvers (such as change of perfusate temperature or change of anesthetic) warrant is also critical, because it permits dynamic change of the frame of reference.
4. The ability to monitor and easily switch between multiple feature sets including monopolar and bipolar absolute and relative power as well as asymmetry and coherence, either as raw or Z-transformed values using self-norms or population norms, makes CIMON a powerful research tool and clinical instrument. Continuous automatic checking and warnings based upon off-screen feature sets minimize errors due to poor feature selection.
5. The calculation of multivariate features across each of the cortical regions associated with the major arterial perfusion fields can serve as a sensitive indicator of hemodynamic changes and regional cerebral dysfunction in addition to more localized changes [27].
6. Automatic on-line calculation of all QEEG features in close to real-time facilitates correlations to be perceived between discrete QEEG feature changes and specific surgical or anesthetic maneuvers. This real-time capability has been found to be especially important while monitoring evoked potentials during neurosurgical procedures [42].
7. Automatic artifacting set separately to exclude muscle (high frequency) and movement (low frequency) types of artifact has been shown to increase the reliability of data collected. This function as well as the ability to view feature headmaps and the raw EEG simultaneously should decrease false

alarms from EEG changes that are due to artifact. For example, slow waves in the EEG caused by the surgeon moving the patient's head or body.

8. Statistically defined automatic warning systems based upon monopolar and bipolar univariate features and/or multivariate features should eventually reduce the technical and EEG expertise needed to monitor effectively. Warning features are monitored whether or not they are currently being viewed.

9. Monitoring should also be made easier by the automatic spike detection algorithm. It has been our experience that significant EEG slowing associated with developing ischemia is often preceded by the appearance of multiple and continuous sharp waves.

The preceding list of advantages highlights the clinical and research possibilities of CIMON. Clearly much research has to be accomplished during intraoperative CPB monitoring before the true clinical utility of this instrumentation can be evaluated properly. Our early experience suggests that it represents a future generation of monitoring device that may help decrease the incidence of CNS dysfunction during CPB surgery.

Notes

1. Cadwell Laboratories, Kennewick, Washington.
2. The authors wish to thank Henry Merkin and MeeLee Tom for their aid in collecting this QEEG data.
3. Supported by funds from Cadwell Laboratories, Kennewick, Washington.
4. By Dr. Laverne Gugino at Brigham and Women's Hospital, Boston, MA.
5. The authors wish to thank Rita Heino, MD and Linda Aglio, MD for their help in collecting the data presented within this section.

References

1. Sotaniemi KA. Cerebral outcome after extracorporeal circulation: Comparison between prospective and retrospective evaluations. Arch Neurol 1983; 40:75.
2. Fulan AJ, Jones SC. Central nervous system complications related to open heart surgery. In: Furlan AJ (ed). The Heart and Stroke. Berlin Heidelberg, Springer-Verlag, 1987; p. 287.
3. Breuer AC, Furlan AJ, Hanson MR, Lederman RJ, Loop FD, Cosgrove DM, Greenstreet RL, Estafanous FG. Central nervous system complications of coronary artery bypass graft surgery: Prospective analysis of 412 patients. Stroke 1983; 14:682.
4. Sotaniemi KA, Mononen H, Hokkanen TE. Long-term cerebral outcome after open-heart surgery: A five-year neuropsychological follow-up study. Stroke 1986; 17:410.
5. Kopf GS, Hume AL, Durkin MA, Hammond GL, Hashim SW, Geha AS. Measurement of central somatosensory conduction time in patients undergoing cardiopulmonary bypass: An index of neurologic function. Amer J Surg 1985; 149:445.
6. Shaw PJ, Bates D, Carthidge NEF, Heaviside D, Desmond JG, Shaw DA. Early neurological complications of coronary artery bypass surgery. Br Med Jr 1985; 219:1384.
7. Hammeke TA, Hastings JE. Neuropsychologic alterations after cardiac surgery. J Thorac Cardiovasc Surg 1988; 96:326.

8. Smith PLC, Newman SP, Ell PJ, Treasure T, Joseph P, Schneidau A, Harrison MJG. Cerebral consequence of cardiopulmonary bypass. Lancet 1986; iv:823.

9. Aberg T, Ronquist G, Tyden H, Brunnkvist S, Bergstrom K. Cerebral damage during open-heart surgery. Scand J Cardiovasc Surg 1987; 21:159.

10. John ER, Prichep LS, Chabot RJ and Isom WO. Monitoring brain function during cardiovascular surgery. In: Refsum H (ed). Brain and Heart, Heart and Brain. Berlin Heidelberg, Springer-Verlag, 1989 (in press).

11. Taylor KM. Brain damage during open-heart surgery. Thorax 1982; 37:873.

12. Henriksen L. Evidence suggestive of diffuse brain damage following cardiac operations. Lancet 1984; iv:816.

13. Kolkka R, Hilberman M. Neurologic dysfunction following cardiac operation with low-flow, low-pressure cardiopulmonary bypass. J Thorac Cardiovasc Surg 1980; 79:432.

14. Astrup J, Siesjo BK, Symon L. Thresholds in cerebral ischemia – The ischemic penumbra. Stroke 1981; 12:723.

15. Glaria AP, Murray A. Comparison of EEG monitoring techniques: An evaluation during cardiac surgery. Electroenceph Clin Neurophysiol 1985; 61:323.

16. Sarnquist FH. Neurological outcome after' low flow low pressure' cardiopulmonary bypass. In: Hilberman M (ed). Brain Injury and Protection during Heart Surgery. Boston, Martinus Nijhoff Publishing, 1988; p. 13.

17. Fish KJ. Microembolization: Etiology and prevention. In: Hilberman M (ed). Brain Injury and Protection During Heart Surgery. Boston, Martinus Nijhoff Publishing, 1988; p. 67.

18. Bjork VO, Ivert T. Early and late neurological complications after prosthetic heart value replacement. In: Becker R, Katz J, Polonius MJ, Speidel H (eds). Psychopathological and Neurological Dysfunctions Following Open-Heart Surgery. New York, Springer-Verlag, 1982; p. 3.

19. Minami K, Sagoo KS, Breymann T, Fassbender D, Schwerdt M, Korfer R. Operative strategy in combined coronary and carotid artery disease. J Thorac Cardiovasc Surg 1988; 95:303.

20. Sotaniemi KA. Clinical and prognostic correlates of EEG in open-heart surgery patients. J Neurol Neurosurg Psychiatry 1980; 43:941.

21. Sundt JM, Sharbrough FW, Piepgras DG, Kearns TP, Messick JM, O'Fallon WM. Correlation of cerebral blood flow and EEG changes during carotid endarterectomy. Mayo Clin Proc 1981; 56:533.

22. El-Fiki M, Fish KJ. Is the EEG a useful monitor during cardiac surgery? A case report. Anesthesiology 1987; 67:575.

23. Russ W, Kling D, Sauerwein G, Hempelmann G. Spectral analysis of the EEG during hypothermic cardiopulmonary bypass. Acta Anaesthesiol Scand 1987; 31:111.

24. Salerno TA, Lynn RB, White CN, Charrette EJ. Cerebral surveillance during cardiac surgery. Can J Surg 1979; 22:325.

25. Chiappa KH, Burke SR, Young RR. Results of electroencephalographic monitoring during 367 carotid endarterectomies: Use of a dedicated minicomputer. Stroke 1979; 10:381.

26. McFarland HR, Pinkerton JA, Frye D. Continuous electroencephalographic monitoring during carotid endarterectomy. J Cardiovasc Surg 1988; 29:12.

27. Jonkman J, Poortvliet DCJ, Veering MM, deWeerd AW, John ER. The use of neurometrics in the study of patients with cerebral ischemia. Electroenceph Clin Neurophysiol 1985; 61:333.

28. Prior PF. EEG monitoring and evoked potentials in brain ischaemia. Br J Anaesth 1985; 57:63.

29. Murray A, Glaria AP, Pearson DT. Monitoring EEG frequency and amplitude during cardiac surgery. Anaesthesia 1986; 41:173.

30. Bolsin SNC. Detection of Neurological damage during cardiopulmonary bypass. Anaesthesia 1986; 41:61.

31. Bashien G, Bledsoe SW, Townes BD, Coppel DB. Tools for assessing central nervous system injury in the cardiac surgery patient. In: Hilberman M (ed). Brain Injury and protection during Heart Surgery. Boston, Martinus Nijhoff Publishing, 1988; p. 109.

32. Maynard DE, Jenkinson JL. The cerebral function analysing monitor: Initial clinical experience, application and further development. Anaesthesia 1984; 39:678.

33. Steele ER, Albin MS, Monts JL, Harman PK. Compressed spectral array EEG monitoring during coronary bypass surgery in a patient with vertebrobasilar artery insufficiency. Anesth Analg 1987; 66:271.

34. Bolsin SNC. Is the EEG a useful monitor during cardiac surgery. Anesthesiology 1988; 68:956.

35. Malone M, Prior P, Scholtz CL. Brain damage after cardiopulmonary by-pass: Correlations between neurophysiological and neuropathological finding. J Neurol Neurosurg Psychiatry 1981; 44:924.

36. Fish KJ. Is the EEG a useful monitor during cardiac surgery? Anesthesiology 1988; 68:956.

37. John ER, Prichep LS, Ahn H, Easton P, Fridman J, Kaye H. Neurometric evaluation of cognitive dysfunctions and neurological disorder in children. Progr Neurobiol 1983; 21:239.

38. John ER, Prichep LS, Easton P. Normative data banks and neurometrics. Basic concepts, methods and results of norm constructions. In: Gevins AS, Remond A (eds). Methods of analysis of Brain Electrical and Magnetic Signals. EEG Handbook. Amsterdam, Elseiver Science Publishers, 1987; p. 449.

39. Rabiner LR, Gold B. Theory and application of digital signal processing. Englewood Cliff NJ, Prentice-Hall, 1975.

40. John ER, Prichep LS, Fridman J, Easton P. Neurometrics: Computer-Assisted differential diagnosis of brain dysfunctions. Science 1988; 239:162.

41. Prichep LS, John ER. Neurometrics: Clinical applications. In: Lopes da Silva FH, Storm van Leeuwen W, Remond A (eds). Handbook of Electroencephalography and Clinical Neurophysiology. (Revised Series), vol. 2. Amsterdam, Elsevier Science Publishers, 1980; p. 153.

42. John ER, Chabot RJ, Prichep LS, Ransohoff J, Epstein F, Berenstein A. Real-time intraoperative monitoring during neurosurgical and neuroradiological procedures. J. Clin. Neurophysiol 1989; 6:125.

PART THREE

Psychological damage

13. Impairment in basic cognitive functioning: attention, concentration, mental flexibility

HEINZ-JÖRG MEFFERT and BERNHARD DAHME

A. Theoretical assumption

The research about organic brain problems in cardiac surgery patients and the use of neuropsychological tests as diagnostic measurements is based on the general hypotheses:

1. Because of a cardiac abnormality, cerebral damage exists preoperatively in the sense of a (chronic) hypoxic cerebropathy, resulting in a global, unspecific restriction of brain functions. Successful surgery improves the oxygen supply to the brain and consequently improves cognitive functions.
2. The intraoperatively restricted blood flow through the cerebrum during extracorporeal circulation (ECC) leads to a temporary reversible deterioration of cognitive functioning.

This chapter presents a selection of the most common neuropsychological tests for the measurement of specific basic cognitive functions as well as results from psychological investigations with heart-surgery patients, gained by means of these instruments. Relations between these results and the psychopathology of cardiac-surgery patients are only considered insofar as they allow statements and give evidence about the validity of the neuropsychological instruments and test results. (See Chapter 4 of this volume).

B. Problems of measuring basic cognitive functioning

As problematical as the definition of a borderline between basic and higher cognitive functions is the demarcation of basic cognitive functioning itself. An attempt to exactly measure specific basic cognitive functions such as attention, concentration and mental flexibility throws light on this problem. Available neuropsychological tests almost never evaluate specific isolated mental abilities but rather mostly evaluate various partial brain functions, based on different complexity levels: ". . . psychological tests are not pure measures

186

of ability. Many of them involve primary motor and sensory functions and a variety of higher mental abilities, difficult to define" [1]. This statement, overall, still applies for today's most common neuropsychological tests, and especially for those used in clinical investigations with hospitalized patients.

Attention and concentration especially, but mental flexibility, too, have to be regarded as basic mental abilities, which are necessary requirements for the performance of most tests, without being, at the same time, their definite diagnostic aim. Only exceptionally special tests for the assessment of attention and concentration, either separately or as parts of test-batteries, have been performed with heart-surgery patients (especially various versions of letter-cancellation tests, see below). Attention and concentration as requirements, on the other hand, often influence various diagnostic claims like the assessment of psychomotor abilities or capability of orientation, and therefore confound the test scores. Various study reports exist in which different investigators use identical neuropsychological tests, some of them reporting on the patients' psychomotor ability, others reporting on the patients' attention and concentration ability.

Any investigator planning a clinical neuropsychological research program is confronted with the dilemma of choosing from a steadily increasing, nearly immense, variety of tests, the best one, according to the cognitive functions which a test is described as assessing.

A literature-overview concerning neuropsychological investigations with heart-surgery patients throws light on the consequences deriving from this dilemma: discordant technical terms, unclear abbreviations, missing descriptions and references, the use of test battery sumscores, mostly combining measures of basic and higher cognitive functions, and the attribution of different brain functions to identical tests lead to confusion instead of clarification. In addition, there are the doubts about many tests' objectivity and reliability in a test-theoretical sense, a questionable resistance against training effects and, as a general difficulty in clinical field research, the problem of standardized test settings.

All those problems impede a systematic analysis of this research area; therefore in the following, only those neuropsychological tests and those results will be reported which either proved valid in various independent investigations, or which support underlying theories, or which are of special interest for future research.

C. Neuropsychological tests

In order to diagnose perioperative disturbances of attention, concentration and mental flexibility in heart-surgery patients, only those tests are suitable which can be applied in the hospital with physically ill and mentally stressed patients. Such tests must not require complicated technical equipment but must permit quick performance in rather uncomfortable surroundings. Most of the tests, which meet these criteria are paper and pencil tests. All the psychometric tests described in this chapter satisfy these conditions and have been used in cardiac surgery research programs.

Tests for attention and concentration

1. Digit span [2, 3]

The Digit Span is one subtest of the Wechsler Adult Intelligence Scale (WAIS). It consists of two parts. In both parts, a series of numbers of increasing length are read to the patient. In the first part the patient's task is to repeat orally the numbers in the original order. In the second part, the task is to repeat the digits in the reverse sequence. Test scores are the number of items remembered correctly in each part. Some investigations only used the second part of the test (Digits Backwards).

The Digit Span test assesses audioverbal memory in addition to attention and concentration. It was used in numerous investigations [4–16].

2. Benton visual retention test [17]

The most common version of this test consists of 10 drawings of abstract geometrical figures, which are presented to the patient for 10 seconds each. Following each single presentation, the patient is requested to draw the figure he has just seen from memory. The test score is the number of correct reproductions of the rough structure of the figure, not taking into account the quality of the patient's drawing.

Besides concentration and attention, the Benton Test assesses disturbances of short term memory. Numerous researchers have applied this test (or a similar version) [7, 9–13, 18–20].

3. Letter cancellation test

There are numerous versions of this test, which generally affords the patients prompt, reliable and steady discrimination of similar details. The German version [21] requests the subject to cross out, from a great number of identical letters (d) marked with different but similar signs, those which are marked with a specific sign. This test assesses several independent quantitative mental ability scores, giving information about quantity and correctness, as well as the oscillation of attention and concentration during a given period of time.

This test (or similar versions) indeed are the most specific instruments to measure these abilities; but in comparison with other instruments they were performed only rarely in research with heart surgery patients [6, 9, 14, 22–25].

188

Test for the assessment of mental flexibility

1. Trailmaking test [26]

The trailmaking test is part of the Halstead-Reitan Test Battery and was used frequently to diagnose minor mental lesions in heart-surgery patients. The test consists of two parts, A and B, with Part A used as a control form of Part B. In the more sensitive Part B, 25 circles are distributed on a sheet of paper, containing the numbers 1 to 13 and the letters A to L in random order. The task is to connect, as fast as possible, the numbers and letters, beginning with 1 and keeping the order in both series, i.e. 1A, 2B, 3C, etc. until L13. If the patient makes a mistake, this is mentioned to him and he is requested to correct himself. The test score is the total time required to perform the test.

The test assesses mental flexibility but also perceptual speed, psychomotor speed, visual-spatial organization, attention and concentration. It was used in a number of investigations with heart-surgery patients [8, 15, 16, 22–25, 27–30].

2. Stroop colour and word test [31]

This test requires the patient to name, as fast as possible, the colour of colour-names (blue, green, yellow, red) printed so that the printed colour never corresponds to the printed colour name. The test is divided into three parts: reading the colour name, recognizing the printed colour and naming the colour. If a colour is named incorrectly, the patient is requested to correct himself. The test score is the total time including corrections.

Clinical studies proved the Stroop Test to be a very effective instrument for the assessment of psychopathological symptoms in general and of organic brain dysfunction, especially for the assessment of mental flexibility but also for concentration and discrimination ability. Studies with heart-surgery patients using this test were only done by Marien [9], Prüssmann-Balck [14] and, using a similar version of this test, by Sotaniemi et al. [11, 12].

3. Digit symbol [2, 3]

The Digit Symbol is also a subtest of the Wechsler Adult Intelligence Scale (WAIS). This test requires associating numbers with shapes. The numbers 1 to 9 are associated with special simple shapes. The task for the patient is to connect the correct symbols within 120 seconds to a given random order of numbers. The test score is the number of correct associations.

The Digit Symbol test assesses mental flexibility with respect to speed and efficiency of performance. This test was used, either in this or similar versions, with heart surgery patients by Gilberstadt and Sako [5], Heller *et al.* [7], Frank *et al.* [27], Mass [30], Smith *et al.* [22], Shaw *et al.* [15, 16], Newman *et al* [23, 24] and Treasure *et al* [25].

4. Remschmidt perseveration test [32]

This instrument is probably the purest test of mental flexibility that has been developed. The task for the patient is to write the capital letter S for 30 seconds, as fast as possible. Then under the same conditions, the patient writes the mirror-image of the capital letter S, and finally, again for 30 seconds as fast as possible, the letter and its mirror-image alternately. The test score is the total number of signs in each series.

Besides mental flexibility, the best score is a measure of concentration, attention and visuomotor coordination ability and psychomotor speed. Low test scores in the third part of the test (alternating letters and signs) refer to perseverative tendencies as a symptom of an organic brain syndrome. The Remschmidt Perseveration Test, to the authors' knowledge, has only been applied to heart surgery patients by Marien [9].

D. Preoperative neuropsychological findings of heart-surgery patients

1. Preoperative status

The aim of most heart surgery studies using neuropsychological tests is to detect changes (deterioration or improvement) in organic brain functioning after the surgery. Therefore they used pre and post comparisons, mostly stressing the pre-post differences and not giving much attention to the preoperative test values. In general, available preoperative findings confirm the theory that brain functions, especially of cardiac valve replacement patients and patients with congenital cardiac lesions, are already restricted preoperatively. Zaks *et al.* [4] found cardiac patients to have worse basic (and higher) cognitive functions than the normal population. Corresponding results were published by Gilberstadt and Sako [5], comparing preoperative cardiac and general surgery patients, as well as internal patients, finding worse basic (and higher) cognitive functions in the first group. Burzig [20] found similar results for cardiac patients when compared to patients with skin diseases. These results are supported by investigations using EEG which find more EEG-abnormalities in cardiac patients compared to the normal population [6, 7]. In contrast to those findings, coronary artery bypass patients do not differ in their preoperative cognitive functions from peripheral vascular surgery patients [16]. Comparable results can be concluded from Treasure *et al.* [25] reporting no preoperative differences between bypass patients and those undergoing other major surgery.

There are only a few statistically valid comparisons between different cardiac diagnosis groups concerning cognitive functions. It has been suggested that valve patients, and especially patients having mitral valve lesions, because of their longer duration of illness and their long lasting restricted oxygen supply to the brain, show worse cognitive functions. Results from Maass [30] comparing mitral valve and coronary artery bypass patients confirm this hypothesis. The reason for the small number of investigations finding significant preoperative differences between cardiac diagnosis groups is based on the general (and probably correct) idea that the effects of extracorporeal circulation (ECC) on cognitive functions are much stronger than the effects of the basic cardiac disease.

2. Pre-post surgery comparisons

The literature shows a characteristic perioperative course: an early postoperative deterioration of basic cognitive function (compared to preoperative measures), and later a reasonable increase, sometimes exceeding the preoperative level. The time of testing during the perioperative course obviously is decisive for the significantly different findings in the literature. Those authors who checked their patients preoperatively and not before an interval of half a year postoperative – or even later – nearly exclusively report improvements in the patients' cognitive functioning [10, 13, 27].

As regards these results, it should be mentioned that these pre-post comparisons were not the focus of these studies, but were side results.

Early postoperative investigations up to a fortnight after surgery, generally show a significant deterioration of the patients' attention, concentration and mental flexibility [15, 16, 22, 23, 25, 28, 30]. However, late postoperative results (from about 4 months after surgery) show a significant improvement in the respective values, exceeding the preoperative measures [13, 27, 28, 30]. (Intermediate values show less definite results). It can be concluded that about 3 to 4 weeks after surgery, basic cognitive functions generally have stabilized so that they roughly correspond to the preoperative level (with some slightly lower or higher). This is supported by two very detailed studies, both investigating patients about 3 weeks after heart surgery [9, 14]. While Marien, at this interval, found slightly deteriorated measures for attention and concentration compared to the preoperative results and unchanged mental flexibility values, Prüssmann-Balck found almost identical measures for attention and concentration, but improved mental flexibility as compared to preoperative scores.

Previous inspection of the course of the mean values verifies the theoretical assumptions about the pre-postoperative course of basic cognitive functions. But because mean values can level existing differences between those patients who improve and those who become worse, it is necessary in order to verify the underlying theory, to crosscheck these results in terms of selected correlations between postoperative neuropsychological test results and other postoperative measures of cognitive and psychic functions.

In this context, a very detailed study of Sotaniemi et al. [11, 12] is of great interest. They divided their sample of valve patients by means of early postoperative EEG and clinical neurological outcome into a complicated and non-complicated group and were able to demonstrate a significant difference in basic and cognitive functions between both groups in the long term post-operative course. This discrepancy became especially striking at five years after the surgery with respect to higher mental functioning. It was also apparent in the patient's performance on a recognition test similar to the Benton Test measuring concentration and attention.

E. Validity of instruments and test-results of basic cognitive functioning

While basic cognitive functions of heart surgery patients (following corre-sponding literature findings) cannot be clearly differentiated with respect to heart disease, sex and age, they obviously correlate with psychopathological dysfunctions and neurological problems. Juolasmaa *et al.* [10], Tienari *et al.* [13], Sotaniemi *et al.* [11, 12] and Shaw *et al.* [15, 16] universally agree that patients which postoperative cerebral complications, demonstrated by EEG and/or other neurological diagnostic measures, showed worse basic mental test results at some time during the postoperative course than patients without such complications. Åberg and Kihlgreen [33] proved similar correlations for more complex cognitive functions. Prüssmann-Black [14] found numerous signifi-cant correlations between deteriorated basic cognitive test results, especially concerning mental flexibility and concentration, and psychiatric ratings of the degree of psychopathological disorders.

The independent measurement of organic brain dysfunctions, by means of neuropsychological tests as well as psychiatric rating scales, e.g., the Hamburg Rating Scale for Psychic Disturbances (HRPD) [34], rating among other cognitive functions disturbances of vigilance, orientation, attention and formal thinking, enables a well founded statement about the validity of neuropsy-chological tests for basic cognitive functioning. The inspection of the correlations between the two sets of scores, neuropsychological test results and psychiatric rating measures, with regard to cognitive functioning clearly shows their similar direction.

There is open discussion about whether the results of the neuropsycho-logical tests are preoperatively influenced by the patients' moods. Prüssmann-Balck [14] found correlations especially between depressive and dysphoric moods, fears, anxiety, aggression, hostility and resignation as rated by a psychiatrist, and reduced mental flexibility, and, less obvious, lacking concentration. These correlations were preoperatively stronger than post-operatively. In contrast to these findings, there were no such correlations between neuropsychological test results and respective factors of the patients' personality structure [20]. These results go well together with findings of Newman *et al.* [24] They found no differences in neuropsychological test results one year after operation between those patients complaining about cognitive deficits (attention, concentration, memory, etc.) and those who did not complain, but had higher levels of assessed depression, and to a minor extent, higher levels of state anxiety, both especially affecting concentration in the complaining group.

These results lead to the conclusion that a correlation between the personality structure of cardiac surgery patients and their basic mental abilities, if it exists, is based upon the influences of the perioperative situational and emotional stress. This mental stress may express itself in unconscious mood disorders and is correlated with basic mental dysfunctions. Nevertheless, the question remains open of whether a common organic brain etiology exists for lack of drive and deteriorated basic cognitive functioning.

F. Conclusions

This chapter dealt with neuropsychological tests for the assessment of disturbances of attention, concentration and mental flexibility applied to open-heart surgery patients. Concordant findings of various investigations from different countries, using identical or comparable test instruments, demonstrate as well a characteristic perioperative course of basic mental functioning, as positive correlations with psychiatric and neurological findings, thus proving the validity of test instruments and results. The findings support – without enlightening their etiology – the theoretical assumptions of postoperatively reduced but reversible basic cognitive function.

References

1. Meyer V. Psychological effects of brain damage. In: Eysenck HJ (ed). Handbook of Abnormal Psychology. London, Pitman Medical Publishing Co., Ltd., 1960.
2. Wechsler D. The Measurement of Adult Intelligence. Baltimore, Williams and Wilkins, 1958.
3. Wechsler D. Der Hamburg-Wechsler-Intelligenztest für Erwachsene (HAWIE). Bern, Huber, 1974.
4. Zaks MS. Disturbances in Psychologic Functions and Neuropsychiatric Complictions in Heart Surgery. A Four-Year Follow-up Study, Cardiology: An Encyclopaedia of the Cardiovascular System III. New York, McGraw-Hill, 1959.
5. Gilberstadt H, Sako Y. Intellectual and personality changes following open-heart surgery. Arch Gen Psychiatry 1968; 16:210.
6. Lehmann HJ, Grahmann H, Hauss K, Rodewald G, Schmitz Th. Akute organische psychosyndrome nach herzoperationen. Der Nervenarzt 1968; 39:529.
7. Heller SS, Kornfeld DS, Frank KA, Hoar PF. Postcardiotomy delirium and cardiac output. Amer J Psychiat 1979; 136:337.
8. Kilpatrick DG, Miller WC, Allain AN, Huggins MB, Lee WC, Jr. The use of psychological test data to predict open-heart surgery outcome: a prospective study. Psychosom Med 1975; 37/1:62.
9. Marien R. Cerebrale Vorschädigung und die psychopathologischen Erscheinungen in den ersten Tagen nach Herzoperationen. Unpublished Dissertation, Hamburg, 1978.
10. Juolasmaa A, Outakoski J, Hirvenoja R, Tienari P, Sotaniemi K, Takkunen J. Effect of open-heart surgery on intellectual performance. J of Clin Neuropsychol 1981; 3:181.

11. Sotaniemi K A, Juolasmaa A, Hokkanen T E. Neuropsychologic outcome after open-heart surgery. Arch Neurol 1981; 38:2.

12. Sotaniemi K A, Mononen H, Hakkanen T E. Long-term cerebral outcome after open-heart surgery. A five year neuropsychological follow-up study. Stroke 1986; 17:410.

13. Tienari P, Outakoski J, Juolasmaaa A, Hirvenoja R, Takkunen J, Sotaniemi K, Järvimäki V. Psychiatric complications following open-heart surgery: a prospective study. Psychiatria Fennica (Supplementum), 1981; p. 63.

14. Prüssmann-Balck K. Zusammenhänge zwischen neuropsychologischen Auffälligkeiten und psychologischem/psychiatrischem Status bei Patienten mit Herzklappenvitien vor und nach cardiochirurgischen Eingriffen. Unpublished Dissertation, Hamburg, 1985.

15. Shaw P J, Bates D, Cartlidge N E, French J M, Heaviside D, Julian D G, Shaw D A. Early intellectual dysfunction following coronary bypass surgery. Q J Med 1986; 58:59.

16. Shaw P J, Bates D, Cartlidge N E, French J M, Heaviside D, Julian D G, Shaw D A. Neurologic and neuropsychological morbidity following major surgery: Comparison of coronary artery bypass and peripheral vascular surgery. Stroke 1987; 18:700.

17. Benton A L, Der Benton-Test, Handbuch, Deutsche Bearbeitung von O. Spreen, 4, Aufl. Bern, H. Huber Verlag, 1972.

18. Lair Ch, Biddy R L. Some psychological correlates associated with open-heart surgery. Alab J Med Sci 1968; 5/4:458.

19. Kornfeld D S, Heller S S, Frank K A, Moskowitz R. Personality and psychological factors in postcardiotomy delirium. Arch Gen Psychiat 1974; 31:249.

20. Burzig G. Testpsychologische und psychopathologische Untersuchungen an Herzfehlerkranken zur Frage einer hirnorganischen Beteiligung. Nervenarzt 1979; 50:631.

21. Brickenkamp R. Test d2, Handbuch, 5. Aufl., Hogrefe, Göttingen, Toronto, Zürich, Verlag für Psychologie, 1962.

22. Smith P L C, Treasure T, Newman S P, Joseph Ph, Ell P J, Schneidau A, Harrison M J. Cerebral consequences of cardiopulmonary bypass. The Lancet 1986; 1:823.

23. Newman S P, Smith P, Treasure T, Joseph P, Ell P, Harrison M. Acute neuropsychological consequences of coronary artery bypass surgery. Curr Psych Res Rev 1987; 6:115.

24. Newman St, Klinger L, Venn G, Smith P, Harrison M, Treasure T. Subjective reports of cognition in relation to assessed cognitive performance following coronary artery bypass surgery. J Psychosom Res 1989; 33:227.

25. Treasure T, Smith P L C, Newman S, Schneidau A, Joseph Ph, Ell P, Harrison M J G. Impairment of cerebral function following cardiac and other major surgery. Eur J Cardio-Thorac Surg 1989; 3:216.

26. Reitan R M. Trail Making Test. Manual for administration, scoring and interpretation. Department of Neurology, Section of Neuropsychology, Indianapolis, Indiana University Medical Center, 1958.

27. Frank K A, Heller S S, Kornfeld D S, Malm J R. Long-term effects of open heart surgery on intellectual functioning, Thorac and Cardiovasc Surg 1972; 64:811.

28. Savageau J A, Stanton R A, Jenkins D, Klein M D. Neuropsychological dysfunction following elective cardiac operation, I. Early assessment. J of Thorac and Cardiovasc Surg 1982a; 84:585.

29. Savageau J A, Stanton B A, Jenkins C D, Frater R W M. Neuropsychological dysfunction following elective cardiac operation, II. A six-month reassessment. J of Thoracic and Cardiovasc Surg 1982b; 83:595.

30. Maass R. Eine neuropsychologische Follow-up-Studie an Patienten vor und nach offenen Herzoperationen. Unpublished Diplomarbeit, Hamburg, 1985.

31. Stroop J T. Studies of interference in serial verbal reactions. J Exp Psychol 1935; 18:643.

32. Remschmidt H. Experimentelle Untersuchungen zur sogenannten epileptischen, Wesensänderung. In: Fortschr d Neur, Psych und ihrer Grenzg 1970; 38:524.

33. Åberg T, Kihlgren M. Effect of open-heart surgery on intellectual function. Scand J Thoracic and Cardiovasc Surg Suppl. 1974; 15.

34. Götze P, Dahme B, Wessel W. Die Hamburger Schätzskala für psychische Störungen nach Herzoperationen (HRPD). Eur Arch Psachiatr Neurol Sci 1985; 234:308.

14. The use of neuropsychological tests as criteria of brain dysfunction in cardiac surgery research

A. E. WILLNER

The use of neuropsychological tests to assess cognitive changes in cardiac surgery patients rests upon certain assumptions:

1. There may be considerable brain dysfunction in cardiac surgery patients before surgery

Patients are referred for surgery because of serious cardiac problems. Since the heart's main function is pumping blood, and the brain needs more blood than any other organ, many cardiac surgery patients may have sustained brain dysfunction before surgery.

2. Cardiac surgery may sometimes compromise brain functioning even though it is necessary to preserve life and enhance cardiac functioning

This may occur because of the various unphysiological parameters of the surgery: e.g., non-pulsatile blood flow, untoward effects of blood filters and oxygenators, etc. and the stressful nature of the surgery.

Methodological differences can also influence experimental results. For example, the question, "Do patients suffer cognitive impairment after cardiac surgery?" can be answered in two different ways that yield different results.

One method requires testing patients pre-and postoperatively and determining whether their mean score changes significantly [1–6]. Typically it increases postoperatively; this indicates no postoperative decline in test score for the whole group but it does not reveal whether the scores of a subgroup decline substantially.

This possibility can be evaluated by making comparisons patient-by-patient [7–27]. In most recent studies, a postoperative drop of one standard deviation is taken as a significant drop. Thus, if 20% of the patients show a significant postoperative loss, this finding is not obscured by the scores of the majority who show an improvement. Essentially the two approaches answer different questions. The first shows whether cardiac surgery results in an improvement in cognitive functioning for the average patient. The second identifies patients who suffer cognitive losses so that the reasons can be investigated. For example, are the cognitive losses related to aspects of the patients' cardiac condition and/or perioperative conditions? Such investigations can identify conditions which require further study [9, 14–20, 23–27].

The writer can provide an example [28, 29]. In 1982, cardiac surgeons at his hospital came to him with a problem. They had used one arterial line filter (filter A) in cardiac surgery for several years but had shifted to a new one (filter B) because it had smaller pores and presumably could filter out more unwanted particulate matter from the blood. Recently however, ECRI, an organization that monitors medical equipment, had sent out an urgent hazard warning, stating that the new filter seemed related to instances of postoperative brain damage. The surgeons said they noticed no difference in patients who had surgery with either filter. They were not sure, however, that they would notice such brain dysfunction if it occurred. Since they knew that patients were tested both before and after cardiac surgery, they asked the writer to look into this matter. Fifty-six patients were studied. The first 12 had arterial filtration during cardiopulmonary bypass with filter A, the next 34 with filter B, and the last 10 again with filter A. Cognitive impairment was defined as a postoperative score on the CLAT [30] analogy test (described below) at least one standard deviation lower than the preoperative score. The filter A group had a 5% incidence of cognitive impairment as compared to a 24% incidence in the filter B group, $p < 0.05$. Moreover, the preoperative to postoperative change in CLAT scores correlated significantly ($p < 0.5$) with bypass time for filter B, but the correlation was almost exactly zero for filter A (i.e., the longer the bypass time, the lower the CLAT score for filter B patients only). Finally evidence was presented, from an earlier study of cardiac surgery patients, indicating that cognitive impairment was stable over a 5 year period and related to poor outcome during that period [29]. Conclusions were as follows:

1) Patients having surgery with filter B had significantly more cognitive impairment than did those with filter A.
2) Impaired abstraction is related to a parameter of the cardiopulmonary bypass pump (bypass time).
3) This cognitive impairment has long-standing consequences.

What is the clinical significance of such a finding? If a substantial proportion of patients suffers impaired cognitive functioning postoperatively, does this represent a transitory deviation which soon returns to normal or does it have more long lasting meaning? Savageau et al. [31] found that a substantial proportion of patients was cognitively impaired at discharge from the hospital, and a similar proportion impaired six months later, but these were usually not the same people [32]. They described their finding as evidence that the cognitive impairment seen after surgery was short-lived and of little consequence. Willner [29] criticized this study on the basis of the unreliability of the cognitive tests used. Sotaniemi [20], however, had more telling findings. He investigated patients preoperatively, and at several intervals postoperatively. He found impairment immediately postoperatively with improvement at one year, but then the patients who had shown presumably transient impairment post-operatively were definitely impaired five years later. Sotaniemi concluded that while the findings of post-operative impairment disappeared after the first year, they were a signal of vulnerability, in view of the patients' condition five years postoperatively. One might find a similar situation in examining patients during a transient ischemic attack and again a day later. Although one might conclude that the t.i.a. was a temporary effect with no lasting meaning, it may, in fact, often be a harbinger of future troubles. Sotaniemi's findings also recall Meyendorf's paper [33] noting that many symptoms reported after open heart surgery had also been reported in the earlier (pre-cardiac surgery) literature going back as far as 1817. Meyendorf regarded cardiac surgery as an experimental technique which could immediately reveal psychopathology which could otherwise take years to become evident. Perhaps Meyendorf's observation further illuminates the nature of Sotaniemi's finding.

Recently, increasingly lengthy batteries of tests have been used as criteria for cognitive impairment [7, 8, 13–15, 21, 26, 27]. These tend to provide more sensitive and stable measures than those derived from a small number of tests. There are some problems however. On how many tests must the patient have an abnormal postoperative score to be rated as impaired? Several studies have used a battery of 8 to 10 tests. If the patient's score drops by one standard deviation on one test, two tests, or three tests, is his performance impaired postoperatively? The usual decision has been that impaired performance on at least two tests is enough to classify him as impaired. Typically no rationale is offered as to why two were chosen rather than, for example, one or three. This issue will remain unresolved until explicit reasons are given and concensus reached for how many tests in a large battery must be abnormal to call a patient impaired.

Most research into the psychological and neuropsychological implications of cardiac surgery has involved small samples of patients studied with a wide variety of measuring instruments. This has produced considerable controversy about whether discrepant findings resulted from differences in the basic phenomena investigated or from the use of different tests. The Multicenter International Study [34] attempted to remedy this situation by using a "common yardstick", e.g., the same six neuropsychological tests, in all centers participating in the study. One result is that these six tests are well represented among the plethora of tests used in cardiac surgery research, since all International Study centers used an identical test battery and other studies used very different batteries. Table 1 shows the tests used in 41 studies, arranged in order of frequency of use. The International Study is listed as 7 studies, one for each participating center whose data was available for analysis in 1989. Data

Table 1. Number of cardiac surgery studies using each of several neuropsychological tests

Test	Studies using test
WAIS Digit Symbol	19
Trail-Making Test	18
WAIS Block Design	13
WAIS Digit Span	12
Benton Visual Retention	11
CLAT Analogy Test	10
Åberg Figure Rotation	9
Bethune-Williams Visual Memory	8
Wechsler Memory [45] Visual Reproduction	4
Wechsler Memory-Logical Memory	4

from the two remaining centers were delayed and will be included in future analyses.

Examination of Table 1 shows that six of the eight tests used most often in studies of the effect of cardiac surgery on cognitive functioning, were tests used in the International Study. These tests and their frequency of use were: WAIS [35] Digit Symbol 19 studies, Trail-Making [36] Part B 18, WAIS [35] Block Design 13, Conceptual Level Analogy Test [30] (CLAT) 10, Figure Rotation [9, 37–39] Test 9, Bethune-Williams [40, 41] Visual Memory 8. The most frequently used tests not in the International Study battery were the WAIS [35] Digit Span 12 and the Benton [42] Visual Retention 11. The data in Table 1 suggest that the use of a standard test battery in the International Study can help promote more uniform use of tests in cardiac surgery research.

Using a standard test battery is not enough, however: there is also the question of the sensitivity of the tests. Clearly, some tests are more effective than others. What are the requirements for tests to assess cognitive function in cardiac surgery research? Certain standards are listed below that seem relevant for tests used to document postoperative cognitive changes.

1. The tests can be administered quickly

In many countries, e.g., the USA, only a short time is available for preoperative testing, typically about 60 to 90 minutes.

2. The task should not be too demanding for a patient convalescing from cardiac surgery

Obviously, one must avoid having the patient perform strenuous tasks too soon after the surgery. In addition, one must consider what kinds of tasks need to be administered, even if they are frequently used neuropsychological tests, and even if the patient had no difficulty doing them preoperatively. The Trail-Making Test [36], a much used neuropsychological test, will serve as an example. In this test, the patient is presented with many circles scattered over a sheet of paper, each encircling a number or a letter. The task is to draw a line connecting the circles in the following order: 1, A, 2, B, 3, C, etc. The task can be done more quickly when one is free to use large arm movements. Cardiac surgery requires that the sternum be cut, and patients may vary widely, a week after surgery in the discomfort felt in carrying out such large arm movements. This additional source of variance postoperatively is probably responsible for the reduced size of test-retest correlations for the Trail-Making Test in cardiac surgery samples.

3. Complexity of the task

Complex tasks typically require preserved functioning in many areas of the brain whereas simple tasks require adequate functioning in a more delimited area. If a task requires several intact abilities for correct solution, impairment of any one results in poor performance. Consequently, complex tasks are more sensitive than simple ones at detecting impairment which may be present anywhere in the brain.

4. Level of difficulty

The items must encompass a wide enough range of difficulty so that they can detect losses in very bright people who are still functioning quite well; they must also be easy enough so that they can detect further losses in people who were rather limited preoperatively. (A loss in a very bright person is still a loss, even though the test is not sensitive enough to measure it. Similarly, a loss in a person of limited ability is important even though the test is too difficult to detect it). The test battery should therefore include a wide range of easy and difficult items so that it can assess these changes.

5. The nature of the task does not change upon retesting

In certain tasks one is required to learn a principle, e.g., the Halstead-Reitan Categories Test [43], or the Wisconsin Card Sort Test [44]. When the test is readministered postoperatively, the patient can remember the principle rather than having to relearn it. If the ability to learn the principle is impaired postoperatively, such a test may not indicate so.

6. Type of stimulus material

Both visual-spatial and verbal stimuli are useful. Roughly speaking, visual-spatial material tends to be processed in the right cerebral hemisphere and verbal material in the left.

7. Objectivity of scoring

Objectively scorable test items provide increased reliability.

8. Patient response required

Multiple-choice formats tend to be easier, since the patient is not required to recall the correct answer but only to select it from among several alternatives. They also facilitate objective scoring. Fill-in or short answer tasks tend to be more difficult because the patient must supply the correct answer rather than only select it.

9. Standard deviation units

Presenting scores in standard deviation units makes possible comparisons: 1) within different abilities of the patient and 2) between different patients and groups of patients. Standard deviation units (standard scores) are often used in cardiac surgery research to compare patients' abilities. However, almost all investigators use the standard deviation of the experimental sample to calculate the standard score. Although that procedure allows comparing the patients' functioning across several variables, it does not allow comparing patients across several studies. Since different studies may have quite different standard deviations, standard scores derived from those standard deviations are not comparable. There is a simple solution to this problem, one which is not often used however. Since the tests have their own standardizing samples and standard deviations, one could use those. In that case the standard scores would all be comparable. One could use the preliminary standard deviation for a newly developed test until more formal scores were available.

Reference

1. Campbell DE, Raskin SA. Cerebral dysfunction after cardiopulmonary bypass: aetiology, manifestations and interventions. Perfusion 1990; 5(4):251.
2. Townes BD, Bashein G, Hornbein TF, Coppel DB, Goldstein DE, Davis KB, Nessly ML, Bledsoe SW, Veith RC, Ivey TD, Cohen MA. Neurobehavioral outcomes in cardiac operations: a prospective controlled study. J Thor Cardiovasc Surg 1989; 98:774.
3. Fish KJ, Helms KN, Sarnquist FH, van Steennis C, Linet OI, Hilberman M, Mitchell RS, Jamieson SW, Miller DG, Tinklenberg JS. A prospective randomized study of the effects of prostacyclin on neuropsychological dysfunction after coronary artery surgery. J Thorac Cardiovasc Surg 1987; 93:609.
4. Patrick RT, Kirklin JW, Theye RA. The effects of extracorporeal circulation on the brain. In: Allen JG (ed). Extracorporeal Circulation. Springfield, Ill., Charles C. Thomas, 1958.
5. Walsh G, Hearn S, O'Reilly W. A comparison of psychological test results in patients post cardiopulmonary bypass using membrane and bubble oxygenators. Proceed Amer Acad Cardiovasc Perfusion 1986; 7:35.

6. Frank A, Heller S, Kornfeld D. A survey of adjustment to cardiac surgery. Arch Intern Med 1972; 130:735.

7. Klonoff H, Clark C, Kavanagh-Gray D, Mizgala H, Munro I. Two-year follow-up study of coronary bypass surgery: psychologic status, employment status, and quality of life. J Thorac Cardiovasc Surg 1989; 97:78.

8. Shaw PJ, Bates D, Cartlidge NE, French JM, Heaviside D, Julian DG, Shaw DA. Early Intellectual dysfunction following coronary bypass surgery. Q J Med 1986; 255:59.

9. Åberg T, Kihlgren M. Cerebral protection during open-heart surgery. Thorax 1977; 32:525.

10. Tufo HM, Ostfeld AM, Shaekelle R. Central nervous system dysfunction following open-heart surgery. JAMA 1970; 212:1333.

11. Lee WH, Brady MP, Rowe JM, Miller WC. Effects of extracorporeal circulation upon behavior, personality and brain function. Ann Surg 1977; 173:1013.

12. Sotaniemi KA. Brain damage and neurological outcome after open-heart surgery. J Neurol Neurosurg Psychiatry 1980; 43:127.

13. Shaw PJ, Bates D, Cartlidge N, French JM, Heaviside D, Julian DG, Shaw DA. Neurologic and neuropsychological morbidity following major surgery; comparison of coronary artery bypass and peripheral vascular surgery. Stroke 1987; 18:700.

14. Smith PLC, Newman SP, Ell PJ, Treasure T, Joseph P, Schneidau A, Harrison MJG. Cerebral consequences of cardiopulmonary bypass. Lancet 1986; 1:823.

15. Shaw PJ, Bates D, Cartlidge N, French JM, Heaviside D, Julian DG, Shaw DA. Long-term intellectual dysfunction following coronary artery bypass graft surgery: a six month follow up study. Q J Med 1987; 239:259.

16. Juolasmaa A, Outakoski J, Hirvenoja R, Tienari P, Sotaniemi KA, Takkunen J. Effect of open heart surgery on intellectual performance. J Clin Neuropsych 1981; 3:181.

17. Sotaniemi KA, Juolasmaa A, Hokkanen ET. Neuropsychological outcome after open heart surgery. Arch Neurol 1981; 38:2.

18. Aris A, Solanes H, Camara ML, Junque C, Escartin A, Caralps JM. Arterial line filtration during cardiopulmonary bypass. J Thorac Cardiovasc Surg 1986; 91:526.

19. Malone P, Prior P, Scholtz CL. Brain damage after cardiopulmonary bypass: correlations between neurophysiological and neuropsychological findings. J Neurol Neurosurg Psychiatry 1981; 44:924.

20. Sotaniemi KA, Mononen H, Hokkanen TE. Longterm cerebral outcome after open heart surgery. Stroke 1986; 17:410.

21. Venn G, Klinger L, Smith P, Harrison M, Newman SP, Treasure T. Neuropsychological sequellae of bypass twelve months after coronary artery surgery. Br Heart J 1987; 57:565.

22. Pugsley W. The use of Doppler ultrasound in the assessment of microemboli during cardiac surgery. Perfusion 1989; 4:115.

23. Larmi TKI, Karkola P, Kairaluoma MI, Sutinen S, Partanen-Talsta A. Calcium microemboli and microfilters in valve operation. Ann Thorac Surg 1977; 24:34.

24. Kolkka R, Hilberman M. Neurologic dysfunction following cardiac operation with low-flow low-pressure cardiopulmonary bypass. J Thorac Cardiovasc Surg 1980; 79:332.

25. Groom RC, Hill A, Vinansky RP, Speir AM, Macmanus Q, Lefrak EA. Hollow fiber membrane and bubble oxygenation: A comparison of psychometric test results. Proceed Amer Acad Cardiovasc Perfusion 1985; 6:70.

26. Newman S. The incidence and nature of neuropsychological morbidity following cardiac surgery. Perfusion 1989; 4:93.

27. Treasure T, Smith PLC, Newman S, Schneidau A, Joseph P, Ell P, Harrison MJG. Impairment of cerebral function following cardiac and other major surgery. Eur J Cardio Thor Surg 1989; 3:216.

28. Garvey JW, Willner A, Wolpowitz A, Caramante L, Rabiner CJ, Weisz D, Wisoff GB. The effect of arterial filtration during open heart surgery on cerebral function. Circulation 1983(Suppl. II); 68:125.

29. Willner AE, Caramante LL, Garvey JW, Wolpowitz A, Weisz D, Rabiner CJ, Wisoff BG. The relationship between arterial filtration during open heart surgery and mental abstraction ability. Proceed Amer Acad Cardiovasc Perfusion 1983; 4:56.

30. Willner A E. Conceptual Level Analogy Test. New York, Cognitive Testing Service, 1971.
31. Savageau J A, Stanton B A, Jenkins CD, Klein MD. Neuropsychological dysfunction following elective cardiac operation. I. Early assessment. J Thorac Cardiovasc Surg 1982; 84:585.
32. Savageau J A, Stanton B A, Jenkins CD, Frater R W M. Neuropsychological dysfunction following elective cardiac operation. II. A six month reassessment. J Thor Cardiovasc Surg 1982; 84:595.
33. Meyendorf R. Psychopathology in heart disease aside from cardiac surgery: A historical perspective of cardiac psychosis. Comprehen Psychiatry 1979; 20:326.
34. Rodewald G and Willner A E. Introduction. In: Willner A E, Rodewald G (eds). Impact of Cardiac Surgery on the Quality of Life: Neurological and Psychological Aspects. New York, Plenum Press, 1990; p. 1.
35. Wechsler D. The Measurement and Appraisal of Adult Intelligence. Baltimore, Williams and Wilkins, 1958.
36. Reitan R M. Trail Making Test: Manual for Administration, Scoring and Interpretation. Indianapolis, Indiana University Medical Center, 1958.
37. Åberg T, Kihlgren M. Effect of open-heart surgery on intellectual function. Scand J Thor Cardiovasc Surg 1974(Suppl 15):1.
38. Åberg T, Kihlgren M. Cerebral protection during open-heart surgery: a comparison between a disc oxygenator and two bubble oxygenators. Thoraxchirurgie und Vaskulare Chirurgie 1977; 25:146.
39. Åberg T, Kihlgren M. The use of psychometric testing as a quality criterion in open-heart surgery. In: Speidel H and Rodewald G (eds). Psychic and Neurological Dysfunction After Open-heart Surgery. Stuttgart, Georg Thieme Verlag, 1980; p. 107.
40. Bethune D W. Psychometric testing in the evaluation of the postoperative cardiac patient. In: Longmore D B (ed). Towards Safer Cardiac Surgery. Boston, GK Hall Medical Publishers, 1981; p. 613.
41. Bethune D W. The assessment of organic brain damage following open-heart surgery. In: Speidel H and Rodewald G (eds). Psychic and Neurological Dysfunctions After Open-heart Surgery. Stuttgart, Georg Thieme Verlag, 1980; p. 100.
42. Benton A L. The Revised Visual Retention Test (4th ed.) New York: Psychological Corporation, 1974.
43. Halstead W C. Brain and Intelligence. Chicago, Univ. Of Chicago Press, 1947.
44. Grant D A, Berg E A. A behavioral analysis of degree of reinforcement and ease of shifting to new responses in a Weigl-type card-sorting problem. J Exper Psych 1948; 38:404.
45. Wechsler D. A standardized memory scale for clinical use. J of Psych 1945; 19:87.

15. Neuropsychological dysfunction before and after cardiac surgery

A.E. WILLNER

Improvements in cardiac surgical technique and equipment, and closer approximations to physiological conditions, have led to a sharp reduction in postoperative mortality and morbidity [1]. Major neurological morbidity has also been reduced to 5% or less [2]. Whether there has been a corresponding reduction in postoperative neuropsychological impairment is still controversial. Several authors [1–8] report little postoperative neuropsychological impairment and Klonoff, in a well-controlled study, found no evidence of neuropsychological impairment at all [9]. However, other researchers have demonstrated significant neuropsychological impairment after cardiac surgery [10–36]. How may we account for such discrepant findings?

The discrepancy in kinds of tests and measuring techniques used could account for much of the difference. Differences in experimental design could also play a major role. Thus, some studies have examined differences between preoperative and postoperative mean scores, while others were focused primarily on patients whose test scores have fallen off sharply after the surgery. Some authors have used the same test before and after surgery; others have used alternate forms of the test. Still another variation concerns the time of testing, and especially the length of the interval between surgery and postoperative testing. Finally, the definition of impairment as well as length of the test battery used has varied considerably among investigators.

In an effort to clarify these issues, a Multicenter International Study [37] was initiated in 1985. To promote consistency in measurement all centers in the Multicenter International Study, used the same tests ("a common yardstick"), to avoid the problem. This proved only a partial solution. Other variations in experimental procedure needed to be controlled as well. The ways in which differences in experimental design can influence findings were discussed further in chapter 14 on neuropsychological testing. The following experimental procedure was used in the Multicenter International Study: pre- and postoperative scores were compared for each patient to permit detection of impairment even if only in a minority of patients. An extended follow-up study of the patients is being conducted routinely to ascertain whether cognitive impairment is transitory or more permanent. Impairment was defined as a significant drop in at least one of the three tests used in the battery. Requiring abnormal performance in two-thirds of the tests seemed too stringent a criterion.

The data presented here from the Multicenter International Study investigate the relationships between preoperative and postoperative cognitive scores and several cardiac variables. The data were obtained from testing 498 cardiac surgery patients at seven centers in the United States, Western Europe and South America. The patients were tested preoperatively, and one day before hospital discharge. Of the data gathered in the study (psychiatric, neurological, neuropsychological and medical-surgical), we are concerned here only with the neuropsychological and the medical-surgical.

Methods

Study sample

In all, 498 cardiac surgery patients from seven centers in Europe, North and South America were included in the study. The patients were distributed as follows: Hamburg, Germany 121; Oulu, Finland 101; New York, USA 91; Bad Krozingen, Germany 79; Kiel, Germany 55; Sao Paulo, Brazil 29; and Evanston Illinois, USA 22. The data from the two remaining centers in Milan Italy and Bogota Colombia were incomplete and were not included at this time. All patients had to be at least 25 years old. The mean age was 56.3 (standard deviation 9.6, range 41–83 years). The patients from the United States were the oldest, (75% of patients not from the U.S. were 50 years or younger.) Eighty-one percent were male.

Cardiologic status before and after surgery

The following surgical procedures were performed: Coronary Artery Bypass Graft 435 (88%), Cardiac Valvular surgery 42 (9%), both CABG and valve surgery 16 (3%) and other 1 (0%). In 45% of CABG patients the internal thoracic artery was used, and in 15% of the cases an isolated arterial replacement was used. On the average, 3.1 peripheral coronary anastomoses were performed (standard deviation 0.4, minimum = 1, maximum = 8). In 46 cases (10%) an endarterectomy was carried out. Only 30 patients had previous coronary bypass grafting; seventeen had cardiac surgery two or more times previously.

Angina pectoris was found in 380 of 451 patients undergoing coronary artery bypass surgery. The types of angina were as follows: chronic stable 224 (59%), recent onset 16 (4%), progressive 85 (22%), unstable (15%).

Other medical history problems

Myocardial infarctions were recorded in 258 of 398 (65%), Hypertension in 153 of 428 (36%), Diabetes 61 of 498 (12%), previous surgical procedures 97 of 498 (19%). The incidence of cerebrovascular disease was 32 of 498 (6%), which consisted of 8 previous strokes, 8 cerebral emboli, 8 TIA and 10 asymptomatic bruits for a total of 34 findings in 32 patients.

Cardioplegia

Surgery was accomplished with cardioplegia in 457 cases. Of these, 307 (67%) were crystalloid, 99 (22%) used blood, and 51 used other materials.

Mortality rate and clinical outcome

Four hundred eighty eight of 498 patients were discharged from the hospital. The 2% mortality rate was accounted for by the remaining 10 patients. Three deaths occurred during surgery for technical reasons (one was declared equipment failure).

A total of 45 pathophysiological events were seen in 33 patients (7%) of the populations. Most common were hypertension and low cardiac output syndrome.

Equipment used for extracorporeal circulation

Bubble oxygenators
These were used in 225 patients (46% of the sample).

Membrane oxygenators
These were used in 273 patients (54% of the sample). Three types of membrane oxygenators were used:

Membrane sheet oxygenator	144 patients (29%)
Hollow fiber membrane	120 patients (24%)
Silicone membrane	9 patients (2%)

Arterial line filters

No filter 130 cases (26%)	
Filter #4 176 cases (35%)	25 micron pore, nylon material
Filter #14 79 cases (16%)	40 microns, nylon
Filter #20 113 cases (23%)	40 microns, polyester

Neuropsychological examination procedures

Six neuropsychological tests were used: the Conceptual Level Analogy Test (CLAT) [38, 39], the WAIS Block Design [40], the WAIS Digit Symbol [40], the Trail-making Test [41], the Figure Rotation Test [11, 32–34], and the Bethune Williams Visual Memory Test [35, 36]. These tests were selected by the neuropsychology subcommittee of the International Consortium, chaired by Prof. Ralph Reitan. The tests were considered measures of verbal abstraction (CLAT), alertness, speed of response, flexibility in thinking, visual memory (Trail Making Test), visual-spatial abstraction (WAIS Block Design), symbolic association of number and shapes, speed and efficiency of performance (WAIS Digit Symbol), visual-spatial ability (Figure Rotation Test), and visual memory (Bethune-Williams Visual Test). Patients were required to be examined both preoperatively and postoperatively.

Only the first three tests listed were used in the data analyses below. Of the remaining three tests, the Figure Rotation Test and the Bethune-Williams Visual Memory Test were excluded because they bore little relationship to the physical medical criteria of the study. The Trail-making Test was excluded because of concerns with its reliability as a measure of change in cardiac surgery patients, due to acute postsurgical factors.

The three tests used in the data analysis were the CLAT, WAIS Digit Symbol and WAIS Block Design. The CLAT is a 42 item analogy test which is designed to be free of solution by word association. The words in the CLAT are simple enough to be understood by 10 year old children. Since it is a multiple choice test, all the items are scored objectively. The CLAT is described in Willner [31] and has been used in several cardiac surgery studies. The WAIS Block Design and Digit Symbol are two subtests of the Wechser Adult Intelligence Scale. On the Block Design the patient is required to arrange blocks into patterns of increasing difficulty, as illustrated on cards. The Digit Symbol Test requires the patient to learn associations between numbers and symbols, and to copy the correct symbol for each number as quickly as he can.

Some results of the study are indicated below; they are initial findings since the study is still in progress.

Figure 1 shows patients grouped by age at the time of surgery into columns labelled: 30s, 40s, 50s, 60s and 70s. The columns are divided by crosshatching into three ranges of CLAT analogy test scores: devastated (random performance), low scores, and average to high performance. The scale at the left indicates the percent of patients who achieved each level of performance. The ordinate on the right shows the CLAT scaled score. There is a highly significant drop (p < 0.001) in CLAT score with age, as might be expected. The whole curve is substantially below the average normative score (a scaled score of 10), indicating the inroads of the patients' cardiac illness on their cognitive functioning. Willner [42] has described a similar difference between elderly symptomatic volunteers and elderly psychiatric patients.

Figure 2 shows the relationship between cardiac diagnosis and preoperative CLAT score. The patients are divided into 3 diagnostic groups: those

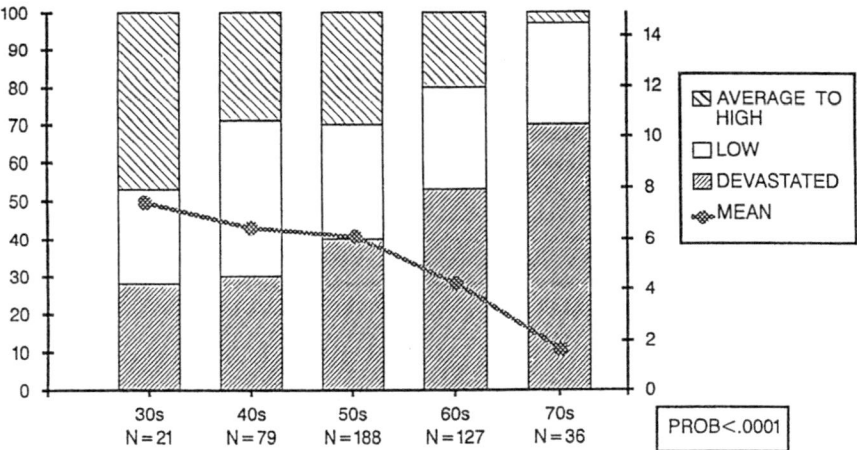

Fig 1. Preoperative CLAT scaled score as a function of age.

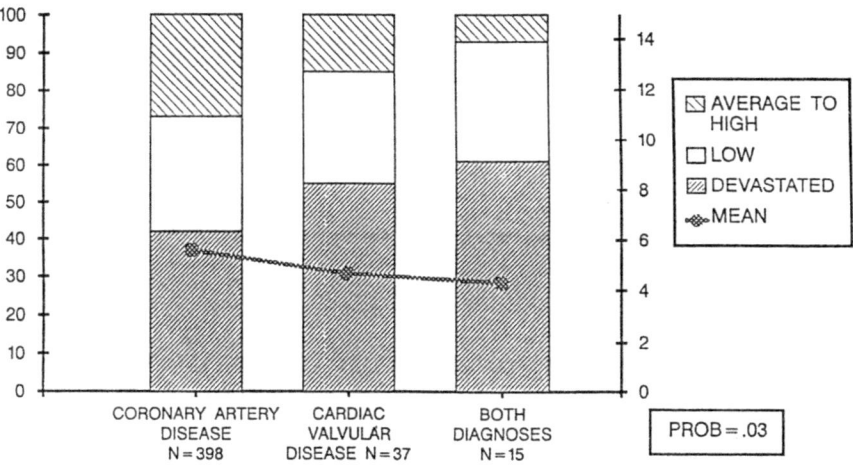

Fig 2. Preoperative CLAT scaled score as a function of diagnosis.

who will have coronary bypass surgery (coronary artery disease), those who will have cardiac valvular surgery (cardiac valvular disease), and those who will have both surgeries (both diagnoses). The crosshatching again indicates the magnitude of the CLAT score. The mean scores for each group are indicated; there is a significant relationship (p = 0.03) between CLAT score and preoperative cardiac diagnosis in these patients.

Figure 3 shows a significant relationship (p = 0.005) between patients' sex and pre-operative CLAT score; women have significantly lower preoperative CLAT scores. Since women have bypass surgery later than men do, this finding might be an epiphenomenon of age. This possibility was investigated, however, and the data did not support it. A second consideration took into account that the ratio of men to women is quite different for

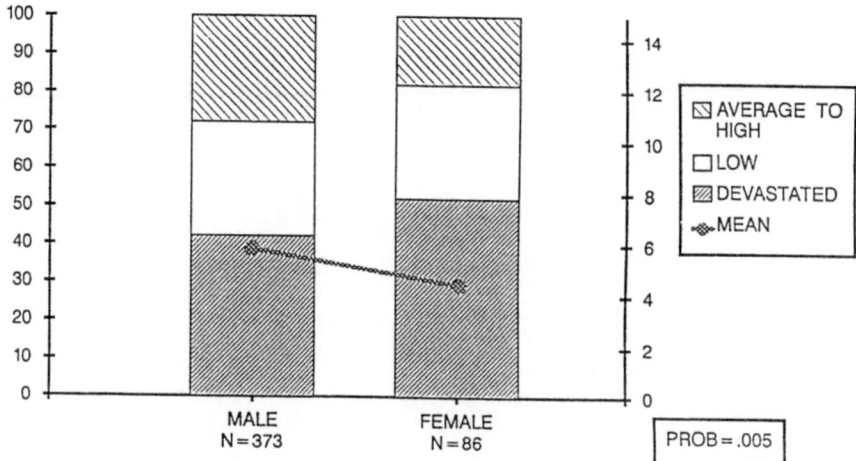

Fig 3. Preoperative CLAT scaled score as a function of sex.

coronary bypass and cardiac valvular surgeries. The significant sex difference might pertain to one type of surgery and not the other. Figure 4 shows
the relationship between pre-operative CLAT scores and sex, investigated
separately for both types of surgery. CLAT scores of the 395 male and female
coronary bypass patients were not significantly different, whereas the 37
cardiac valvular surgery patients did show a significant difference (p = 0.001).
Apparently women's pre-operative CLAT scores are lower than mens', but only
for women with cardiac valvular disease.

Not only were there relationships between pre-operative CLAT scores and
several variables related to cardiac status, but there were also significant

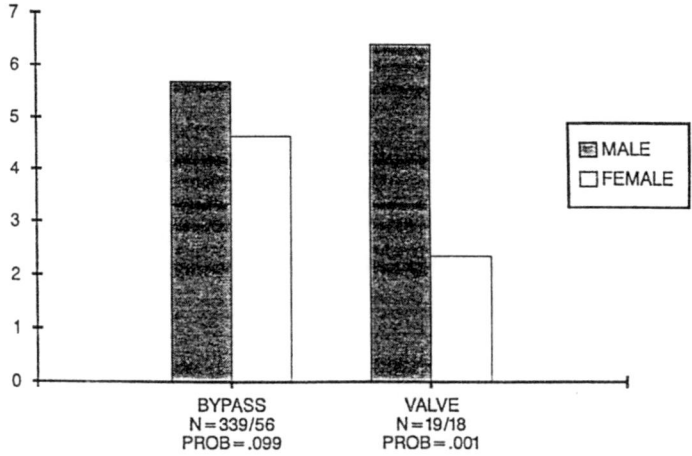

Fig 4. Preoperative CLAT scaled score as a function of sex.

correlations between a post-operative drop in CLAT scores (preoperative minus post-operative) and several parameters of extra-corporeal perfusion such as:

– bypass pump time ($p < 0.01$)
– venous oxygen saturation ($p = 0.05$)
– hematocrit level ($p < 0.05$)

One problem with the use of the CLAT was that it is too sensitive a measure in this population. About 35% of the patients had such low pre-operative scores that there was no room for them to drop one standard deviation post-operatively. This was not the case for two other tests: the WAIS Block Design and WAIS Digit Symbol. A battery of these three tests proved useful for detecting cognitive losses: the CLAT was especially useful for higher func-tioning patients, and the Block Design and Digit Symbol for lower functioning patients.

Figures 5 and 6 show that the relationship between venous oxygen saturation and drop in post-operative cognitive test scores improved when the battery of three tests was used, as opposed to when the CLAT was the sole cognitive measure. (For the battery, a drop of at least one standard deviation in the score of any of the three tests was evidence of diminished cognitive functioning. For the CLAT, the drop must perforce be on the CLAT). Figure 5 shows a significant ($p = 0.0501$) relationship between the drop in CLAT score and the level of venous oxygen saturation during surgery. The seven columns (from left to right) show increasing levels of venous oxygen saturation. The darker crosshatching in each column shows, for that level of oxygen saturation, the proportion of patients whose CLAT scores dropped. Figure 6 shows the same comparison except that the measure of cognitive function is a drop in any one of the three test scores. The relationship between

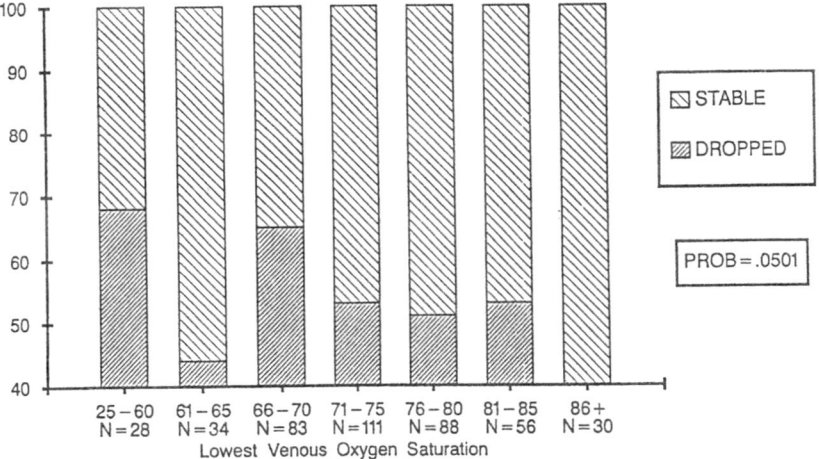

Fig. 5 Drop on CLAT as a function of lowest venous oxygen saturation.

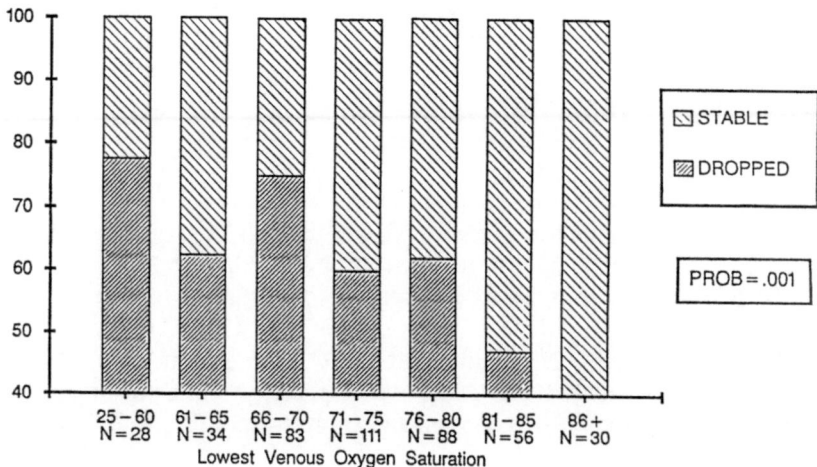

Fig.6. Drop on CLAT/WAIS as a function of lowest venous oxygen saturation.

drop in cognitive functioning and level of venous oxygen saturation was significant (p < 0.001).

Figure 7 shows the correlation between drop in cognitive test score and hematocrit level. The size of the correlation is represented by the length of the bar. The strongest correlation is between a drop in any of the 3 tests and hematocrit level (p < 0.01), followed by drops in the CLAT (p > 0.05), Digit Symbol (p < 0.05), and Block Design (N.S.). Similarly, Figure 8 shows the correlations between the cognitive tests and venous oxygen saturation. The strongest correlation is between a drop in any of the 3 test scores and oxygen saturation (p < 0.001), followed by drops in Block Design (p < 0.05), CLAT (p < 0.0501) and Digit Symbol (N.S.). The corresponding correlations for

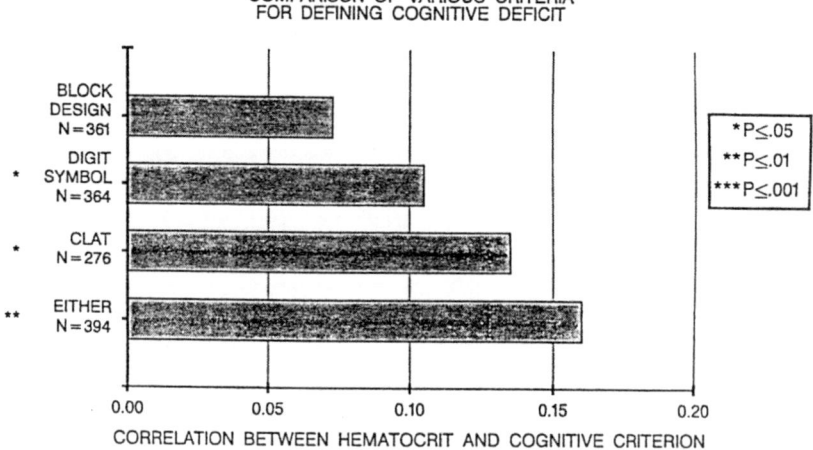

Fig. 7. Relationship between neuropsychological test scores and hematocrit.

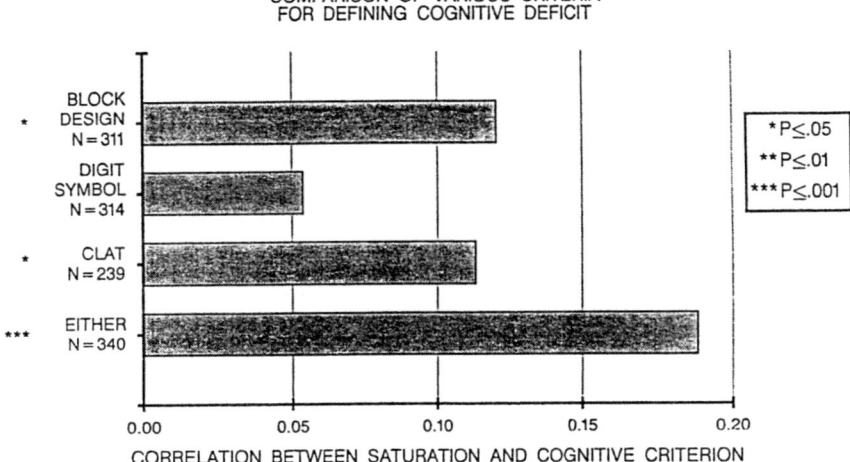

Fig. 8. Relationship between neuropsychological test scores and venous oxygen saturation.

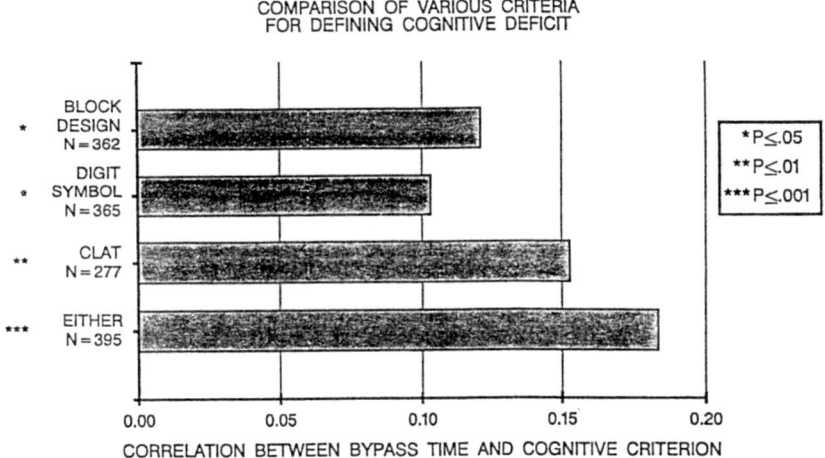

Fig. 9. Relationship between neuropsychological test scores and bypass time.

bypass time are shown in Figure 9. The strongest correlation is with a drop in any one of the 3 test scores ($p < 0.001$), and next drops in the CLAT ($p < 0.01$), Block Design ($p < 0.05$), and Digit Symbol ($p < 0.05$).

In Figure 10, we see a comparison of the correlations of the criteria for cognitive deficit with: hematocrit level, venous oxygen saturation level, and bypass time.

These results suggest that several parameters of the perfusion pump are related to post-operative drop in cognitive test scores. Two parameters which have often been considered are oxygenators and arterial line filters. Patients

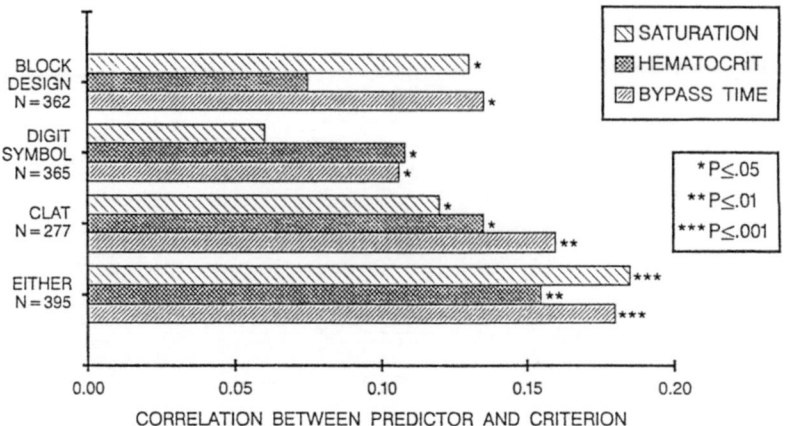

Fig. 10. Comparison of several measures for defining cognitive deficit as predictors of perfusion values..

cannot survive cardiac surgery while their hearts are artificially stopped without a source of oxygen. However several features of oxygenators have been cited as potentially deleterious to cognitive functioning. Although arterial line filters are not required for patients' survival, most surgeons use them to filter out unwanted particles each time the blood goes through the pump before it returns to the body.

In this study the surgeons used whatever oxygenators and/or filters they preferred; we had no control over this. Figure 11 shows the combinations of

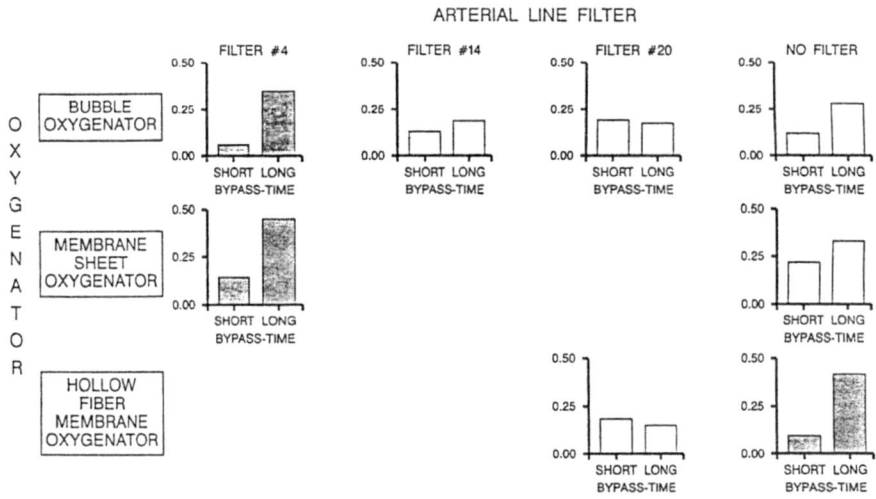

Fig. 11. Drop on at least one of 3 tests as a function of oxygenator, filter, and bypass time.

oxygenators and filters investigated. Across the top of the figure are four arterial line filter conditions: Filter 4, Filter 14, Filter 20, and no filter. Listed down the left side of the figure are three types of oxygenators: Bubble Oxygenators, Membrane Sheet Oxygenators, and Hollow Fiber Membrane Oxygenators. Since there are four columns and three rows, there can be a maximum of twelve oxygenator and filter combinations in this chart. We actually had enough data to investigate eight of these combinations. Each cell in Figure 11 represents a combination of oxygenator and filter (or no filter). The labels beneath the two bars in each cell indicate whether bypass time was short or long (as compared with the median bypass time). The height of each bar within the cell indicates the proportion of patients who showed a cognitive drop (on any of the 3 cognitive tests). Solid shaded bars indicate significant differences between the proportions of cognitively impaired patients who had long vs. short bypass times. Figure 11 shows that three combinations of oxygenator and filter conditions are associated with a significantly larger incidence of cognitive impairment as bypass time increases. Specifically, the incidence of cognitive drop is significantly higher in patients who have surgery with:

– bubble oxygenators and filter #4
– membrane sheet oxygenators and filter #4
– hollow-fiber membrane oxygenator and no filter.

Discussion

There are at least two major components in the relationship between cognitive test scores and variables related to cardiac surgery: those related to the patient's condition before the surgery, and those related to aspects of the surgery itself. The variables studied in Figures 1–4 belong to the former category since they relate to the patient's preoperative CLAT analogy test score, and several aspects of the patient's pre-surgical condition (age, cardiac diagnosis, sex, and interaction between cardiac diagnosis and sex). The patient's preoperative CLAT score is negatively related to age, diagnosis of cardiac valvular disease, and female sex (for patients with cardiac valvular disease). It is likely that cognitive functioning declines with age, especially in patients with severe cardiac illness. It is also likely that patients with cardiac valvular disease have less effective cognitive function than those with coronary artery disease; the former is a more chronic and debilitating condition. The meaning of the finding that among cardiac valvular disease patients, females have poorer cognitive function than males is unclear.

The variables depicted in Figures 5–11 refer to relationships between several cognitive measures and aspects of the surgery itself. Figure 5 shows a relationship between a drop of at least 1 S.D. in the CLAT and the lowest level of venous oxygen saturation in the bypass pump. Figure 6 shows a corresponding relationship between a drop of at least 1 S.D. in any of the three tests used and venous oxygen saturation. Presumably, the drop in cognitive functioning is related to the effect of reduced oxygen saturation in the blood.

Figures 7, 8, 9 and 10 show correlations of a drop in cognitive functioning with hematocrit level, venous oxygen saturation, and bypass time. Presumably, lowered hematocrit level, lowered venous oxygen saturation, and increased bypass time are all related to a drop in cognitive functioning mediated by the effects of reduced oxygen supply to the brain.

Figure 11 shows the effects of oxygenator and filter used in the bypass pump, and bypass time, upon drop in cognitive functioning postoperatively. For three of the eight combinations of oxygenators and filters studied, cognitive drop increased significantly with longer bypass time. The history of cardiac surgery has shown a sharp drop in mortality. This was accomplished by replacing earlier surgical techniques with newer techniques associated with lower mortality. Occasional newly introduced measures that increased mortality were identified and discarded. A similar progression has been observed with obvious neurological damage. Fortunately, both mortality and obvious neurological impairment have been reduced to low levels. This improvement was facilitated by the easy observability of the outcome. The same, however, does not apply to more subtle neuropsychological damage. Since the surgical team doesn't observe the problem, they have little reason to deal with it. Similarly, it is difficult to document any improvement or worsening in the problem. This study aims at identifying tests which can detect subtle neuropsychological damage, so that it can be reduced to a minimum. Beyond this practical clinical purpose there is another aim. In many diseases, the patient can be only studied after pathological symptoms occur since one cannot predict the occurence. In the case of cardiac surgery, however, the patient can be studied both before and after the event. This helps to differentiate between impairments present before and after surgery. Hopefully, studies such as this one will spell out changes in cardiac surgery so that the incidence of cognitive problems will fall to the low levels of mortality and major neurological complications. Then presumably, this kind of experimental investigation will become unnecessary with the decline of neuropsychological damage, facilitated by the use of sensitive neuropsychological criteria.

References

1. Campbell DE, Raskin SA. Cerebral dysfunction after cardiopulmonary bypass: aetiology, manifestations and interventions. Perfusion 1990; 5(4):251.
2. Townes BD, Bashein G, Hornbein TF, Coppel DB, Goldstein DE, Davis KB, Nessly ML, Bledsoe SW, Veith RC, Ivey TD, Cohen MA. Neurobehavioral outcomes in cardiac operations: a prospective controlled study. J Thor Cardiovasc Surg 1989; 98:774.
3. Fish KJ, Helms KN, Sarnquist FH, van Steennis C, Linet OI, Hilberman M, Mitchell RS, Jamieson SW, Miller DG, Tinklenberg JS. A prospective randomized study of the effects of prostacyclin on neuropsychological dysfunction after coronary artery surgery. J Thorac Cardiovasc Surg 1987; 93:609.
4. Patrick RT, Kirklin JW, Theye RA. The effects of extracorporeal circulation on the

brain. In: Allen J G (ed). Extracorporeal Circulation. Charles C. Thomas, Springfield, Ill, 1958.

5. Walsh G, Hearn S, O'Reilly W. A comparison of psychological test results in patients post cardiopulmonary bypass using membrane and bubble oxygenators. Proceed Amer Acad Cardiovasc Perfusion 1986; 7:35.
6. Frank A, Heller S, Kornfeld D. A survey of adjustment to cardiac surgery. Arch Intern Med 1972; 130:735.
7. Savageau J A, Stanton B A, Jenkins C D, Klein M D. Neuropsychological dysfunction following elective cardiac operation. I. Early assessment. J Thorac Cardiovasc Surg 1982; 84:585.
8. Savageau J A, Stanton B A, Jenkins C D, Frater R W M. Neuropsychological dysfunction following elective cardiac operation. II. A six month reassessment. J Thor Cardiovasc Surg 1982; 84:595.
9. Klonoff H, Clark C, Kavanagh-Gray D, Mizgala H, Munro I. Two-year follow-up study of coronary bypass surgery: psychologic status, employment status, and quality of life. J Thorac Cardiovasc Surg 1989; 97:78.
10. Shaw P J, Bates D, Cartlidge N E, French J M, Heaviside D, Julian D G, Shaw D A. Early intellectual dysfunction following coronary bypass surgery. Q J Med 1986; 255:59.
11. Åberg T, Kihlgern M. Cerebral protection during open-heart surgery. Thorax 1977; 32:525.
12. Tufo H M, Ostfeld A M, Shaekelle R. Central nervous system dysfunction following open-heart surgery. JAMA 1970; 212:1333.
13. Lee W H, Brady M P, Rowe J M, Miller W C. Effects of extracorporeal circulation upon behavior, personality and brain function. Ann Surg 1977; 173:1013.
14. Sotaniemi K A. Brain damage and neurological outcome after open-heart surgery. J Neurol Neurosurg Psychiatry 1980; 43:127.
15. Shaw P J, Bates D, Cartlidge N, French J M, Heaviside D, Julian D G, Shaw D A. Neurologic and Neuropsychological morbidity following major surgery; comparison of coronary artery bypass and peripheral vascular surgery. Stroke 1987; 18:700.
16. Smith P L C, Newman S P, Ell P J, Treasure T, Joseph P, Schneidau A, Harrison M J G. Cerebral consequences of cardiopulmonary bypass. Lancet 1986; 1:823.
17. Shaw P J, Bates D, Cartlidge N, French J M, Heaviside D, Julian D G, Shaw D A. Long-term intellectual dysfunction following coronary artery bypass graft surgery: a six month follow up study. Q J Med 1987; 239:259.
18. Juolasmaa A, Outakoski J, Hirvenoja R, Tienari P, Sotaniemi K A, Takkunen J. Effect of open heart surgery on intellectual performance. J Clin Neuropsych 1981; 3:181.
19. Sotaniemi K A, Juolasmaa A, Hokkanen E T. Neuropsychological outcome after open heart surgery. Arch Neurol 1981; 38:2.
20. Aris A, Solanes H, Camara M L, Junque C, Escartin A, Caralps J M. Arterial line filtration during cardiopulmonary bypass. J Thorac Cardiovasc Surg 1986; 91:526.
21. Malone P, Prior P, Scholtz C L. Brain damage after cardiopulmonary bypass: correlations between neurophysiological and neuropsychological findings. J Neurol Neurosurg Psychiatry 1981; 44:924.
22. Sotaniemi K A, Mononen H, Hokkanen T E. Longterm cerebral outcome after open heart surgery. Stroke 1986; 17:410.
23. Venn G, Klinger L, Smith P, Harrison M, Newman S P, Treasure T. Neuropsychological sequellae of bypass twelve months after coronary artery surgery. Br Heart J 1987; 57:565.
24. Pugsley W. The use of Doppler ultrasound in the assessment of microemboli during cardiac surgery. Perfusion 1989; 4:115.
25. Larmi T K I, Karkola P, Kairaluoma M I, Sutinen S, Partanen-Talsta A. Calcium microemboli and microfilters in valve operation. Ann Thorac Surg 1977; 24:34.
26. Kolkka R, Hilberman M. Neurologic dysfunction following cardiac operation with low-flow low pressure cardiopulmonary bypass. J Thorac Cardiovasc Surg 1980; 79:332.
27. Groom R C, Hill A, Vinansky R P, Speir A M, Macmanus Q, Lefrak E A. Hollow fiber

membrane and bubble oxygenation: a comparison of psychometric test results. Proceed Amer Acad Cardiovasc Perfusion 1985; 6:70.

28. Newman S. The incidence and nature of neuropsychological morbidity following cardiac surgery. Perfusion 1989; 4:93.

29. Treasure T, Smith PLC, Newman S, Schneidau A, Joseph P, Ell P, Harrison M J G. Impairment of cerebral function following cardiac and other major surgery. Eur J Cardio Thor Surg 1989; 3:216.

30. Garvey J W, Willner A, Wolpowitz A, Caramante LL, Rabiner CJ, Weisz D, Wisoff G B. The effect of arterial filtration during open heart surgery on cerebral function. Circulation 1983(Suppl. II); 68:125.

31. Willner A E, Caramante LL, Garvey J W, Wolpowitz A, Weisz D, Rabiner CJ, Wisoff B G. The relationship between arterial filtration during open heart surgery and mental abstraction ability. Proceed Amer Acad Cardiovasc Perfusion 1983; 4:56.

32. Åberg T, Kihlgren M. Effect of open-heart surgery on intellectual function. Scand J Thor Cardiovasc Surg 1974(Suppl 15); p. 1.

33. Åberg T, Kihlgren M. Cerebral protection during open-heart surgery: a comparison between a disc oxygenator and two bubble oxygenators. Thoraxchirurgie und Vaskulare Chirurgie. 1977; 25:146.

34. Åberg T, Kihlgren M. The use of psychometric testing as a quality criterion in open-heart surgery. In: Speidel H and Rodewald G (eds). Psychic and Neurological Dysfunction After Open-heart Surgery. Stuttgart, Georg Thieme Verlag, 1980; p. 107.

35. Bethune D W. Psychometric testing in the evaluation of the postoperative cardiac patient. In: Longmore D B (ed). Towards Safer Cardiac Surgery. Boston, G K Hall Medical Publishers, 1981; p. 613.

36. Bethune D W. The assessment of organic brain damage following open-heart surgery. In: Speidel H and Rodewald G (eds). Psychic and Neurological Dysfunctions After Open-heart Surgery. Stuttgart, Georg Thieme Verlag, 1980; p. 100.

37. Rodewald G and Willner A E. Introduction. In: Willner A E, Rodewald G (eds). Impact of Cardiac Surgery on the Quality of Life: Neurological and Psychological Aspects. New York, Plenum Press, 1990; p. 1.

38. Willner A E. Conceptual Level Analogy Test. New York, Cognitive Testing Service, 1971.

39. Willner A E. The use of cognitive tests to assess impairment in cardiac surgery patients: with emphasis on the CLAT analogy test. In: Willner A E, Rodewald G (eds). Impact of Cardiac Surgery on the Quality of Life: Neurological and Psychological Aspects. New York, Plenum Press, 1990; p. 155.

40. Wechsler D. The Measurement and Appraisal of Adult Intelligence. Baltimore, Williams and Wilkins, 1958.

41. Reitan R M. Trail Making Test: Manual for Administration, Scoring and Interpretation. Indianapolis, Indiana University Medical Center, 1958.

42. Willner A E. Relationship between psychopathology and cognitive functioning in elderly persons. Psych Reports 1987; 60:1150.

PART FOUR

Psychopathology

16. Emotional reactions to cardiac surgery

P. GÖTZE, B. DAHME, G. HUSE-KLEINSTOLL and
H.-J. MEFFERT

1. Introduction

When cardiac surgery first began, serious psychopathological disturbances, even culminating in psychoses, were prevalent. Since cardiac surgery has become routine and serious physical damage the exception, emotional reactions, in particular anxiety but also sadness and hostility, are receiving increased attention.

Since Janis' paper [1] on preoperative anxieties and their effects on postoperative development, numerous research papers on this subject, particularly in connection with cardiac surgery, have been published [2–5]. The results of the individual studies are contradictory or, allow only limited comparison due to the methods applied. Summarizing the existing literature, it can be stated that the following questions should always be taken into consideration when examining preoperative anxiety and coping with anxiety:

- On which theoretical model is the perception, the analysis and the interpretation of data based?
- How is the anxiety perceived and measured?
- Does the patient describe his anxiety himself or does the examiner form his own assessment?
- Is a differentiation made between the patient's trait anxiety and his state anxiety?
- How is coping with the anxiety perceived?

Whatever applies to anxiety generally also applies to sadness and hostility. In the following descriptions the emphasis is, however, placed on anxiety, it being the predominant emotional reaction and the one which has, so far, been studied the closest.

220

2. Preoperative state

2.1. Anxiety, depressive reactions and hostility

2.1.1. Anxiety
The patient's psychic condition is determined by anxieties, both conscious and subconscious (masked)

1. Those that the patient consciously perceives and can communicate to the doctor, nursing staff, other patients and relatives.
2. Those that the patient cannot perceive because they appear subconsciously "masked" in his experiences and behaviour.

2.1.1.1. Conscious anxieties. The most important conscious anxieties are related to three areas [6,7]:

– to the cardiac ailment leading to surgery
– to the anaesthesia and operation
– to thoughts relating to the period after surgery (Table 1).

Table 1. Preoperative anxieties.

---
1. Anxieties concerning the illness itself
   – anxiety regarding the true nature of the illness that may be revealed through surgery.

2. Anxieties directly connected with the anaesthesia and the operation
   – fear of surrendering onself
   – fear of losing self-control
   – fear of surgery procedure
   – fear of pain in case of insufficient anaesthesia
   – fear of injuries
   – fear of death

3. Anxieties concerning the period after surgery
   – fear of painful wounds
   – fear of loss of control, dependency, separation, isolation
   – fear of death
   – fear of loss of organs/functions
   – fear of the unknown
   – fear of surgery failure
   – fear of psychological consequences
   (e.g. postoperative role changes in career and family)

This division is artificial and purely made for a clearer survey as the afore-mentioned anxieties in the patient's preoperative experiences and behaviour do not appear independently of each other, but constitute a complex framework of development and conditions. A further important aspect is that the preoperative anxieties listed in the table blend with any other real and neurotic anxieties existing in the patient's life.

We would like to draw special attention to two anxiety complexes in Table 1 (items 1 and 2) as, in our opinion, they receive too little attention compared with surgery and anaesthesia anxieties. They refer to the question of anxieties relating to the illness itself: Is the illness leading to surgery chronic or acute? What importance does the illness have for the patient in his psychosocial experience and feelings about his body? Is the illness already integrated within a framework of psychophysical and psychosocial equilibrium and, therefore, practically ego syntonic or "indispensible", so that the surgery is perceived as a frightening interference rather than a help, or is the illness ego dystonic representing a constant source of worry, even leading to fear of death? What are the psychosocial consequences of the approaching operation in e.g. career and family, particularly from the aspect of a possibly unclarified postoperative role change resulting in a different level of efficiency and an altered perception of self-estimation dependent on the immediate environment [8].

2.1.1.2. Subconscious or "masked" anxieties. Preoperative experience and behaviour are frequently so radically altered that the character of the emotion can only be revealed by a thorough analysis (Table 2). These are anxieties which predominantly occur subconsciously masked, and which the patient does not spontaneously communicate but which the doctor can only deduce through observation and questioning. The subconsciously masked anxieties relate to the same areas as the consciously experienced anxieties (Table 1). These anxieties are revealed as follows:

Table 2. How does the patient experience and express his partially subconscious "masked" anxieties? (both pre- and postoperative)

1. Changes in the emotional areas
   - increased irritability culminating in states of anxiety and dysphoria

2. Changes in perception capability
   - increased tension
   - narrowed awareness, concentration and orientation
   - filtering and distortion of environmental experiences

3. Development of functional/psychosomatic symptoms
   - psychic functional disorders and psychosomatic reactions

4. Changes in contacts with the environment
   - inner withdrawal (alienation behaviour)
   - dependency (devotional behaviour)
   - strong fluctuations between withdrawal and dependency desires and behaviour (ambivalent) expressing considerable self-insecurity.

A. Changes in the emotional area: Patients reveal a range of emotions from anxiety and insecurity to hostility and distrust. If the examiner is aware of the disorder, the patient may himself realize it upon questioning. The problem for these patients, who are often performance oriented, is how to save their endangered concept of themselves. Almost all examiners report these changes in the emotional area.

B. Changes in psychic sensitivity: The above mentioned anxieties effect a change in the patient's perception of environment and self [9–13].

C. The development of functional psychosomatic symptoms: Anxious patients generally develop preoperative functional disorders and psychomotoric symptoms which are not an expression of the existing organic changes [9, 14, 15].

D. Changes in the relationship between the patient and his environment: It can frequently be observed that the patient not only outwardly withdraws from his psychosocial relationship in an anxiously-depressed and insecure manner, but also inwardly (stress-alexithymia by Möhlen and Davies-Osterkamp 1979 or the secondary alexithymia by Freyberger 1977) [16, 17]. Alternatively, he reveals compensatory behaviour of an almost clingingly-euphoric, over-conformistic dependant nature (see "Symbiotic" by Kimball 1969, Götze 1980) [14, 18].

2.1.2. Depressive reactions

In the postoperative period, every other cardiac patient exhibits considerable psychophysical instability. Feelings of depressive tension and anxiety tension dominate with constrictions in experiences and behaviour, as well as a reduction in brain organic efficiency.

Besides the feeling of anxiety, most authors mention depressive and dysphoric moods. Kimball [14], for instance, differentiates four groups: "adjusted", "symbiotic", "denying anxiety", and "depressive". These group names denote the different psychic coping styles with regard to affective problems connected with surgery.

We have the impression, however, that the term depressive mood in the preoperative state is not entirely accurate. A depressive mood takes time to develop. The time period between diagnosis and surgery is, however, in most cases of cardiac surgery too short. We should therefore, perhaps not speak of a depressive mood in this connection, but rather of a "depressive reaction".

2.1.3. Hostility (dysphoric moods)

The emotional reaction of hostility does not appear on its own in the preoperative phase. Regardless of how the psychopathological symptoms were perceived, almost all authors mention symptoms which could best be described as psychopathological symptoms of a tense, anxious, dysphoric-based mood.

The mood character is always very changeable. Almost every third patient is affected by this mood in the preoperative phase. The emphasis placed on the different syndromes within these moods depends predominantly on the individual patient's primary personality and his psychosocial situation.

2.2. Coping with preoperative anxiety

2.2.1. Psychoanalytical theory – defense mechanism

The types of preoperative anxieties mentioned, as well as coping with them, belong in the context of psychoanalytical hypotheses to the Theory of Anxiety and Defense Mechanisms [19, 20] which we would like to go into briefly:

All anxieties originate in the ego, being the integrative, psychic instance coordinating the various personal needs, wishes, demands and ideals with those demands made by the environment. Anxiety originates in the ego as a feeling of being threatened, and the necessary anxiety defenses are, also present in the ego. As many of these processes remain subconscious, the patient can only consciously experience that part of the anxiety that was not repressed, or not totally repressed. In this connection it is important to note that the anxiety experienced is dependent on the manner and intensity of the sources, the quality, of the ego-functions and the stability of the anxiety defenses. The anxiety defenses are dependent here on the development and health of the ego-functions. In accordance with the psychoanalytic ego-Psychology [21, 22] the term ego-functions describes all of the individuals's abilities to deal with his environment while maintaining his self-confidence. In addition to the sections of early childhood and later experiences, the ego-functions also include inherent characteristics. These are always further influenced by the individual's momentary physical constitution. The ego functions can therefore be so detrimentally disturbed due to e.g. lack of oxygen, medications, strong pain or the inability to move, that the ability to defend against anxiety is reduced.

As the anxiety experienced by the patient is a result of previous insecurity and anxiety defenses, disproportionately strong state anxiety denote an incomplete ability to repress anxiety. Should it lead to a flood of anxiety and a breakdown of the anxiety defenses, extreme cases develop a psychosis.

Besides the perception of conscious and nearly conscious anxiety symptoms, we are more easily able to recognize the subconscious character of anxiety and anxiety defences in some patients' preoperative conditions and behaviour with the aid of psychoanalytical insight. We frequently observe a denial of reality, a regression into early-childhood experience and behaviour patterns, as well as idealization of doctors and nursing staff as an expression of subconscious anxiety defenses. In connection with denial, idealization and regression, we often see a tendency towards a positive portrayal of the ego and the environment, with a harmonisation of family and career [23]. In the preoperative stage a change also often occurs whereby the anxiety is experienced through the body in the sense of a secondary hypochondria, and a projection of anxieties into the environment, e.g. in the simplest form: "I am not anxious, but my wife is afraid that I could die". This projected form often denotes a character of delegation, especially if the partner actually experiences strong anxieties, and the patient is noticeably reticent about helping the partner cope with those anxieties.

In the preoperative situation, these forms described are most frequently mobilized plus the predominantly complex anxiety defense processes, and are defined as defense mechanisms [20]. They represent the subconscious part of coping with anxiety. In extreme cases the patient is no longer aware of his anxiety.

2.2.2. IL Janis' "work of worrying" concept

Among the analysts it was particularly KA Menninger [24], Helene Deutsch [25], Jessner *et al.* [26] and Janis [1] who dealt with the peculiarities of pre- and postoperative stress. In "Psychological Stress: Psychoanalytical and Behavioural Studies of Surgical Patients" Janis describes the patient's preoperative coping with anxiety as a "work of worrying". In addition, he discovered that patients whose preoperative anxiety level he assessed as average, by means of an in-depth psychological interview, reported fewer emotional disturbances and physical complaints in the postoperative events compared to patients with high or low anxiety levels. He, therefore, assumed a U-shaped connection between the preoperative anxiety level and the condition in the postoperative events. Only one author discovered this connection (curved line) between the patient's preoperative increase in anxiety compared with a later recovery time [27]. Janis was, however, less involved with the manner of coping with anxiety than with its effectiveness. His work group reported that therapeutic support for the patient in creating a constructive attitude towards surgery lead to a decrease in dosage of anaesthesia, analgesics and sedatives, and also had a beneficial influence on the patient's postoperative condition [28].

2.2.3. Taxonomy of coping with anxiety by N Haan

Norma Haan [13] did not use the term defense mechanism in her taxonomy of different ego processes. She was of the opinion that defense mechanisms are described as factors of traits, rather than as dynamic processes of coping with anxiety in analytical literature. In her taxonomy she attempts to portray the integration of demands determined by development as a conformistic and maturation process. She divides 10 general ego-processes according to the level of intersubjective reality into three groups which she names "coping", "defense", and "fragmentation". All of the ego-processes show a retention of feelings of self-confidence. Haan makes no evaluations within the taxonomy. The choice of the ego-processes takes place according to individual and situational aspects of the demand-coping relationship. Haan describes this relationship as follows: "This person will cope if he can, defend if he must, and fragment if he is forced . . ." Viewed analytically this taxonomy, in our opinion, still implies a hierarchy in the sense that the experienced or observed anxiety is less if a person shows coping processes as opposed to defense or even fragmentation processes.

2.3. Psychometric measurement of preoperative anxieties

2.3.1. Self ratings and expert ratings

When examining preoperative psychic conditions, we cannot dispense with simultaneous self and expert ratings for reasons of content and method. From the psychoanalytical viewpoint, it should be noted that the amount stated in the self-assessments are influenced by the patient's defense mechanisms, while the amounts stated in the expert ratings are influenced by the interviewers countertransference feelings [29].

2.3.2. Trait anxiety and state anxiety

A differentiation between trait and state anxiety is of the utmost importance [30]. The preoperative anxieties are named exactly in Table 2, and Table 2 illustrates which changes in feeling, physical condition, mental functions and in contacts with the environment can be experienced by the patient in a state of anxiety. Not all of these phenomena are recognized by the patient as expressions of anxiety. On measuring the patient's state of anxiety, it will be necessary to ask about these phenomena with the aid of the respective tests and questionnaires, in the same way as with lists measuring emotions and complaints.

In contrast, a study of patients showing a readiness to experience anxiety, i.e. trait anxiety, contains (independent of surgery) questions about the nature, frequency and strength of situations which create anxiety, functional disorders and irritation. Trait anxiety should not be compared with neurotic anxiety, but is stronger in patients who exhibit more and increased neurotic anxieties [1]. In addition, trait anxiety is influenced by the quality and the stability of the ego functions. The Spielberger work group came to the following conclusions, while making a differentiation between state and trait anxieties, in their empirical studies of patients undergoing general surgery [2, 27, 31, 32].

1. No changes occur in trait anxiety readiness during the pre- and postoperative period.
2. State anxiety increases greatly one or two days before surgery, and decreases continually after surgery.
3. The amount in which state anxiety decreases from the preoperative to the postoperative period is dependant on the individual level of trait anxiety readiness.

In our own studies with cardiac surgery patients, we found a significantly positive interrelationship between trait anxiety and preoperative state anxiety [8]. Trait and state anxiety are, therefore, not independent of each other in the preoperative stage. This would confirm Spielberger's concept that people with greater trait anxieties generally react with greater state anxieties [30]. In our own studies we also proved that the amount of preoperative and trait anxieties predict the level of postoperative depression. For coping with cardiac surgery and the stressful early postoperative phase, the level of trait anxiety appears to be more significant that the preoperative state anxiety. A possible, partial explanation for this discovery, is that patients with stronger trait anxieties had less stable object relationships. This applied both to the self-assessment in the "Partnership Harmony" section, as well as the external ratings in the "Family Harmony" section [8]. The close connection between low trait anxiety counts and the patient's ability to form positive personal relationships is of great importance for the patient's relationships with doctors and nursing staff while in hospital. Just as good personal relationships have also proved to be supportive in overcoming stress, the positive effects of lower trait anxiety in the same way seem to multiply with regard to an uncomplicated psychic development [33].

2.4. Psychometric measurement of coping with preoperative anxiety

The different uses of the term "coping", whether in the sense of conscious cognitive direction in coping with stress [34], or in the sense of realistic ego processes drawing on individual capabilities [13], or as a compound term uniting all conscious and subconscious coping processes [35, 36], has lead to great confusion. All too often, therefore, "coping" research is concerned with comparing apples with fruit or gardens.

On examining the diagnosis and prognosis instruments used in coping, Prystav [37] misses those instruments developed and published by psycho-analysts. This seems understandable at first sight, as psychoanalytical constructions of anxiety and defense mechanisms were mentioned in the development of numerous instruments such as, e.g. The Coping and Defense Scale by Haan [13], the Stress Questionnaire by Bousein *et al.* [38], the Dealing with Stress Questionnaire by Erdmann and Jahnke [39], The Defense Mechanism Inventory by Gleser and Ihlevitch [40], The Life Style Index by Plutschik *et al.* [41], the Scales by Houston [42] as well as Scales by Davies-Osterkamp and Salm [29, 43].

Developing a Coping Scale is not what we see as an operating psychoanalytical structure to deal with anxieties and defense mechanisms, but rather the interpretation of perceptible and observable anxiety phenomena based on psychoanalytical theory. (Transference, counter-transference, stability of object relationships, etc.).

Psychoanalytical assessment always strives to establish a sound evaluation of the anxiety, the source of anxiety, the amount of real and unreal threats, defense mechanisms as well as the effectiveness and economy of coping processes. Particularly interactive communication factors in the interview give important indications of the quality of object relationships, and the possibilities of coping with anxiety within the patient's personal environment relationship. The variability of the above mentioned influences requires complex adaptability processes in different situations by the individual. This complexity cannot be expressed in psychological scales. In addition, data collection and evaluation is made by separate people when applying classical psychological methods, which leads to the evaluator not being able to grasp certain subtle and individual significances observed and interpretations made by the interviewer.

We are also of the opinion that a false impression is often created, whereby prognoses regarding efficient or inefficient adaptability behaviour could be infered merely from different styles of coping [43]. The proposal to describe the coping processes instead of coping traits does not solve the problem, because without knowing further details which direct the coping process nothing can be stated regarding the effectiveness, economy, or the therapeutic relevance of the interventions [13, 44, 45].

The perception and measurement of coping patterns is also difficult in view of the interpretation of the situations creating anxiety, since both the rational as well as the symbolic significance of an event define the demands made on the individual to cope (first detailed studies on this subject by K Menninger and H Deutsch [24, 25].

Finally, surgery represents both stress and an attempt to cope with the illness, so that a combination of threat and hope always exists. In this connection, Lipowski [46] differentiates between four types of illness implications which can come to the fore or could interfere: threat, loss, profit and indifference.

There are, therefore, many unsolved problems when studying coping with anxiety, particularly from the aspect of making comparisons in connection with differing definitions and theoretical assumptions on the part of the examiner.

2.5. Therapeutic support for preoperative coping with anxiety

The type and intensity of the manifested state anxieties experienced by the patient, as well as the various influences which contribute to stabilization or destabilization in coping with anxiety, are therapeutically of great importance for the clinical doctor. Since the 50s, therapeutically orientated programmes to prepare for surgery have been developed such as systematic desensitization, muscle relaxation, model films, operant modification of behaviour, detailed surgery information on tape, informative and supportive group and individual discussions, etc. (Further literature in Davies-Osterkamp [2]).

Because of the very different methods, the results of the individual studies are not comparable and difficult to investigate, as definite postoperative reference data is either arbitrary or, in most cases, missing altogether.

One exception was the Langer *et al.* [28] studies of various forms of therapy attempting to reduce psychological stress in surgery patients. The most effective form proved to be selective emphasis on the positive aspects of surgery, contrasted with worrying aspects in the sense of coping with anxiety by making a fresh evaluation. Postoperative anxiety, flexibility in behaviour, as well as the use of analgetics and sedatives served as the criteria. This method of anxiety reduction is very similar to the form of coping in low anxiety patients, who successfully overcome their anxiety and experience a favourable postoperative development by ignoring and denying preoperative anxieties in favour of emphasizing the expected positive results of surgery [47].

As a result of her own studies of cardiac surgery, Salm [48], however, is of the opinion that patients who experience intense anxieties before surgery need not necessarily exhibit a poor postoperative condition. She presumes that the time available in the preoperative period can be of great significance in terms of the possibility of dealing with the anxiety thoroughly in the sense of coping by being prepared. Regardless of the type of therapy, therefore, and the comparability of the individual studies, it is obvious that positive effects are always emphasized so that one already reads of artifacts in literature. Meffert [49] found a clear explanation for this: "It is possibly not the effects of the anxiety reducing measures that are important for the patient, but the effect of a believable offer of a helpful relationship. Believable meaning that the doctor or psychologist makes a serious offer of therapy and wholeheartedly supports the specific anxiety reduction measures embedded in the relationship. The resultant differences in the degree of successful anxiety reduction would then be a function of the relationship offer, in the sense that success is dependant on how wholeheartedly the examiner is behind his offer of help, and how well he manages to reconcile his offer with the patient's wishes and expectations. Meffert places emphasis, therefore, on a specific relationship and not on a specific method of therapeutic action that would influence all patients equally favourably. This agrees with the results of an empiric study by Träger et al. [50] on preoperative, informative discussions. Taking the current stand of research into consideration, a provisional consequence can be drawn from a psychoanalytical point of view: namely, supporting the patient in his own defense mechanism is of central importance in therapy where complex conscious and subconscious preoperative anxieties appear [2, 51]. H Deutsch was already leaning in this direction in 1942 as a result of her psychoanalytical individual case study of preoperative situations.

"It is not the freedom from anxiety or its presence before an operation which gives the favorable prognosis, but the inner assimilation of the anxiety signal which arises in the patient who expects an operation; its goal is the building up of inner defenses" [52].

Besides considering individual processes of coping with a situation in preoperative anxiety therapy, individual protective resources relevant to the therapy must be recognized and mobilized. This, however, only seems possible if the patient feels his relationship with the doctor or psychologist is trustworthy and reliable [49].

If coping with the anxiety is ineffective, the doctor or psychologist, together with the nursing team and, if possible, also the relatives, should strongly consider a "holding function" procedure, e.g. taking over the patient's functions and compensating for deficits (orientation, acceptance of inadequate expression, offers of contact, easing medication, etc.).

Further assistance in coping with anxiety can follow indirectly if the strain is reduced by, e.g. shortening or lengthening the preoperative period, eliminating pain, providing information and distraction, etc. Each individual must

be examined for stress and resources in order to select the appropriate therapeutic action.

3. Early postoperative state

3.1. Anxiety, depressive reactions and hostility

Most patients are mostly psychologically stable on the first postoperative
day – possibly due to the after effects of anaesthesia and the realization that
one has "survived" the operation. On the second and third postoperative day,
however, an accentuated deterioration in condition appears. While some
patients at this time do indeed react with relief and a decrease in anxiety, almost
every other patient exhibits more or less vehement anxiety, depressive sadness
or dysphoria, and partly anxious paranoia.

They also exhibit types of behaviour and experience that appear substu-
porous (most likely as an expression of repelled subconscious anxieties) as
well as cognitive disturbances within a framework of organic psychosyndrome
culminating in pronounced paranoid-hallucinatory psychoses. These are mostly
described as "post-cardiotomy delirium" or as "transient psychosis", which
also include acute brain organic psychosyndromes. Emphasis in early studies
of psychopathology in cardiac patients was placed on the perception and
classification of cerebral disturbances and psychotic symptoms. Today,
however, types of experiences and behaviour which appear more neurotic,
are increasingly coming to the fore.

3.2. Cluster and factoranalytical measurement

In cardiac surgery in the 60s and 70s, however, dysphoric reactions [53–56],
anxiety reaction [57, 14], as well as depressive reactions [54–59] had already
been pointed out. It should also be noted here that sadness was always included
within the depressive reactions summary. Within the framework of an
international multi-centre study, emotional reactions were again examined
cluster – and factor analytically with, among other things, the aid of a newly
developed psychiatric rating scale (HRPD-Hamburg Rating Scale for Psychic
Disorders) [60–63]. The Hamilton Anxiety and Depression Scales (HAMA,
HAMD) were also used.

The HRPD contains a list of 36 items.

In a further step of test construction, these 36 items were condensed to 8
symptom scales (by factor analysis/principle components and Varimax rotation).
These were

1. Disorientation
2. Impaired thinking/concentration
3. Paranoid-hallucinatory symptoms

4. Anxiety
5. Depression
6. Hostility
7. Loss of control
8. Resignation

Then 8 HRPD scales were formed by summing up the item ratings with substantial loadings (0.40 or more) in the respective factors.

The *Factor IV Anxiety* consists of the items:

anxious	0.84
internally restless, tense	0.81
narrowed thinking	0.57
hopeless	0.52
depressed/sad	0.46
secondary hypochondria	0.46

The *Factor V Depressive Symptoms* consists of the items:

affective inflexibility	0.77
feeling of inadequacy	0.72
depressed/sad	0.64
blunted affect	0.58
apathetic	0.55
slowed thinking	0.47

The *Factor VI Hostility* consists of the items:

suspicious/hostile	0.98
aggressive thoughts or behaviour	0.75
sullen/irritated/dysphoric	0.72
diminished social interest	0.41

Statistical classification of Patients into Symptomatic of Syndrome Groups (N = 99):

In order to obtain objective, homogeneous symptomatic subgroups, we applied methods of cluster analysis (especially K means algorithm 5). By the K means algorithm we tried to get subgroups (clusters) with maximal symptom homogenity within groups and maximal symptom variance between groups. Six subgroups resulted from this analysis. For comparison with the new results of the current international study, we concentrated upon the symptom profiles (mean raw scores) of the 2nd postoperative day (for more details Götze *et al.*) [62].

(1) About 1/4 of all patients had no signs of psychopathological symptoms at all (N = 28);
(2) about 1/3 of the patients had distinct, but clinically unremarkable, signs of anxious and depressive mood (N = 32);

(3) a further 1/4 of the patients suffered from a psycho-organic syndrome with disturbances in orientation, concentration, memory and reasoning, associated with depressive mood (N = 23);
(4) 4 patients manifested a severe psycho-organic syndrome;
(5) 8 patients manifested aggressive hostility and paranoid-hallucinatory symptoms mainly at the 2nd post-operative day after a rather symptom free first post-operative day;
(6) 4 patients suffered from a severe, generalized delirious syndrome with maximum severity on the 3rd and 4th post-operative day.

We are able to present results of a new but small sample of 58 patients who underwent open heart surgery in Hamburg University Hospital during the last years who participated in the current International Multi-Center Study mentioned before. All patients had been rated on the 36 HRPD symptom items. The ratings were summed up into the respective 8 symptom scales mentioned above for each patient. These data were submitted to a cluster analysis. Again, 6 clusters or homogeneous subgroups came out of these analyses.

(1) Nearly half of the patients had no clinical signs of psychic disturbances (N = 22).
(2) About the same number of patients had slight cognitive impairments accompanied by depression and anxiety (N = 23).
(3) 8 patients showed symptoms of mild anxiety, depression and impaired concentration/reasoning.
(4) 2 patients manifested remarkable anxiety, depression and hostility accompanied by mild disturbances in concentration and orientation.
(5) 2 patients suffered from a psycho-organic syndrome with more severe disorientation and disorders in concentration, anxiety and depression.
(6) 1 patient suffered from a severe delirious syndrome, even with the experience of loss of self-control.

The emotions of anxiety, hostility (dysphoria) and depression could be clearly isolated in the factor analysis. These emotions appear in a different mixture in the individual clusters in the cluster analysis, although with respectively differing emphasis.

We can infer, therefore, that there are obviously no emotions which can appear separately in the postoperative phase.

In constructing and analyzing the Hamburg Rating Scale of Psychic Disturbances (HRPD) we offered a psychometric and diagnostic tool for research into psychic disturbances after open heart surgery. The scientific usefulness of this tool still has to be further evaluated.

3.3. Hamilton anxiety scale and Hamilton depression scale

Results from Speidel [64] as well as from Strauss and Paulsen [65], measuring pre- and postoperative psychometric developments of emotional conditions in cardiac surgery patients, paying particular attention to anxiety, have been submitted. Speidel reported about an international sample (N = 300) of a multicenter research project (Willner and Rodewald [66]); Strauss and Paulsen about a regional German sub-group (N = 71) of the same study.

The amount of anxiety was rated by psychiatrists and clinical psychologists using the Hamilton Anxiety Scale [67]. The HAMA measures both psychic and somatic anxiety. Psychic anxiety is created by symptoms such as anxious moods, tension and fears and insomnia; somatic anxiety by symptoms such as gastrointestinal symptoms, cardiovascular symptoms, respiratory symptoms, etc. Generally a total score is calculated.

Using careful interpretation and taking the premises discussed in the preoperative situation into consideration, the Hamilton Depression Scale [68] can be used to measure depression and sadness, which appear equally in the few early days of postoperative development, and the total HAMD some can be interpreted as a measurement for sadness.

The HRPD Factor 4 Anxiety and the amount of anxiety rated by the patient himself using the State-Trait-Anxiety Scale [69] were used as reference data; the reference data for sadness was the HRPD Factor 5: masked depression. Hostility is measured by the HRPD Factor 6.

The results are not always clear. In general, however, the results of the total group [64], as well as the partial samples [65], show an even development: HAMA and HAMD scores for anxiety and sadness increase from the preoperative week to the early postoperative period and decrease towards the time of discharge, and decreasing approximately one week later to the beginning figures, sometimes lower.

HRPD factors for masked depression and hostility show similar results. In contrast to the HAMA scores, the HRPD Anxiety scores show different results, whereby anxiety decreases in the early postoperative period. The fact that both HAMA factors (psychic and somatic anxiety) show an identical development (anxiety increases in the early postoperative stage) speaks against the assumption that HAMA and HRPD-Anxiety deal with differing aspects of anxiety. Further hypotheses and interpretation should not be made before the final evaluation of the international study is available.

Is is also surprising that the HAMA expert-rating scores and the Spielberger state-anxiety self-rating scores are not correlated. One could assume, with Strauss and Paulsen [65], either that both procedures measure different aspects of anxiety, or that the self-ratings of anxiety are overlaid by mergers. A conclusive evaluation here should also not be made until the study is completed.

3.4. Therapeutic aspects

Numerous psychological and situational risk factors for psychic disturbances after cardiac surgery are named in the literature. For instance, marriage, family and career problems, cases of cardiac deaths in the family and environment, long waiting periods, postponement of surgery as well as a lack of future perspectives. Fear of surgery and the individual psychic defense mechanism, in particular, seem to play an important role in the development of postoperative psychic stability [70]. In this connection the following appears to be significant: Flemming and Meffert [71] who in a comparison of extreme groups, discovered that high and low anxiety patients, in particular, are endangered regarding postoperative psychic disturbances. There is obviously a combination of anxiety denial with personality orientation, especially ego-structure factors, such as pronounced frustration tolerance and other stress coping resources of decisive protecting significance in individual patients. In the event of insufficient defense mechanisms, outbreaks of anxiety can certainly occur postoperatively. This can be observed in coronary patients especially.

What has already been stated about the preoperative situation is also valid for the postoperative period. Here, too, Freyberger [72] states that in combination with somatic interventions, a supportive psychotherapeutic procedure with the aspect of satisfying regressive needs, the possibility of a positive transference relationship and the stabilization of individual defense mechanisms appropriate to the situation are of central importance. Symptom oriented therapeutic procedures have also proved effective [73]. In situation orientation disturbances, as well as in slightly paranoid-hallucinatory reactions, repeated clarification and constant encouragement of an almost suggestive manner is extremely helpful. Repeated dispensation of sedatives (Diazepam) or neuroleptica (Haloperidol) can be of temporary therapeutic help, particularly for symptoms of paranoid anxiety tendencies as well as for disphoric disturbances. Patients with strong cognitive disturbances should be treated promptly (a longer period) with neuroleptica and/or Benzodiazepines taking the heart-circulatory functions into consideration.

During rehabilitation, the therapist should focus his attention on the patient's psychosocial situation and condition. One can mostly observe that the patient suffers less as the result of physical impairments as from partnership, family, career problems, as well as from altered role behaviour and self-confidence. The cardiologist, and especially the patient's personal physician, can be extremely helpful in coping with psychic and social rehabilitation. In this situation, the patient mostly needs a (unspoken) "relationship" and not a physical examination.

4. Late postoperative situation

Katamnestic studies have drawn attention to the fact that weeks, months and sometimes years after surgery, anxiety, depression, sadness and hostility/dysphoria can be in the foreground of the patient's condition. One reason for this is certainly because the patients can verbalize their moods after longer periods after the operation and do not need somatic defenses as much as in the preoperative period which was experienced as a threat. It also means that the patient in the late postoperative situation can perceive himself and others in a differentiated manner. The frequently occuring phenomenon of increased anxiety and depression weeks after surgery can be an expression of considerable difficulties for some patients to adapt suitably to the altered postoperative and future situation. The patient sees himself confronted both with his own, mostly high expectations, as well as with the existing psychophysical impairments. Also included here is the strong fear of failure, combined with problems in career, family and partnership which applies particularly to the coronary patient of advanced years.

References

1. Janis IL. Psychological stress. Psychoanalytic and behavioral studies of surgical patients. New York, Wiley, 1958.
2. Davies-Osterkamp S. Angst und Angstbewältigung bei chirurgischen Patienten. Med Psychol 1977; 3:169.
3. Beckmann D, Davies-Osterkamp S, Scheer JW (eds). Medizinische Psychologie. Berlin, Heidelberg, New York, Springer, 1982.
4. Tewes U (ed). Angewandte Medizinpsychologie. Fachbuchhandlung für Psychologie, Verlagsabteilung Frankfurt, 1984.
5. Tolksdorf W. Der präoperative Stress. Berlin, Heidelberg, New York, Tokyo, Springer, 1985.
6. Corman HH, Hornick EJ, Kritchman M, Terestma N. Emotional reactions of surgical patients to hospitalization, anesthesia and surgery. Amer J Surg 1958; 96:646.
7. Dony M. Psychologische Aspekte im Bereich der Anästhesie. In: Beckmann D, Davies-Osterkamp S, Scheer JW (eds). Medizinische Psychologie. Berlin, Heidelberg, New York, Springer, 1982.
8. Huse-Kleinstoll G, Boll A, Götze P. Angst und Angstbewältigung vor und nach operativen Eingriffen. In: Götze P (ed). Leitsymptom Angst. Berlin, Heidelberg, New York, Tokyo, Springer, 1984.
9. Scheffer MB, Greifenstein FE. The emotional responses of patients to surgery and anesthesia. Anesthesiology 1960; 21:502.
10. Andrew JM. Recovery from surgery, with and without preparatory insruction, for three coping styles. J Personal Soc Psychol 1970; 15:223.
11. Lazarus RS. Psychological stress and the coping process. New York, McGraw Hill, 1966.
12. Epstein S. Versuch der Theorie der Angst. In: Birbaumer N (ed). Psychophysiologie der Angst. Fortschritte der klinischen Psychologie 3. München, Urban and Schwarzenberg, 1977.
13. Haan N. Coping and defending. Processes of self-environment organization. New York, Academic Press, 1977.
14. Kimball ChP. Psychological responses to the experience of open heart surgery. Amer J Psychiat 1969; 126:348.
15. Galster JV, Druschky KF. Bedingungen für Indikatorfragen zur Einschätzung des Patientenverhaltens. Ein Versuch der Quantifizierung der präoperativen psychischen Situation des chirurgischen Patienten. In: Rügheimer E (ed). Jahrestagung der Deutschen Gesellschaft für Anästhesiologie und Widerbelebung 1974, Erlangen, Perimed, 1975.
16. Möhlen K, Davies-Osterkamp S. Psychische und körperliche Reaktionen bei Patienten der offenen Herzchirurgie in Abhängigkeit von präoperativen psychischen Befunden. Z Psychosom Med Psychoanal 1979; 25:128.
17. Freyberger H. Psychosomatik des erwachsenen Patienten. In: Freyberger H (eds). Psychosomatik des Kindesalters und des erwachsenen Patienten. Klinik d Gegenw, Bd XI, 1977.

18. Götze P. Psychopathologie der Herzoperierter. Stuttgart, Enke, 1980.
19. Freud S. (1936) Hemmung, Symptom und Angst, GW, Band 14, 4.Aufl. Frankfurt, Fischer, 1968.
20. Freud A (1936). Das Ich und die Abwehrmechanismen. München, Kindler, 1973.
21. Hartmann H (1964) Ich-Psychologie. Stuttgart, Klett, 1972.
22. Blank C, Blanck R (1974). Angewandte Ich-Psychologie. Klett-Cotta, 1978.
23. Guth W, Werner W, Müller V, Volkmer E. Zur Psychopathologie der Herzoperierten. Med Klin 1978; 73:1812.
24. Menninger KA. Polysurgery and polysurgical addiction. Psychoanal Quarterly 1934; p. 173.
25. Deutsch H. Some psychoanalytic observations in surgery. Psychosomatic Med 1942; 4:105.
26. Jessner L, Blom GE, Waldvogel S. Emotional implications of tonsillectomy and adenoidectomy on children. Psychoanal Study Child 1952; 7:126.
27. Auerbach SM. Trait-state anxiety and adjustment to surgery. J Consult Clin Psychol 1973; 40:264.
28. Langer EJ, Janis IL, Wolfer JA. Reduction of psychological stress in surgical patients. J Exp Soc Psychol 1975; 11:155.
29. Davies-Osterkamp S, Salm A. Ansätze zur Erfassung psychischer Adaptationsprozesse in medizinischen Belastungssituationen. Med Psychol 1980; 6:66.
30. Speilberger CD. Anxiety as an emotional state. In: Spielberger CD (ed). Anxiety, current trends in theory and research. New York, Academic Press, 1972.
31. Speilberger CD, Auerbach SM, Wadsworth AP, Dunn TM, Taulbee ES. Emotional reactions to surgery. J Consult Clin Psychol 1973; 40:33.
32. Martinez-Urrutia A. Anxiety and pain in surgical patients. J Consult Clin Psychol 1975; 43:437.
33. Llynch JJ. Das gebrochene Herz. Rowohlt, Reinbek, 1971.
34. Lazarus RS, Launier L. Stress-related transactions between person and environment. In: Pervin LA, Lewis M (eds). Perspectives in International Psychology. New York, Plenum, 1978.
35. Heim E. Coping oder Anpassungsvorgänge in der psychosomatischen Medizin. Z Psychosom Med Psychoanal 1979; 25:251.
36. Heim E, Augustiny K, Blaser A. Krankheitsbewältigung (Coping)- ein integriertes Modell. Psychother Med Psychol 33, Sonderheft 35–40, 1983.
37. Prystav G. Psychologische Copingforschung: Konzeptbildungen, Operationalisierungen und Messinstrumente. Diagnostica 1981; 27:189.
38. Boucsein W, Erdmann G, Janke W, Albrecht D. Der Belastungsfragebogen, BELA. ärztliche Praxis 1978; p. 37.
39. Erdmann G, Janke W. Der situative Reaktionsfragebogen. ärztliche Praxis 1978; 39:1240.
40. Gleser GC, Ihilevich D. An objective instrument for measuring defense mechanisms. J Counseling Clin Psychol 1969; 33:51.
41. Plutschik R, Kellerman H, Conte HR. A structural theory of egodefenses and emotions. In: Izard C (ed). Emotions in personality and psychopathology. New York, Plenum, 1979.
42. Houston BK. Dispositional anxiety and the effectiveness of cognitive coping strategies in stressful laboratory and classroom situations. In: Spielberger CD, Sarason IG (eds). Stress and anxiety, Vol 4. Washington, Hemisphere, 1977.
43. Davies-Osterkamp S, Salm A. Psychische Bewältigungsprozesse in kardiologischen Belastungssituationen. In: Langosch W (ed). Psychische Bewältigung der chronischen Herzerkrankung. Berlin, Heidelberg, New York, Tokyo, Springer, 1985.
44. Folkman S, Schaefer C, Lazarus RS. Cognitive processes as mediators of stress and coping. In: Hamilton V, Warburton DM (eds). Human stress and cognition; an information processing approach. London, Wiley, 1979.
45. Roskies E, Lazarus RS. Coping theory and the teaching of coping skills. In: Davidson PO, Davidson SM (eds). Behavioral medicine: Changing health life-styles. New York, Brunner and Mazel, 1980.
46. Lipowski ZL. Psychological aspects of disease. Ann Int Med 1969; 71:1197.

236

47. Cohen D, Lazarus R. Active coping processes, coping dispositions and recovery from surgery. Psychosom Med 1973; 35:375.
48. Salm A. Angstverarbeitung und Stimmungsverläufe vor und nach Herzoperationen. In: Tewes U (ed). Angewandte Medizinpsychologie. Fachbuchhandlung für Psychologie. Frankfurt, Verlagsabteilung, 1984.
49. Meffert H-J. Angstreduktion bei chirurgischen Patienten – kritische überlegungen und Fallbeispiele zur medizinpsychologischen Forschung für Klinik und Praxis. In: Tewes U (ed). Angewandte Medizinpsychologie. Fachbuchhandlung für Psychologie, Frankfurt, Verlagsbuchhandlung, 1984.
50. Träger H, Flemming B, Nordmeyer J, Meffert H-J, Bleese N, Krebber H-J. Psychological effects of preoperative doctor-patient-communications. In: Becker R, Katz J, Polonius M-J, Speidel H (eds). Psychopathological and neurological dysfunctions following open-heart surgery. Berlin, Heidelberg, New York, Springer, 1982.
51. Davies-Osterkamp S. Psychologische Vorbereitung chirurgischer Patienten. In: Basler H-D, Florin J (eds). Klinische Psychologie und körperliche Krankheit. Stuttgart, Berlin, Köln, Mainz, Kohlhammer, 1985.
52. Kennedy J A, Bakst H. The influence of emotions on the outcome of cardiac surgery: a predictive study. Bull New York Acad Med 1966; 42:811.
53. Quinlan D M, Kimball C P, Osborne F. The Experience of Open Heart Surgery IV. Disorientation and Dysphoria Following Cardiac Surgery. Arch Gen Psychiat 1974; 31:241.
54. Rabiner C J, Willner A E, Fishman J. Psychiatric complications following coronary bypass surgery. J Nerv Ment Dis 1975; 160:342.
55. Meyendorf R. Psychische und neurologische Störungen bei Herzoperationen. Prä-und postoperative Untersuchungen. Fortschr Med 1976a; 94:315.
56. Meyendorf R. Hirnembolie und Psychose. Unter besonderer Berücksichtigung der Basalganglienapoplexie bei Herzoperationen mit extrakorporaler Zirkulation. J Neurol 1976b; 213:163.
57. Rimon R, Lehtonen J, Scheinin T M. Psychiatric disturbances after cardiovascular surgery. Acta Psychiat Scand (Suppl) 1968; 203:125.
58. Egerton N, Kay J H. Psychological Disturbances Associated with Open Heart Surgery. Brit J Psychiat 1964; 110:433.
59. Jakubik A. Mental Disorders in Patients after cardio-surgical Operations. Acta Med Pol 1972; 13:103.
60. Götze P, Dahme B. Hamburg Rating Scale for Psychic Disturbances – HRPD. In: Becker R, Katz J, Polonius MJ, Speidel H (eds). Psychopathological and neurological dysfunctions following open-heart surgery. Berlin, Heidelberg, New York, Springer, 1982; p. 77.
61. Dahme B, Götze P, Wessel M. Brief psychiatric inventory for assessment of psychopathological disorders after open heart surgery. In: Becker R, Katz J, Polonius MJ, Speidel H (eds). Psychopathological and neurological dysfunctions following open-heart surgery. Berlin, Heidelberg, New York: Springer, 1982; p. 68.
62. Götze P, Dahme B, Wessel M. Die Hamburger Schätzskala für psychische Strörungen nach Herzoperationen (HRPD). Eur Arch Psychiatr Neurol Sci 1985; 234:308.
63. Götze P, Dahme B, Lamparter U, Falck S. Methods, constructions and clinical application of the Hamburg Rating Scale for Psychic Disturbances (HRPD). In: Willner AE, Rodewald G (eds). Impact of cardiac surgery on the quality of life. New York, Plenum Press, 1990; p. 9.
64. Speidel H. Psychiatric issues: Simple frequencies pre- and postoperatively. In: Willner AE, Rodewald G (eds). Impact of cardiac surgery on the quality of life. New York, Plenum Press, 1990; p. 27.
65. Strauss B, Paulsen G. Psychiatric methods of the International Study: Hamilton Depression and Anxiety Scales. In: Willner AE, Rodewald G (eds). Impact of cardiac surgery on the quality of life. New York, Plenum Press, 1990; p. 19.
66. Willner A E, Rodewald G (eds). Impact of cardiac surgery on the quality of life. New York, Plenum Press, 1990.
67. Hamilton M. The assessment of anxiety states by rating. Brit J Med Psychol 1959; 32:50.

68. Hamilton M. Development of a rating scale for primary depressive illness. Brit J Soc Clin Psychol 1967; 6:278.
69. Spielberger C-D, Gorsuch R, Lushene R, Vagg P, Jacobs G. Manual for the state trait anxiety inventory. Palo Alto, Cons Psycholog Press, 1983.
70. Lazarus HR, Hagens JH. Preventions of psychosis following open-heart surgery. Amer J Psych 1968; 124:1190.
71. Flemming B, Meffert H-J. The role of personality traits for psychic disturbances after open-heart surgery. In: Speidel H, Rodewald G (eds). Psychic and neurological dysfunction after open-heart surgery. Stuttgart, New York, Thieme, 1980; p. 169.
72. Freyberger H. Psychotherapeutic strategies in patients treated in intensive care units. In: Speidel H, Rodewald G (eds). Psychic and neurological dysfunctions after open-heart surgery, Stuttgart. New York, Thieme, 1980; p. 200.
73. Götze P, Dahme B, Huse-Kleinstoll G, Meffert H-J, Speidel H. Therapiemöglichkeiten psychopathologischer Syndrome nach Herzoperationen. Verh Dtsch Ges Inn Med 1979; 85:1372.

17. Adjustment disorder in cardiac surgery patients

PEKKA TIENARI

Some problems experienced by cardiac surgery patients are basically psycho logical rather than organic in nature. They can relate, of course, to possible cerebral damage, but even more often to psychological stress related to the operation and the illness. They can influence illness behavior very much in both immediate and long-term recovery.

Surgery on chronic heart patients with valvular disease, also led to problems in adaptation, as persons with life-long illness had to cope with new-found health. Previous psychiatric and psychological research on valvular and congenital repair surgery has only a limited relevance to coronary artery bypass surgery patients. They have generally not been burdened by long-standing heart failure. Their frequently type A behavior stands in contrast to the passivity of the chronically ill cardiac patient [1].

Adjustment disorder

Adjustment disorder is defined thus in the DSM-IIIR [2]: "The essential feature of this disorder is a maladaptive reaction to an identifiable psychosocial stressor, or stressors, that occurs within three months after onset of the stressor and has persisted for no longer than six months". "The severity of the reaction is not completely predictable from the intensity of the stressor. People who are particularly vulnerable may have had a more severe form of the disorder following only a mild or moderate stressor, whereas others may have only a mild form of the disorder in response to a marked and continuing stressor". As an example of the stressors, a psychological reaction to a physical illness is given. "Symptoms of the disorder are varied. Each specific type presents a predominant clinical picture; many of the types are partial syndromes of specific disorders. For example, Adjustment Disorder with Depressed Mood is an incomplete depressive syndrome that develops in response to a psychological stressor".

"Diagnostic criteria for Adjustment Disorder [2] (DSM IIIR):

239

A) A reaction to an identifiable psychosocial stressor (or multiple stressors) that occurs within three months of onset of the stressor(s).
B) The maladaptive nature of the reaction is indicated by either of the following: (1) impairment in occupational (including school) functioning or in usual social activities or relationships with others; (2) symptoms that are in excess of normal and expectable reaction to the stressor(s).
C) The disturbance is not merely one instance of a pattern of over-reaction to stress or an exacerbation of one of the mental disorders previously described.
D) The maladaptive reaction has persisted for no longer than six months.
E) The disturbance does not meet the criteria for any specific mental disorder and does not represent Uncomplicated Bereavement".

The types of Adjustment Disorder are: Adjustment Disorder with Anxious Mood, with Depressed Mood, with Disturbance of Conduct, with Mixed Disturbance of Emotions and Conduct, with Mixed Emotional Features, with Physical Complaints, with Withdrawal, with Work (or Academic) Inhibition, and not Otherwise Specified.

A computerized literature search did not produce any publications using the diagnostic concept of Adjustment Disorder in relation to cardiac surgery. The best possibility seems to be to discuss the main aspects of Adjustment Disorder: Impairment in occupational functioning and symptoms of depression and anxiety.

Clinical viewpoints

At the onset of illness, effective care of the patient generally requires that he admits to being ill and accepts the limitations involved therein. He is thus expected to adopt the "sick role" [3], which implies the blessing of society for the patient to relinquish his ordinary tasks and duties. At the same time, he is expected to wish to recover and to accept the help of doctors and other nursing staff. Apart from this transient passivity, increased dependence and diminished responsibility, the patient must adapt to special arrangements and various discomforts if his illness becomes prolonged. He must, at least partly, entrust his care in the hands of strangers, endure the pain and stress of his symptoms and therapeutic procedures, and tolerate fear, tension and uncertainty. While recovering, the patient is expected to adopt a role opposite to that ascribed to him at the onset of the illness. He is expected to relinquish passivity and dependence, albeit initially still co-operating with the nursing staff, and to resume his usual activities as a responsible citizen. In the case of chronic or incurable illness, the patient is expected to maintain simultaneously both the dependence on the nursing personnel required for treatment and as much independence and personal initiative as his condition allows.

It is not unusual that the stress and associated symbolic significance of a severe disease may exceed the patient's psychic resources and mobilize excessive anxiety and regression. As the disease persists, the patient naturally tries to adapt to it in different ways. The longer the patient is ill without his condition deteriorating markedly, the better he usually learns to control the anxiety and depression the illness originally aroused. This seems to be the case particularly in chronic heart diseases. At times, the patient may adapt too well to prolonged illness from the point of view of his recovery. The condition of being ill, cared for and exempted from adult responsibilities, may have proved so useful to the patient, both as a source of regressive gratifications and as a defence against various difficulties, that his motivation to recover may have flagged or died out completely [4].

Preoperative adjustment

By far the most commonly reported and analyzed preoperative emotional state is anxiety or fear. Various authors have invited attention to the state vs. trait distinction in anxiety measurements. When considering preoperative emotion, one is usually referring to the transitory state resulting from the threatening surgery being expected, and therefore measures of state, rather than of more enduring traits, are appropriate.

Despite the complexity of the preoperative measures and diversity of the post-operative parameters, it is possible to conclude that high preoperative anxiety implies a poor postoperative outcome, and that low preoperative anxiety predicts a good outcome. There may be certain predisposing individual characteristics, especially trait anxiety, that determine the degree of preoperative anxiety reached. These features may be useful in identifying patients at risk for postoperative problems.

There are numerous models relating preoperative anxiety and postoperative outcome. At one extreme there is the psycho-physiological explanation, which suggests that experienced anxiety triggers a neuro-endocrine chain preoperatively, which then has a deleterious effect on the postoperative recovery pattern. At the other extreme there is the behavioral-communicational explanation, which postulates that the patient's manifest distress influences both the preoperative measures of anxiety and the postoperative assessments, as well as the responses of the nursing and medical staff with regard to the patient's physical state [5].

Kimball [6] traced long-term life adjustment for 15 months. The patients were preoperatively assigned to four categories on the basis of psychiatric interviews. 1) "Adjusted". Patients whose life course had been relatively smooth and successful in the family and occupational dimensions, and who expressed a moderate degree of anxiety, were optimistic about the future and felt in control of their life. 2) "Symbiotic". Patients who had experienced illness in childhood, had advanced through life with this illness as a major factor in their interpersonal relations, came to surgery at a time when dependent relationships were threatened, and demonstrated a fair amount of rigidity and inflexibility in their daily lives. 3) "Denying anxiety". Patients who disclaimed having

242

any feelings of anxiety, but, nevertheless, exhibited symptoms and signs of anxiety during the interview. These were individuals with notably restricted affect, marked tremulousness, and monosyllabic responses to questions. They also presented a relatively recent history of heart disease. 4) "Depressed". These were individuals who were utterly and hopelessly depressed. They did not care. They did not expect much from surgery. Many of them were only having surgery to please their surgeon. Their previous life was portrayed as a long period of chronic illness, increasing despondency and reduced interest in anything and everything.

Three fourths of the adjusted group had a benign convalescence and recovery. The symbiotic patients showed delayed convalescence and a poor long-term response. The anxious patients had 25% surgical mortality, frequent arrhythmias and variable long-term outcomes. The depressed patients did poorly, showing the highest death rate (79%) and either no improvement or deterioration in the survivors.

Tienari et al. [7, 8] discovered that increased preoperative anxiety was significantly associated with postoperative psychiatric complications and with poor psychosocial recovery after 12 months [9]. Fleming et al. [10] also demonstrated that high preoperative anxiety is a predictor for postoperative disturbance. Fleming et al. [11] claim that, contrary to the sensitization – repression concept, from an ego-psychological point of view, the highly anxious, or the sensitizers, have less developed ego functions, whereas the low-anxiety patients, or the repressers, have a functioning defence mechanism. Heller et al. [12] identified the postoperative high risk group as the patients who were disorganized and highly anxious and showed a paranoid tendency.

Sokol et al. [13] demonstrated that women had significantly higher mean scores of preoperative anxiety and depression than men. Postoperatively, however, there was a small sex-bound difference in the mean scores.

The findings of Möhlen et al. [14] also suggest that the styles of coping with the forthcoming operation and the emotional behavior shortly before it are predictive of both the postoperative psychological reaction and the long-term outcome. The patients who showed an aggressive, hostile reaction immediately after the operation and had a good bodily recovery were identified as the ones emotionally withdrawn or depressedly inhibited in the preoperative interview. They seemed able to preconceive the full significance of the operation. One year after the operation they appeared well balanced and less depressive than preoperatively. The patients who showed a rationalizing and technically oriented coping style preoperatively exhibited unstrained anxiety and paranoid ideation shortly after the operation. One year later they judged themselves more depressed, more restless, and mentally less stable. They also considered themselves to be medically and psychologically poorly supported by their family doctors. They had endeavoured to cope with the threatening event by avoiding any emotional involvement in it. Depression, restlessness and mental lability might be indicative of an inability to cope with chronic disease.

In summary, the patient's thoughts during the preoperative period are considered important for predicting the adequacy of postoperative coping. A high level of preoperative fear or anxiety is predictive of a poor postoperative outcome. Thus, the more fearful the patient is preoperatively, the more likely he is later on to show more emotional confusion, to experience more pain and to have a slower recovery compared with the patients who are less anxious about their surgery [5].

Depressive symptoms

Another important category where psychic factors tend to prolong illness consists of the patients who were already depressed at the onset of their illness or became depressed during its course. This type of depression does not usually take the form of obvious psychic symptoms, but rather of fatigue, lassitude, weakness, nondescript pain, lack of appetite and insomnia [15]. These symptoms tend to merge with those seen after the onset of the disease and may easily lead both the patient and the doctor to the erroneous conclusion that the somatic disease has taken a chronic course. It is naturally not always easy to determine whether the symptoms of a somatic pathologic process are being insidiously replaced by the somatic correlates of depression, or whether it is the depression itself that paralyses or weakens the patient's physiological potentials for recovery and prolongs his convalescence from somatic illness.

Bech et al. [16] noticed that psychic or cognitive symptoms on the Hamilton Anxiety Scale rather than somatic symptoms of anxiety explained the score variation before and after cardiac surgery. On the Melancholia Scale, symptoms such as depressed mood, psychic anxiety, pains, emotional and intellectual retardation were more predominant than symptoms of guilt, motor retardation or suicidal impulses.

Blacher [17] described patients who became depressive immediately after heart surgery. Nearly all of them shared a history of having lost a close object, who either had died from complications of a minor surgical procedure or illness, or had suffered from a disease similar to the one the patient had, but had not had any surgical help available at that time. Discussion of this problem of guilt over survival with the patient almost invariably resulted in a rapid remission of symptoms.

Eriksson [18] found that test measures of depression and anxiety were significantly lower postoperatively than preoperatively. Clinically, the signs of depression did not change as much. Depressive symptoms were quite common: 38.6% showed clinical signs of depression preoperatively and 31.3% continued to be depressed clinically after 7.5 months. In Horgan et al. [19] series, appr. 50% of the subjects had abnormally high scores on anxiety and depression preoperatively, the corresponding postoperative percentage being appr. 30%.

Preoperative depression correlates with poor outcome [6, 10, 12]. Heller et al. [1] recommend that elective surgery should be postponed until the depression has been treated. A severely depressed person is an increased risk post-operatively because of poor cooperation and compliance in the immediate postoperative period. The physiological changes associated with severe major depression can probably also contribute to the increased morbidity and mortality in these patients.

Occupational functioning

Kimball [20] replicated his earlier finding that those evaluated "adjusted" preoperatively had a greater likelihood of return to work than others.

Tienari et al. [21] reported that those with a poor psychosocial recovery after one year had even preoperatively considered the time to prepare for the operation too short and thought their own attitude towards the treatment to be of no significance, while the psychiatrist also evaluated their tolerance of stress to be poorer than that of the others. Those with a good recovery after 12 months were more satisfied with themselves in the preoperative interview and reported a better social adjustment and more pleasure in their human relations, and the psychiatrist estimated their coping ability was more adequate than in the case of the others.

Ramshaw et al. [22], using discriminant function analysis, demonstrated that the ability to cope with stressful events and low neuroticism were significant predictors of a good outcome. The results of Radley et al. [23] indicated that the adjustment styles employed prior to surgery are not necessarily applicable during the recovery. Specific findings indicated that the different styles of adjustment are consistent with the different expectations of surgery.

In the Finnish sample, those working after follow up 7.5 months after surgery had been away from work for a shorter period preoperatively, expressed their with to return to work in the preoperative interview, and belonged preoperatively more often to the NYHA classes I and II, compared to those not working at the final follow-up [18].

Stanton et al. [24] found that 73% of the patients who had been working during the year before surgery resumed their jobs within six months. Of those not so employed, 18% started working. The patients who expected preoperatively to return to work did so at a rate of 82% as compared with 39% of the others. Educational level and family income were more powerful predictors than occupation or the level of physical exertion required. The results suggested that the determinants for the resumption of work are largely present even before the coronary bypass surgery and that the patients' attitudes and expectations play an important role.

Less favourable results were obtained in a study of a largely blue collar, predominantly white, male population in rural North Carolina [25]. These patients were in good physiological condition, as measured by treadmill testing. Despite a good physical outcome, these patients were functioning poorly, 83% being unemployed 1–2 years after the operation. A number of other manifestations of maladjustment were also reported, including restricted social life, low self-esteem and lack of pleasure from close relationships. Patients with preoperative symptoms of greater than eight months duration did particularly poorly.

Kornfeld et al. [26] reported that those who returned to work were younger and were more likely to be type A preoperatively. They emphasize that it is essential in evaluating postoperative return to work that we distinguish between patients unable to return to work for physical reasons, those afraid to return, those kept from working by employer attitudes and those who choose to retire or accept a disability pension. Therefore, return to work cannot be used as a sole criterion for a successful procedure [1].

Treatment considerations

Tienari et al. [21] pointed out that clinical methods may help to identify preoperatively the patients at risk, on whom more attention should be focused to improve the outcome of the operation. The natural history of each patient undergoing open-heart surgery for valve replacement consists of a series of object losses. They have been suffering from a chronic disease, often for most of their adult lives. More often than not the disease has resulted in variable degrees of disability – but also some gain and value. The patients and their families have been faced with the necessity to adapt to the situation. The operation signifies an overall change. All of the major events – leaving home, adaptation to the hospital ward, leaving it, the operation, transfer to the intensive care unit, transfer back to the hospital ward, leaving the hospital, coming home – have the character of an object loss and a necessity to adapt to something new. When the patient comes to a new situation where the sick role must be abandoned and new tasks taken up, the benefits given by the operation do not work. Problems accumulate before the operation, which then acts as a kind of trigger mechanism. The physical change in the patient interacts with the family.

Pilowski et al. [27] pointed out that a variety of factors affect the degree of success achieved by coronary bypass surgery. The patient's way of perceiving, evaluating and reacting to his own health would seem to be of some relevance for the therapeutic outcome. Thurer et al. [28] found that despite the preoperative information given to many of the patients, most distorted the nature of the procedure in their own thoughts. Patients erroneously described the heart as being cut open and/or being removed from the body.

A preoperative visit from the nursing staff can help develop a trusting relationship. Patients should be told that problems may occur. They should be encouraged to communicate all symptoms and fears to the staff. They should be reassured, that should "confusion" occur, it is a common and temporary problem. Patients who are unprepared may fear that they are "going crazy" or that they have suffered permanent brain damage [1].

The questions asked by the patients should always be taken seriously and answered factually, no matter how childish and unrealistic they may sound. The patient's fears and misconceptions are usually very serious and should never be met with derogatory or arrogant answers or be ignored. Behavior of this kind would reinforce the patients anxiety and also evoke anger, which, in his state of dependence, tends to be turned inwards and leads to depression and lowered self-esteem. It is also important not to promise too much, but to give the patient a realistic view of what can be expected.

While it is important for the patient to have an opportunity to discuss his questions and be fully informed of what will happen to him and how he will feel afterwards, it is still more important that during the conversation he can feel that a personal bond is being formed between him and the people in whose hands he entrusts himself [4].

Heller *et al.* [1] recommend that psychotherapy should focus on: reduction of excessive hostility, the need to derive pleasure from more than work, the importance of recreation and relaxation, and non-competitive and non-perfectionistic attitudes within families. The operation should be viewed as an opportunity to re-think life's priorities and meaning. Steptoe [29] has discussed the long-term influences of psychological factors on cardiovascular functioning. He points out that behavioral interventions are establishing their importance in the armoury of preventive techniques. Many primary risks are themselves behaviors.

Also Pimm and Feist [30] have described the way in which crisis intervention can help coronary bypass patients avoid significant feelings of depression following surgery. Kulik *et al.* [31] demonstrated in a randomized trial that coronary bypass patients who had a roommate that already had the surgery were less anxious preoperatively and were discharged sooner than patients who had a roommate who was also waiting to have surgery.

Subjective acceptance of the loss and the consequence of malfunctioning of the body is achieved through a mental working-through process (a process of mourning). This process of mourning and surrender is greatly facilitated and accelerated if the patient has a chance to talk to somebody about his loss and its meaning to him. The patient is only able to accept his loss and gradually resume his vitality and desire to live if he is first able to think about what he has lost and mourn over it.

Chronically ill patients and invalids who do not have a permanent therapeutic relationship are often lonely, bitter and devoid of initiative. The constant awareness of one's inferiority and deficiency maintains feelings of anger, bitterness and spite. The invalid tends to react to imaginary hostility by aggressively provoking others to react with counteraggression and withdrawal. While thus frightening people away from him, he grows increasingly bitter, isolated and lonely [4].

References

1. Heller S, Kornfeld D. Psychiatric aspects of cardiac surgery. Adv Psychosom Med 1986; 15:124.
2. American Psychiatric Association: Diagnostic and Statistical Manual of Mental Disorder. Third Edition, Revised. Washington D.C., American Psychiatric Association, 1987.
3. Parsons T. The Social System. New York, Free Press, 1964.
4. Tähkä V. The Patient-Doctor Relationship. Sydney, Adis Health Science Press, 1984.
5. Johnston M. Pre-operative emotional states and post-operative recovery. Adv Psychosom Med 1986; 15:1.
6. Kimball CP. Psychological responses to the experience of open-heart surgery I. Am J Psychiatry 1969; 125:348.
7. Tienari P, Outakoski J, Hirvenoja R, Juolasmaa A, Takkunen I, Kampman R. Psychiatric complications following open-heart surgery, a prospective study. In: Becker R, Katz J, Polonius M-J, Speidel H (eds). Psychopathological and Neurological Dysfunctions Following Open-Heart Surgery. Berlin, Heidelberg, Springer-Verlag, 1982.
8. Tienari P, Outakoski J, Hirvenoja R, Juolasmaa A, Takkunen J. Postoperative psychosis in open heart surgery. A longitudinal study on valve replacement patients. Psychiatria Fennica 1984; p. 63.
9. Outakoski J, Juolasmaa A, Hirvenoja R, Tienari P. Biopsychosocial recovery of open heart surgery. A prospective study. Nordisk Psykiatrisk Tidsskrift 1987; 41:91.
10. Flemming B, Meffert H-J. The role of personality traits for psychic disturbances after open-heart surgery. In: Speidel H, Rodewald G (eds). Psychic and Neurological Dysfunctions After Open-Heart Surgery. New York, Theieme Stratton Inc., 1980; p. 169.
11. Flemming B, Dahme B, Götze P, Huse-Kleinstoll G, Meffert H-J, Müller L, Reimer Ch, Speidel H. Patients' fear of cardiosurgery and its significance for the pre- and post-operative state. In: Becker R, Katz J, Polonius M-J, Speidel H (eds). Psychopathological and Neurological Dysfunctions Following Open-Heart Surgery. Berlin, Heidelberg, Springer-Verlag, 1982; p. 281.
12. Heller S, Frank KA, Kornfeld DS, Malm JR, Bowman FO Jr. Psychological outcome following open heart surgery. Arch Intern Med 1974; 134:908.
13. Sokol S, Folks DG, Herrick RW, Freeman AM. Psychiatric outcome in men and women after coronary bypass surgery. Psychosomatics 1987; 28(1):11.
14. Möhlen K, Davies-Osterkamp S, Müller H, Scheld HH, Siefen G. Relationship between preoperative coping styles, immediate postoperative reactions and some aspects of the psychosocial situation of open-heart surgery patients one year after the operation. In: Becker R, Katz J, Polonius M-J, Speidel H (eds). Psychopathological and Neurological Dysfunctions Following Open-Heart Surgery. Berlin, Heidelberg, Springer-Verlag, 1982.
15. Imboden J. Psychosocial determinants of recovery. In: Lipowski ZJ (ed). Advances in Psychosomatic Medicine. Psychosocial Aspects of Physical Illness. Vol 8. Basel, S. Karger, 1972; p. 142.
16. Bech P, Grosby H, Husum B, Rafaelsen L. Generalized anxiety or depression measured by the Hamilton Anxiety Scale and the Melancholia Scale in patients before and after cardiac surgery. Psychopathology 1984; 17:253.
17. Blacher RS. Paradoxical depression after heart surgery: a form of survivor syndrome. The Psychoanal Quart 1978; 47:267.
18. Eriksson J. Psychosomatic aspects of coronary artery bypass graft surgery: A prospective study of 101 male patients. Acta Psychiatrica Scandinavica. Suppl. 340, vol. 77, 1988.
19. Horgan D, Davies B, Hunt D, Westlake GW, Mulleworth M. Psychiatric aspects of coronary artery surgery: A prospective study. Med J Aust 1984; 141:587.
20. Kimball CP, Quinlan D, Osborne F, Woodward B. The experience of cardiac surgery: V. Psychological patterns and prediction of outcome. Psychoter Psychosom 1973; 22:310.
21. Tienari P, Outakoski J, Juolasmaa A, Hirvenoja R. Open-heart surgery: the psychiatric point

of view. In: Krakowski AJ, Kimball CP (eds). Psychosomatic Medicine. NY, Plenum Publishing Corp., 1983; p. 113.

22. Ramshaw JE, Stanley G. Psychological adjustment to coronary surgery. British J of Clin Psychology 1984; 23:101.

23. Radley A, Green R. Styles of adjustment to coronary graft surgery. Soc Sci Med 1985; 20(5):461.

24. Stanton BA, Jenkins CD, Denlinger P, Savageau JA, Weintraub RM, Goldstein RL. Predictors of employment status after cardiac surgery. JAMA 1983; 249(7):907.

25. Gundle J, Bozman R, Reeves JR, Tate S, Raft S, McLaurin LP. Psychosocial outcome after coronary artery surgery. Am J Psychiatry 1980; 137(12):1591.

26. Kornfeld DS, Heller SS, Frank KA, Wilson SN, Malm JR. Psychological and behavioral responses after coronary artery bypass surgery. Circulation 66(suppl III); 1982.

27. Pilowsky I, Spence ND, Waddy JL. Illness behavior and coronary artery bypass surgery. J Psychosom Res 1979; 23:39.

28. Thurer S. The psychodynamic impact of coronary bypass surgery. Int'l J Psychiatry in Medicine 1980; 10(3):273.

29. Steptoe A. Psychological Factors in Cardiovascular Disorder. London, Academic Press Inc. Ltd., 1981.

30. Pimm JB, Feist JR. Psychological Risks of Coronary Bypass Surgery. New York, Plenum Press, 1984.

31. Kulik JA, Mahler HI. Effects of preoperative roommate assignment on preoperative anxiety and recovery from coronary bypass surgery. Health Psychol 1987; 6(6):525.

18. Major depression and adjustment disorder with depressed mood or depressive disorders

CHARLES J. RABINER

Depression is a term that is used to describe everything from a major retreat from reality to a mild case of the "blues". It can be a short-lived reaction to an external event, or it can develop in the absence of an obvious stressor. It can exist along with cognitive deficits or can be seen without difficulties in cognition. In short, depression in its various forms is the most likely presenting problem that patients offer as a reason for seeking psychiatric intervention.

It is not surprising, therefore, that we see a great variety of depressive symptomatology in our work with patients who have recently undergone cardiac surgery. Some patients will have a history of psychiatric illness and may develop an exacerbation in connection with their surgical experience. On the other hand, it is not unusual to see patients with a long history of severe mental illness go through the procedure without a problem. Readers are referred to standard psychiatric texts for a full discussion of Bipolar illness and major depression. This chapter will focus on those depressive conditions one is likely to see in patients undergoing cardiac surgery.

The recognition and diagnosis of a depressive illness in someone recovering from a major surgical procedure is difficult and challenging. The usual indicators one looks for are not apparent. Issues such as sleep impairment, appetite loss and other vegetative signs of depression are hard to evaluate in a patient in a post-recovery state. In addition the entire question of a mood appropriate to the situation is brought into question. Some authors believe that "medical depression is not consonant with primary affective disorder nor with secondary depression" [1]. Klerman [2] suggests that depressive symptoms may be part of the normal reaction to illness. Endicott [3] has suggested the use of alternative criteria from the vegetative measures, and Schwab [4] and Stewart [5] reported that as many as two-thirds of medically ill patients without mood disturbance showed fatigue, sleep disturbance and motor retardation. The prevalence of depression in medically ill patients has been estimated to be between 20–30%. Popkin has reported a 22% incidence in a study of 1072 psychiatric consultations performed at a university hospital [6].

In studies at the Long Island Jewish Medical Center [7], reported on the different prognosis associated with the diagnosis of depression. Early on it appeared that patients displaying what in DSM III would be called Adjustment Disorder with Depressed Mood had a different post-operative course than those patients who had a cognitive component to their depression. We, therefore, think it imperative that an evaluation for depression include a careful examination of the patient's cognition. This requires a full mental status exam but can be augmented by psychological tests. The Conceptual Level Analogy Test described elsewhere in this volume, was particularly useful in testing out early signs of organic impairments.

Types of depression

1. Major depression

This syndrome is the same as seen in the general population except that it occurs during the period following open heart surgery. It may occur prior to surgery, but if it does it is likely that the surgery will be postponed as few surgeons are eager to perform open heart surgery on a profoundly depressed person.

This syndrome is characterized by a dysphoric mood, a loss of interest in usual pastimes, a loss of pleasure in life and is a relatively consistent picture. Symptoms such as poor appetite, sleep disturbances, psychomotor agitation or retardation, loss of energy, feelings of worthlessness, inability to concentrate, and recurrent thoughts of death may be present. There is no evidence of an organic mental disorder and there is no evidence of the bizarre thinking associated with schizophrenia. There may or may not be psychotic features that are mood congruent. History will reveal whether this is a recurrent depression or part of a bipolar illness.

Treatment of these patients is essential and suicide is always a risk. The use of anti-depressant medications, particularly the tri-cyclics, may be contraindicated due to the fragile cardiac status. Medical consultation is strongly advised. Often Electro Convulsive Therapy administered with proper control of the anesthesia by a specialist in that area, will prove to be safer than the administration of anti-depressant medication. If the problem is severe, hospitalization in a psychiatric facility may be necessary before any further surgical procedures can be contemplated.

Fortunately, the incidence of patients about to undergo open heart surgery who present with a major depression is low. The depression often seen following the surgery is more similar to an adjustment disorder with depressed mood. The patients with this disorder have a depressed mood, frequently are tearful and voice feelings of hopelessness. Most of the time, however, these feelings are short lived and last only a few days. The following case report is represented to illustrate the point.

Case report
A 59 year-old pediatrician was very much concerned about developing a

septicemia following surgery. He was extremely anxious throughout the post-operative period. The nurses reported him to be very sluggish. On examination he was noted to hold himself rigid in one position for long periods of time as if he were afraid to move. He was constantly sad and expressed feelings of depression and apathy. He had diminished interest in his surroundings. There was a mild sleep disturbance. As the postoperative period continued, and as the date of discharge came nearer, this picture began to clear. By the time he was discharged he was no longer anxious or depressed.

This case is typical in terms of the course of the patients with Adjustment Disorder with depressed mood. It is important not to rush in and initiate pharmacotherapy, as the symptoms usually clear up within a few days. In general, the depth of the depression is far less than patients with a major depressive disorder and they usually can be readily identified. We feel that these patients have what might be considered to be a grief reaction in relation to their perceived loss as a result of their illness. Repeated psychiatric evaluations over several days will distinguish the different types of depression seen.

This is significant in that major depressions require active intervention while adjustment disorders with depressed mood may not need any more than careful observation. In terms of long term prognosis, a diagnosis of major depression is not a good sign. It may very well be the first manifestation of an organic brain syndrome. Rabiner and Willner [7] found significant differences in mortality rates five years after open heart surgery in those patients who had positive evidence of psychopathology and cognitive disorder when compared to those patients without this disorder. The assumption is that depression and trouble with cognition are the forerunners of an organic brain syndrome, one which can be diagnosed by the use of the CLAT. The following two case vignettes show the combination of depression, organic brain syndrome and mortality often seen in these patients.

Case report

A 61 year-old retired electronics worker was quite depressed for several months preoperatively, with sleep disturbance and a substantial weight loss. Before the surgery he had largely recovered from the depression, but was anxious and pessimistic about his chances of survival. He remarked that his first wife had died in the operating room seven years earlier, following open heart surgery. He had preoperative depression and a devastated CLAT score and therefore was diagnosed as having the PCD syndrome (psychopathology and cognitive disorder). After an aortic valve replacement he became severely depressed and also showed symptoms of an organic brain syndrome. He was unable to recognize the interviewing psychiatrist, was disoriented for a time and showed moderate impairment of attention and memory. He also had periods of marked restlessness, agitation, and dysphoric affect. After hospital discharge he had severe organic and depressive episodes and died ten months postoperatively.

Case report

A 67 year-old retired salesman had no preoperative psychopathology. After an aortic valve replacement, he became moderately depressed and showed signs of an organic brain syndrome, including troubles with memory, attention and concentration. Postoperative retesting was deferred for almost a week because the patient was "mumbling, incoherent and a little deaf." He was thought to have the PCD syndrome. Although he was doing well at 18 month follow-up, he said it took a full year to get back to feeling well. At 5 year follow-up he was moribund, with congestive heart failure, severe liver disorder, and was mentally very slow. He expired soon after.

It can be seen that the above patients have had significantly different courses. It is important to differentiate those patients with "pure" depression from those who have a cognitive disorder along with the depression. The major depressive disorders should be treated along the usual lines with antidepressive medication or electro-convulsive therapy. The adjustment disorders with depression are self limiting, and will do remarkably well if left alone, or given a minimal amount of supportive psychotherapy. Patients who present with signs of organicity along with depression have been labelled as having PCD. These patients have been shown to have a poor outcome when compared to other patients who do not have the PCD syndrome. Here supportive work with the patient, along with the family, can be very helpful in allowing them to adjust to the situation. While definite intervention for these patients remains to be discovered, and awaits future research, family counseling can be crucial in easing the burden of the family and preparing them to accept the likely severe outcome. While we are nowhere near the point where we can predict the future course for an individual patient, we have identified populations at risk, and our therapeutic endeavors should be directed at this group.

Depression in the elderly is a particularly important issue to be considered. As out surgical techniques have improved, many patients who were considered to be poor surgical risks are now accepted for surgery. It is well known that at first glance depression in the elderly may be thought to be dementia. In fact this error is so common, the term "pseudodementia" has been utilized. This term refers to the fact that symptoms such as disorientation, apathy, concentration difficulties and memory loss, which are often associated with dementia, may in fact be caused by a major depressive episode in the elderly. If there is a reasonable chance that these symptoms are the results of a depression, the wisest course is to actively treat the depression. If in fact the depression has caused the symptomatology, the rapid disappearance of the signs of dementia will occur.

Here again, the prognosis is different for those patients who have a cognitive aspect to their depression. These people have a far worse postoperative course as seen in the previously referred to follow-up study.

The evaluation of the emotional state of the patient is not limited to the hospital, but must include an evaluation of the patient after he/she returns home. By far the best prognosis is found in those patients who have been able to return to their former life status, particularly employment. However, this is not surprising since the patients who are more incapacitated have less of a chance of returning to work. For many years psychiatrists have known that the last part of an emotionally ill patient's life to fail is his/her capacity to work. Patients who are severely impaired in their interpersonal relations, nevertheless, may be able to perform at work, and cling to a job tenaciously. It is almost as if they are saying "I can't be ill if I am still working." Unfortunately, many of our cardiac surgery patients can not return to their previous employment. Many choose to retire and face the double threat of surgery and retirement. Others are forced to the sidelines either by a physical impairment or excess physical demands of the job. Therefore, the evaluation of the patient in the post hospital phase must take the above factors into consideration when making a diagnosis. Patients who are undergoing a mourning process for their lost job should be considered to have an adjustment disorder with depressed mood rather than a major depressive disorder. When it is not always easy to distinguish between the two, the passage of time will generally clear the picture. Vocational counseling may be an important part of the overall treatment plan, as some patients unable to return to their former occupation may well be able to do something else. The attitude that they have something to contribute to society, and are not expected to be invalids for the rest of their lives, will go a long way towards helping them cope with whatever losses they have substained.

At the present time we can not say with any certainty why some patients become depressed following cardiac surgery. One interesting idea has been offered by Kenneth Heilman [8] in his chapter on Affective Disorders Associated with Hemispheric Neuropsychology of Human Emotion. He suggests the possibility that since patients with left-hemisphere lesions are aware of their deficits, they then might react to these deficits by becoming depressed. In his studies he found that patients with right-hemisphere lesions were hypoaroused while patients with left-hemisphere disease had an increased arousal response compared with that of normal controls. We await further definitive studies linking specific location of lesions with specific affective changes.

In summary, the key to the understanding of the specific patient with depression symptomatology, is careful differential diagnosis. For those patients who have an adjustment disorder with depressed mood, a period of observation is indicated and zealous intervention is to be avoided. For those patients who have a diagnosible major depressive disorder, active treatment is indicated along with careful evaluation of suicidal potential. Those patients with depression along with a cognitive disorder also require active treatment, but here family counseling should be added in view of the unfavorable prognosis.

References

1. Poplin M, Callies A, Colon E. A framework for the study of medical depression. Psychosomatics 1987; 28:27.

2. Klerman GL. Depression in the medically ill. Psychiatry Clinical North American 1981; 4:301.
3. Endicott J. Measurement of depression in patients with cancer. Cancer 1984; 53 (supp), p. 2243.
4. Schwab JJ, Bialow M, Brown JM *et al.* Diagnosing depression in medical inpatients. Ann Intern Med 1967; 67:695.
5. Stewart JA, Drake F, Winokur G. Depression among medically ill patients. Dis Nervous System 1965; 26:479.
6. Popkin MK, Mackenzie TB, Callies AL. Psychiatric consultation in geriatric medically ill inpatients in a university hospital. Arch General Psychiatry 1984; 41:703.
7. Rabiner CJ, Willner AE. Differential psychopathological and organic mental disorder at follow-up, five years after coronary bypass and cardiac valvular surgery. Psychic and Neurological Dysfunctions After Open-Heart Surgery. Stuttgart, George Thieme Verlag, New York, New York Thieme Stratton Inc., 1980; p. 237.
8. Heilman KM. Neuropsychology of Human Emotion. NY, London, The Guilford Press, 1983.

19. Organic mental disorders in cardiac surgery

K. A. SOTANIEMI

Organic mental disorders have been encountered throughout the history of cardiac surgery. They may occur either in association with neurological defects or as isolated phenomena. These disturbances have formerly been variously called "acute brain syndrome", "toxic psychosis", "metabolic encephalopathy", "postoperative confusion state", "postoperative behavioural disorder", and "abnormal behavioural responses". Although the nomenclature has been heterogenous and the criteria for defining the conditions have not been uniform, the disorders refer to disturbances attributable to organic causes interfering with normal brain function. Generally, these terms have been used to describe a condition which, according to the contemporary classification of mental disorders [1], is defined as delirium. However, the association of postoperative organic mental disorders with cardiac surgery is by no means unique: such disorders are also found for instance after eye surgery, e.g., in postoperative states which require patients to have their eyes closed for several days [2]. However, considering the very special conditions of cardiac patients during the early postoperative period, delirium is a problematic and potentially hazardous complication which needs recognition and treatment.

Dementia is another organic brain disorder occasionally complicating cardiac diseases. The terms "vascular dementia" and "multi-infarct dementia" have been used to describe a condition attributed to the consequences of either cardiac, precerebral or intracerebral vascular diseases causing dementia. Persistent intellectual impairment is one of the most debilitating complications of cardiac surgery. Postoperative intellectual deterioration may have important preoperative determinants but obviously there are a vast number of both intra- and postoperative conditions which are potentially present and often severe enough to result in brain damage and cause dementia or to worsen a preoperatively present intellectual impairment.

This chapter reviews the prevalence, causes, clinical features and treatment of organic mental disorders, specifically delirium and dementia, related to cardiac surgery. First, however, the definitions of the disorders are reviewed very briefly.

The diagnostic criteria for delirium include [1]: clouded consciousness;

255

disturbances in perception, speech, sleep-wakefulness cycle, and psychomotor speed; disorientation and memory impairment; clinical features developing over a short period of time (usually hours to days) and tending to fluctuate; and evidence of a specific organic factor etiologically related to the disturbance. Dementia is diagnosed according to the following criteria [1]: intellectual impairment severe enough to cause social or occupational incompetence; impairment of memory, abstract thinking and other cognitive functions; no clouding of consciousness; and organic causes attributable to the condition. The two conditions do not exclude each other but, by definition, dementia cannot be diagnosed during a delirious state since the consciousness cannot be disturbed during dementia. Another important feature distinguishing these two disorders is the short history of delirium. Delirium appears in hours or days in contrast to months and years for the development of dementia.

The details of the clinical diagnostic criteria as well as the pitfalls in the definitions and in the differential diagnosis have been reviewed recently [2–7].

Delirium related to cardiac surgery

Prevalence of postcardiotomy delirium

Delirium used to be a very common complication after *valvular surgery* in the early 1960s, the reported prevalence values ranging from 41 to 70% [7–9]. More recently, considerably smaller prevalence values have been reported, from 4 to 35% in prospective [10–17] and up to 5 to 13% in retrospective studies [18]. In *coronary artery bypass surgery* (CABS), post-operative delirium has been reported to range from 1 to 31% in the available prospective studies [19–24], whereas the prevalence value in the retrospective evaluations has been claimed to be as low as from 0.3 to 2% [25, 26]. One comparison between valvular and CABS patients [27] revealed acute psychiatric complications in 41% of patients operated on for valvular surgery in contrast to 16% in CABS patients, the difference being statistically significant.

A meta-analysis [28] of 44 studies revealed that the prevalence of postcardiotomy delirium has remained fairly constant at 32% during the past two decades. The authors found no difference in the prevalence reported in studies that used interviews versus chart reviews. Intelligence, sex, preoperative psychiatric illnesses and intraoperative perfusion time did not correlate with postcardiotomy delirium and age correlated with it only slightly. On the other hand, of all the 28 hypothesized risk variables that were tested, preoperative psychiatric intervention had the highest correlation with postcardiotomy delirium. In contrast to these relatively high prevalence values in adults, postoperative organic mental disorders are considered relatively rare in children, the available reports claiming delirium to be virtually non-existent [9, 28–30].

Methodological and terminological heterogeneity makes it difficult to compare older studies with recent ones but, quite obviously, postoperative delirium has become less frequent than it used to be some ten years ago. This is in accordance with the decreasing frequency of severe brain damage and neurological defects generally as has been described in the previous chapters. However, it is important to emphasize that although delirium most commonly is a condition easy to differentiate from a normal postoperative state, reliable information concerning its prevalence and outcome cannot be obtained using chart reviews and retrospective assessment. Regular postoperative surveillance, despite all advances and all the available knowledge concerning the cerebral complications of cardiac surgery, is still principally oriented to recognizing and registering the cardiac and respiratory measures of the patient. Thus, the severity of brain dysfunction still too often has to be disproportionately high to be recognized when compared, for instance, to disorders of cardiac functions, the smallest details of which are monitored with devotion. An example of this methodological and surveillance problem is a report [9] which describes postoperative delirium as occurring in 27% of patients after valvular replacement when judged from chart reviews, in contrast to 70% of patients when judged after an adequate psychiatric interview.

Clinical aspects

Delirium is an acute and transient organic mental disorder. The course of delirium is characteristic, the symptoms appearing rapidly, usually on the second to the fifth day after surgery [9, 10, 15, 31]. Delirium may develop after a lucid postoperative period or appear as a continuation of a drowsy postoperative state [22]. Prodromal symptoms which may or may not progress to real delirium consist of restlessness, motor hyperactivity, anxiety, difficulty in concentrating and thinking clearly, drowsiness, insomnia and transient illusions [2, 5]. Delirium is heralded by confusion, disorientation, agitation, disorders of perception and attention, a disturbed sleep-wake cycle, delusions, disordered consciousness, abnormal psychomotor behaviour (e.g. hyper- or hypoactivity, verbal or non-verbal vocalizations, perseveration and involuntary movements), and hallucinations which are often of the visual type [2, 3, 5, 6, 12, 15, 31]. Delirious symptoms tend to worsen at night and when the eyes are closed. The condition typically fluctuates and patients may have lucid intervals which clearly contrast with the phase of altered mental state. The lucid intervals occur unpredictably and their duration may vary from minutes to hours [5].

Most commonly, the outcome of delirium is favourable and the condition may be self-limiting. However, in contrast to the usual recovery within a few days or not more than one week, the condition may sometimes be prolonged to weeks [2, 5, 6, 10, 12]. Delirium may show transition to chronic brain syndromes such as dementia or amnestic syndrome or to a functional psychosis [5]. Delirium may also have serious consequences in a cardiac patient whose general condition may still at that time be unstable. A delirious patient may develop tachycardia, arrhythmias and severe hyperventilation, all of which may lead to further complications. The patient may be highly anxious and unable to sleep, thus becoming exhausted. All this, together with confusion and paranoia, may severely interfere with cooperation and routine daily activities and therapies, as well as necessary postoperative surveillance and investigations.

Causes of postoperative delirium

A vast number of causes potentially associated with the development of delirium can be recognized [2], including e.g. intoxications, drug and alcohol withdrawal, intracranial and general infections, space occupying lesions of the brain, various metabolic encephalopathies, epileptic and traumatic conditions, cerebro- and/or cardiovascular diseases, hypoxia, haematological diseases and paraneoplastic conditions, to name some of the main factors. In addition to the causes mentioned above, all the pre-, intra- and postoperative determinants of cerebral damage discussed earlier in specific chapters of this book must be taken into account in evaluating the potential causes of delirium in a cardiac surgery patient. However, some aspects of the cardiac surgery patients' post-cardiotomy delirium deserve further consideration.

Old age [17, 20], long duration of perfusion [13, 14, 16], intraoperative hypotension [13, 21, 23], long duration and severity of cardiac disease [13], preoperative mental illness, cognitive disorders and anxiety [15, 31–33] have been mentioned as risk factors for postcardiotomy delirium. These concepts, however, are not uniform: for instance, age and perfusion time were not found to correlate with the development of postoperative delirium in one study comparing a group of 51 CABS patients with a group of 46 valvular surgery patients [26]. In this study, the perfusion times of the CABS patients were even longer than those of the valvular replacement patients and yet the prevalence of postoperative delirium were 16% vs 41%. The authors stressed the differences between the personality types of coronary and valvular disease patients as potential modulators of behavioural responses in exceptional conditions.

In another study involving 421 CABS patients [21], postoperative organic mental disorder could be identified in 49 patients on the fourth post operative day. In two cases, no cause of the encephalopathy could be pointed to, in eight cases one potential cause could be recognized, while from two to five causes of cerebral dysfunction could be stated in the remaining 39 cases. The identified factors of postoperative disorders listed in the order of frequency were hypoxia, medications, fever or sepsis, air in the left ventricular cannula, reoperation within 24 hours, renal failure, ethanol withdrawal and hyperosmolar state. The patients did not show any focal neurological deficits.

Apart from the causes related to the intraoperational conditions mentioned above, particular attention has been paid to drugs associated with the development of postoperative delirium [2, 35, 36], specifically to those with anticholinergic properties. The mechanism of action of anticholinergics is thought to be a central impairment of cholinergic functions [35]. A strong correlation between the occurrence of post-operative delirium and serum concentrations of drugs that block muscarinic receptors has been demonstrated in cardiac surgery patients [37]. Several commonly used drugs, (e.g., antihistamines, mydriatics, tricyclic antidepressants, phenothiazines, chlorpromazine among many others with anticholinergic properties) may thus cause or contribute to delirium. The clinical signs referrring to the presence of muscarinic receptor blocking agents are: dilated pupils; tachycardia, flushed face; dry skin and mucous membranes; urinary urgency coupled with difficulty in initiating micturition; elevated blood pressure; and constipation. This anticholinergic delirium is relieved by physostigmine [5].

In addition to anticholinergics, a vast number of universally used drugs may elicit delirium. Among them are, for instance, digitalis, propranolol, procainamide, clonidine, sodium nitroprusside, lidocaine, quinidine, opiates, benzodiazepines, and indomethacin [2, 5]. Thus, the clarificiation of the etiology of delirium may be very complicated, for instance, cardiac arrhythmia and antiarrhythmic drugs may both cause delirium.

To complicated the etiologic considerations further, delirium has also been associated with the environmental conditions of the postoperative cardiac intensive care unit. One of the environmental determinants of delirium is the hasty and noisy atmosphere of the unit interfering with sleep. Studies of sleep patterns during the postoperative phase have shown marked distortion, sleep deprivation and specifically REM (rapid eye movements) sleep deprivation [38]. In a study with six cardiac surgery patients investigated in the postoperative intensive care unit [38], only one patient showed evidence of REM sleep before the fourth postoperative day. REM sleep suppression continued for several weeks after surgery. It is also to be remembered that REM sleep deprivation may primarily be due to organic brain damage and altered cerebral metabolism related to the intraoperative conditions but, evidently, the environmental conditions at least enhance the sleep distortion. Moreover, annoyance is caused by the manouvres needed for postoperative surveillance, lights, blood sampling, assistance of ventilation and the many other activities typical of an intensive care unit.

Further sleep disturbances may be associated with the medications needed to treat pain and discomfort, e.g., morphine, which is a REM sleep suppressant, and benzodiazepines, which are slow-wave sleep depressants [38]. The risks of withdrawing psychotropic medications must also be kept in mind [39].

Further discomfort to the patient is caused by the monotonous and stereotyped nature of the activities during the intensive care unit phase: there is simultaneous sensory deprivation and overload, which facilitate the development of delirium [14]. Additionally, prolonged immobilization and severe fatigue are likely to favour the onset and worsening of delirium [2].

Thus, the etiology of postoperative delirium in cardiac surgery patients is multifactorial. The conditions related to the operative procedure may elicit derangements in cerebral metabolism, and imbalance of neurotransmitters may be induced with medications, and psychological disturbances may be associated with sensory overload and deprivation, all these factors alone or together facilitating the development of delirium or the increase of its severity.

Treatment of postoperative delirium

Prevention is the best way to treat delirium. Arrangements to avoid sleep deprivation are often simple to accomplish if only paid attention to. Sensory deprivation can be corrected by providing devices helping orientation (e.g. familiar objects, photographs, newspapers, radio, TV, clock, calender, etc. [4, 5]. Special attention should always be paid to the medication initiated and the medication withdrawn. Unnecessary drugs potentially interfering with central cholinergic mechanisms or the sleep pattern should be avoided. The personnel should be made aware of simple preventive measures and to recognize the prodromal symptoms and signs of delirium. When the diagnosis of delirium is set, every effort should be made to define its cause or causes and to eliminate them. Apart from drugs, attention should also be paid to the course of operation and to the patient's neurological and general state. The most commonly recommended medication for the treatment of delirium is haloperidol with the exception of cases in which anticholinergics are the etiological factor [4, 5].

Dementia related to cardiac surgery

The available information concerning the chronic forms of organic mental disorders, specifically dementia, is scarce. No epidemiological studies are available elucidating the prevalence of dementia among patients with cardiac valvular disease or coronary disease, not to mention studies concerning the possible influence of operative treatment on the development of dementia. It is not known whether the correction of prolonged cardiac disease, involving as it does many intraoperatively operant factors which are potentially harmful to the brain, prevents or facilitates the development of dementia. Cardiac disease itself is clearly a risk factor of dementia [40–42] and it has been claimed that some 6% of patients with stroke develop dementia within four years after the cerebrovascular accident [43]. The available long-term studies after cardiac surgery praise the overall benefits of successful cardiac surgery in terms of the quality of life [44, 45], and indeed the clinical neurological [46], EEG [46] and neuropsychological [47] follow-up studies provide no evidence of exceptional intellectual impairment.

These long-term studies have even elicited the question of the possibility of improvement of the higher cerebral functions after the correction of the prolonged cardiac disease [47]. On the other hand, the same studies have shown that intraoperative conditions, e.g, long perfusion times, may have disadvantageous intellectual consequences which manifest themselves only long after surgery. These studies thus highlight not only the price to be paid for the years achieved but also our present lack of knowledge concerning the determinants of the long-term cerebral outcome. Certainly, some patients develop dementia after cardiac operations but the role of the pre-existing preoperative causes and the influence of both the intra- and postoperative cerebral damage and the other treatments applied are poorly outlined. All these aspects pose a major challenge for future research.

Summary

Organic mental disorders are relatively frequent, but fortunately they are most commonly self-limiting and benign complications of cardiac surgery. Both pre-, intra- and postoperative causes of these disorders can be recognized and many of them can be eliminated by simple consideration of the conditions the patient is exposed to, particularly during the immediate postoperative period. However, the continuous occurrence of postoperative organic mental disorders reflects the inadequacy of our present methods for preventing cerebral damage during the substitution of the normal cardiorespiratory functions during cardiopulmonary bypass. Very little is known of the long-term effects of cardiac surgery. Together with biochemical and neurophysiological measures, postoperative organic mental disorders represent the major area of study in the future development of cerebral safety and surveillance in cardiac surgery.

References

1. American Psychiatric Association Committee on Nomenclature and Statistics. Diagnostic and Statistical Manual of Mental Disorders (DSM-III), 3rd ed. Washington, D.C., American Psychiatric Association, 1980.
2. Lipowski SJ. Delirium. Acute Brain Failure in Man. Springfield Ill, Charles C. Thomas.
3. Lipowski ZJ. Delirium updated. Compr Psychiatry 1980; 21:190.
4 Lipowski ZJ. Transient cognitive disorders (delirium, acute confusional states) in the elderly. Am J Psychiatry, 1983; 140:11, p. 1426.
5 Lipowski ZJ. Delirium (acute confusional state). In: Vinken PJ, Bruyn GW, Klawans HL, Frederiks JAM (eds). Handbook of Clinical Neurology. Neurobehavioural Disorders. Amsterdam, Elsevier Science Publishers, 1985; Vol. 2 (46), p. 523.
6. Pitt B. Delirium and dementia. In: Pitt B (ed). Dementia. Edinburgh, Churchill Livingstone, 1987; p. 241.
7. McEvoy JP. Organic brain syndromes. Ann Int Med 1981; 95: 212.
8. Blachly PH, Starr A. Post-cardiotomy delirium. Am J Psychiatry 1964; 121:371
9. Kornfeld DS, Zimberg S, Malm JR. Psychiatric complications of open-heart surgery. N Engl J Med 1965; 273:287.
10. Javid H, Tufo HM, Najafi H, Dye WS, Hunter JA, Julian OC. Neurological abnormalities following open-heart surgery. J Thorac Cardiovasc Surg 1969; 58:502.
11. Heller SS, Frank KA, Malm JR, Bowman FO, Harris PD, Charlton MH, Kornfeld DS. Psychiatric complications of open-heart surgery: A re-examination. N Engl J Med 1970; 283:1015.
12. Tufo HM, Ostfeld AM, Shekelle R. Central nervous system dysfunction following open-heart surgery. J Am Med Ass 1970; 212:1333.
13. Lee, WH Jr, Brady MP, Rowe JM, Miller WC Jr. Effects of extracorporeal circulation upon behaviour, personality and brain function. Ann Surg 1971; 173:1013.

14. Frank, KA, Heller, SS, Kornfeld DS, Malm JR. Long-term effects of open-heart surgery intellectual functioning. J Thorac Cardiovasc Surg 1972; 64:811.
15. Sveinsson IS. Postoperative psychosis after heart surgery. J Thorac Cardiovasc Surg 1975; 70:717.
16. Sotaniemi KA. Brain damage and neurological outcome after open-heart surgery. J Neurol Neurosurg Psychiat 1980; 43:127.
17. Gilberstrand J. Intellectual and personality changes following open-heart surgery. Arch Gen Psychiat 1967; 16:210.
18. Branthwaite MA. Neurological damage related to open-heart surgery. Thorax 1972; 27:748.
19. Kornfeld DS, Heller SS, Frank KA, Edie RN, Barsa J. Delirium after coronary artery bypass surgery. J Thorac Cardiovasc Surg 1978; 76:93.
20. Kolkka R, Hilberman M. Neurologic dysfunction following cardiac operation with low-flow, low-pressure cardiopulmonary bypass. J Thorac Cardiovasc Surg 1980; 79:432.
21. Breuer AC, Furlan AJ, Hanson MR, Lederman RJ, Loop FD, Cosgrove DM, Greenstreet RL, Estafanous FG. Stroke 1983; 14:682.
22. Shaw PJ, Bates D, Cartlidge NEF, Heaviside D, Julian DG, Shaw DA. Early neurological complications of coronary artery bypass surgery. Br Med J 1985; 291:1384.
23. Smith PLC, Newman SP, Ell PJ, Treasure T, Joseph P, Schneidau A, Harrison MJG. Cerebral consequences of cardiopulmonary bypass. Lancet 1986; 1:823.
24. Carella F, Travaini G, Contri P, Guzzetti S, Botta, M., Pieri, E, Mangoni, A. Cerebral complications of coronary bypass surgery. A prospective study. Acta Neurol Scand 1988; 77:158.
25. Gonzales-Scarano F, Hurtig HI. Neurologic complications of coronary artery bypass grafting: case-control study. Neurology 1981; 31:1032.
26. Coffey EE, Massey EW, Roberts KB, Curtis S, Jones RH, Pryor DB. Natural history of cerebral complications of coronary artery bypass graft surgery. Neurology 1983; 33:1416.
27. Rabiner CJ, Willner AE, Fishman J. Psychiatric complications following coronary bypass surgery. J Nerv Ment Dis 1975; 160:342.
28. Smith LE, Dimsdale JE. Postcardiotomy delirium: conclusions after 25 years? Am J Psychiatry 1989; 146:452.
29. Stevenson JG, Stone EF, Dillard DH, Morgan BC. Intellectual development of children subjected to prolonged circulatory arrest during hypothermic open heart surgery in infancy. Circulation 1974; 49, 50: (suppl. 2) 54.
30. Messmer GJ, Schallberger U, Gattiker R, Senning Å. Psychomotor and intellectual development after deep hypothermia and circulatory arrest in early infancy. J Thorac Cardiovasc Surg 1976; 72:495.
31. Layne OL Jr, Yudofsky SC. Postoperative psychosis in cardiotomy patients. N Engl J Med 1971; 284:518.
32. Heller SS, Frank KA, Kornfeld DS, Malm JR, and Bowman FO. Psychological outcome following open-heart surgery. Arch Intern Med 1974; 134:908.
33. Willner AE, Rabiner CJ, Wisoff BG, Hartstein M, Struve FA, Klein DF. Analogical reasoning and postoperative outcome. Arch Gen Psychiatry 1976; 33:255.
34. Rabiner CJ, Willner AE. Psychopathology observed on follow-up after coronary bypass surgery. J Nerv Ment Dis 1976; 163:295.
35. Summers WK. A clinical method of estimating risk of drug induced delirium. Life Sci 1978; 22:1511.
36. Johnson AL, Holister LE, Berger PA. The anticholinergic intoxication syndrome: diagnosis and treatment. J Clin Psychiatry 1981; 41:313.
37. Tune LE, Damlouji NF, Holland A, Gardner TJ, Folstein MF, Coyle JT. Association between postoperative delirium with raised serum levels on anticholinergic drugs. Lancet 1981; 2:651.
38. Orr WC, Stahl ML. Sleep disturbances after open-heart surgery. Am J Cardiol 1977; 39:196.
39. Kales A, Kales J. Evaluation, diagnosis, and treatment of clinical conditions related to sleep. J Am Med Ass 1970; 213:2229.
40. Easton JD, Hart RG, Sherman DG, Kaste M. Diagnosis and management of ischemic

stroke. Part I. Threatened stroke and its management. Current Problems in Cardiology. Chigago, Illinois, Year Book Medical Publishers Inc., 1983; p.1 .

41. Kannel B W, Wolf P A. Epidemiology of cerebrovascular disease. In: Russell R W R (ed). Vascular Disease of the Central Nervous System. 2nd ed. London, Churchill Livingstone, 1983; p. 1.
42. Fields W S. Multi-infarct dementia. Neurologic Clinics 1986;405.
43. Kotila M, Valtimo O, Niemi M-L, Laaksonen R. Dementia after stroke. Eur Neurol 1986; 25:134.
44. Blachly P H, Blachly P J. Vocational and emotional status of 263 patients after open-heart surgery. Circulation 1968; 38:524.
45. Ross J K, Monro J L, Diwell A E, Mackean J M, Marsh J, Barker D J P. The quality of life after cardiac surgery. Br Med J 1981; 282:451.
46. Sotaniemi K A, Mononen H, Hokkanen T E. Long-term cerebral outcome after open-heart surgery. Stroke 1986; 17:410.
47. Sotaniemi K A. Five-year neurological and EEG outcome after open-heart surgery. J Neurol Neurosurg Psychiatry 1985; 48:569.

Index

DEVELOPMENTS IN
CRITICAL CARE MEDICINE AND ANESTHESIOLOGY

1. O. Prakash (ed.): *Applied Physiology in Clinical Respiratory Care*. 1982
ISBN 90-247-2662-X

2. M. G. McGeown: *Clinical Management of Electrolyte Disorders*. 1983
ISBN 0-89838-559-8

3. T. H. Stanley and W. C. Petty (eds.): *New Anesthetic Agents, Devices and Monitoring Techniques*. Annual Utah Postgraduate Course in Anesthesiology. 1983
ISBN 0-89838-566-0

4. P. A. Scheck, U. H. Sjöstrand and R. B. Smith (eds.): *Perspectives in High Frequency Ventilation*. 1983 ISBN 0-89838-571-7

5. O. Prakash (ed.): *Computing in Anesthesia and Intensive Care*. 1983
ISBN 0-89838-602-0

6. T. H. Stanley and W. C. Petty (eds.): *Anesthesia and the Cardiovascular System*. Annual Utah Postgraduate Course in Anesthesiology. 1984 ISBN 0-89838-626-8

7. J. W. van Kleef, A. G. L. Burm and J. Spierdijk (eds.): *Current Concepts in Regional Anaesthesia*. 1984 ISBN 0-89838-644-6

8. O. Prakash (ed.): *Critical Care of the Child*. 1984 ISBN 0-89838-661-6

9. T. H. Stanley and W. C. Petty (eds.): *Anesthesiology: Today and Tomorrow*. Annual Utah Postgraduate Course in Anesthesiology. 1985 ISBN 0-89838-705-1

10. H. Rahn and O. Prakash (eds.): *Acid-base Regulation and Body Temperature*. 1985
ISBN 0-89838-708-6

11. T. H. Stanley and W. C. Petty (eds.): *Anesthesiology 1986*. Annual Utah Postgraduate Course in Anesthesiology. 1986 ISBN 0-89838-779-5

12. S. de Lange, P. J. Hennis and D. Kettler (eds.): *Cardiac Anaesthesia*. Problems and Innovations. 1986 ISBN 0-89838-794-9

13. N. P. de Bruijn and F. M. Clements: *Transesophageal Echocardiography*. With a contribution by R. Hill. 1987 ISBN 0-89838-821-X

14. G. B. Graybar and L. L. Bready (eds.): *Anesthesia for Renal Transplantation*. 1987
ISBN 0-89838-837-6

15. T. H. Stanley and W. C. Petty (eds.): *Anesthesia, the Heart and the Vascular System*. Annual Utah Postgraduate Course in Anesthesiology. 1987 ISBN 0-89838-851-1

16. D. Reis Miranda, A. Williams and Ph. Loirat (eds.): *Management of Intensive Care*. Guidelines for Better Use of Resources. 1990 ISBN 0-7923-0754-2

17. T. H. Stanley (ed.): *What's New in Anesthesiology*. Annual Utah Postgraduate Course in Anesthesiology. 1988 ISBN 0-89838-367-6

18. G. M. Woerlee: *Common Perioperative Problems and the Anaesthetist*. 1988
ISBN 0-89838-402-8

19. T. H. Stanley and R. J. Sperry (eds.): *Anesthesia and the Lung*. Annual Utah Postgraduate Course in Anesthesiology. 1989 ISBN 0-7923-0075-0

20. J. De Castro, J. Meynadier and M. Zenz: *Regional Opioid Analgesia*. Physiopharmacological Basis, Drugs, Equipment and Clinical Application. 1990
ISBN 0-7923-0162-5

21. J. F. Crul (ed.): *Legal Aspects of Anaesthesia*. 1989 ISBN 0-7923-0393-8

DEVELOPMENTS IN
CRITICAL CARE MEDICINE AND ANESTHESIOLOGY

KLUWER ACADEMIC PUBLISHERS – DORDRECHT / BOSTON / LONDON